ABHANDLUNGEN
DER AKADEMIE DER WISSENSCHAFTEN DER DDR
Abteilung Mathematik — Naturwissenschaften — Technik

Jahrgang 1984 · Nr. 1 N

Cellular and Molecular Aspects of the Regulation of the Heart

Proceedings of the Symposium held in Berlin
from 26.—28. August 1982
The Symposium was organized by
The Central Institute of Heart and Circulation Research
of the Academy of Sciences of the GDR
The Society of Cardiology and Angiology of the GDR
The Biochemical Society of the GDR

Edited by
Liane Will-Shahab
Ernst-Georg Krause
Wolfgang Schulze

AKADEMIE-VERLAG · BERLIN 1984

Herausgegeben im Auftrage des Präsidenten
der Akademie der Wissenschaften der DDR
von Vizepräsident Prof. Dr. Heinrich Scheel

Erschienen im Akademie-Verlag, DDR - 1086 Berlin, Leipziger Straße 3—4

Lizenznummer: 202 · 100/068/84
Printed in the German Democratic Republic
Gesamtherstellung: VEB Druckhaus „Maxim Gorki", 7400 Altenburg
LSV 2115, 2025
Bestellnummer: 763 310 4 (2001/84/1 N)
06500

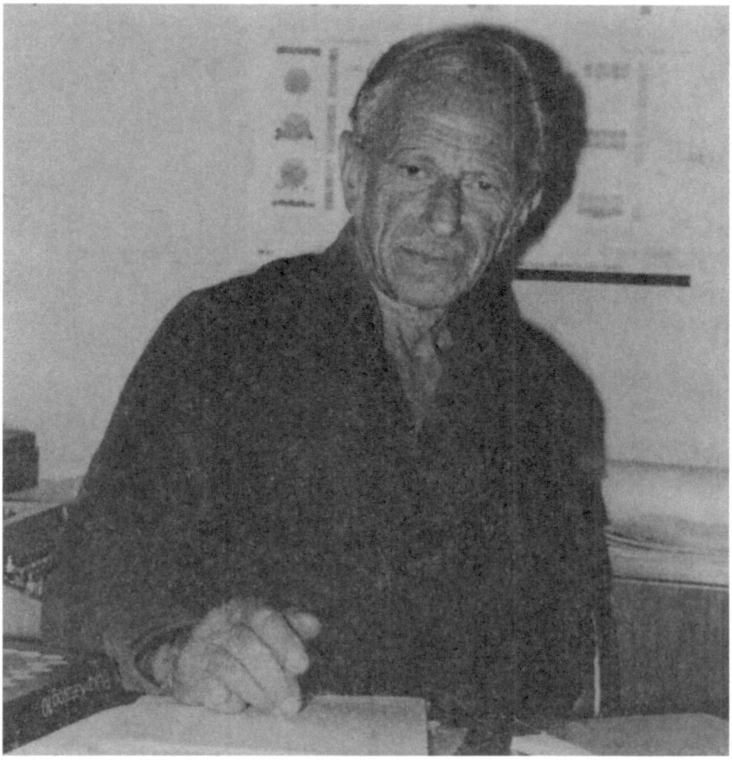

The Symposium was held on the occasion of the 70th birthday of Academician Professor Albert Wollenberger

Preface

Our purpose in selecting the topics of the Symposium was twofold. In the first place, progress in the field of molecular and cellular cardiology has been rapid in the last few years, but there was little opportunity for investigators from different disciplines to meet and discuss matters of common interest in greater depth.

Secondly, and no less important, this Symposium provided a chance to honour Albert WOLLENBERGER as a pioneer in cellular and molecular cardiology. His merits in initiating and pursuing at an early date investigations in the area of cardiac energy metabolism is well known and more lately he has contributed significantly to the elucidation of mechanisms of the neural and hormonal regulation of the heart. Impatient as researcher, he always inspired his coworkers by treading on new paths, by devising new methods and last not least, by keeping on the alert for applications of the results of basic research to practical medicine.

The Proceedings of the Symposium contain contributions of invited speakers and a selection of poster presentations. We express our sincere thanks to all contributors and apologize that on account of space limitations it was necessary for the editors to shorten the text of some of the manuscripts.

H. HEINE
L. WILL-SHAHAB
E.-G. KRAUSE
W. SCHULZE

Albert Wollenberger — Scientific Humanist

RAPOPORT, S. M., President of the Society of Experimental Medicine of the GDR

Dear Ladies and Gentlemen; dear Albert,

I have the great pleasure to speak to you on behalf of the Gesellschaft für Experimentelle Medizin der DDR. As most of you know, this organization constitutes a federation which encompasses 14 societies, among them those of Biochemistry, Pharmacology and Pathophysiology. They represent fields which have been particularly close to the interests of Albert WOLLENBERGER. The Federation as a whole is greatly concerned with the development of interdisciplinary activities. Therefore it is deeply grateful to Albert for the leadership he has given and for the many contributions that he and his coworkers have given to the advancement of science in the GDR, particularly in its interdisciplinary aspects. I also have the honour to convey to you, dear Albert, the best wishes of the Minister of Health, Prof. Ludwig MECKLINGER, who regrets that he is not able to express them to you personally. He wants you to know that the Ministry of Health and many members of the medical profession are grateful to you and proud of your work.

It cannot be my task to recount the details of the results of the work of Albert; instead I should like to view his contributions in a wider respective. If we take a look at the development of medical science in the recent past, we find that increasingly the disciplinary approach is supplemented and even surpassed by the swift growth of organ-centered multidisciplinary research. We thus have a new form of integration of scientific endeavours of various kinds.

Accordingly, cardiac research has grown to be a vigorous field which is the common meeting ground for biochemists, pharmacologists, physiologists, and various other types of specialists. The historic contribution of Albert has been to pioneer this development and to choose his small crew carefully with a view to integrative research.

Albert is not an articulate philosopher, but by his complex multidisciplinary conception of how to study heart function he has proved himself to be a master in the application of dialectics. Both his personal achievements as well as the composition and subject matter of this symposium bear witness to the fertility of Albert's basic conceptions.

But Albert has contributed more than good conceptions. He has been endowed with a deep urge for fundamental understanding, a constant desire to learn techniques and methods as well es an unerring instinct for quality in scientific work. These characteristics have led him to various leading laboratories the world over of which I should like to mention only one, that of LINDERSTRÖM-LANG.

I do this not only because of the scientific training and inspiration which he received there but also because it was a place where he had the good fortunate to meet Gertrud, his better and even more fertile half.

The constant quest for the fundamental understanding of phenomena led Albert to make another contribution of general significance. I have in mind the blending of biochemistry and pharmacology. He has a distinct share in the building of the modern foundations of pharmacology.

Let me say a few more words what Albert has done for science of the GDR. He has represented the GDR in the international scene with dignity, fairness, and firmness and has contributed greatly to its recognition. He has done a great deal to promote international cooperation and has helped to establish close ties with the scientists in the Soviet Union and other socialist countries.

His scientific stature is inseparably linked to his humanistic and socialistic convictions. He has adhered to them from his youth and maintained them even under the overwhelming influence of a capitalistic environment.

Thus his whole life and his present untiring scientific activity are an inspiration to the young generation of scientists.

On the other hand, it was the GDR where Albert found the conditions for his maturation as a scientist and for a wide range of activities as well as for the upbringing of a large happy family.

He emigrated from a fascist Germany and returned to a socialist state with a continuous support of science, governed by humanistic principles, dedicated to peace and offering security.

Let me finally say a few words about Albert as a person. I have known him for 28 years and I am proud to be counted among his friends. But still I find it not easy to encompass his personality in a few sentences. What is its essence? To my mind Albert has the qualities of a Renaissance man in a modern version. He combines a love of all types of culture, including music, painting, sculpture, and literature with a deep love of nature, particularly the mountains, and not to forget his physical culture and prowess with the outlook and attitude of a scientist. This harmonious blend of artistic and scientific gifts, combined with a strong self-contained and self-disciplined character — this is to my mind the essence of the scientific humanist Albert WOLLENBERGER.

Contents

I. Membranes and contractile proteins

LEVITSKY, D. O., M. K. ALIEV, D. S. BENEVOLENSKY and T. S. LEVCHENKO (Moskow): Properties of Ca^{2+}-ATPase in cardiac sarcoplasmic reticulum 15

SUKO, J., B. PLANK, W. WYSKOVSKY and G. HELLMANN (Vienna): Calcium uptake and phosphorylation in sarcoplasmic reticulum: Calmodulin effect in cardiac sarcoplasmic reticulum and stopped flow fluorescence measurement of $Mg \cdot E^{+} - P$ in skeletal muscle sarcoplasmic reticulum 23

ENGLAND, P., D. MILLS, H. T. PASK and S. A. JAECKOCKE (Bristol): The phosphorylation of cardiac contractile proteins 29

SAMUEL, J. L., J. J. MERCADIER, Y. LECARPENTIER, A. M. LOMPRÉ, K. SCHWARTZ and B. SWYNGHEDAUW (Paris): Regulation of cardiac function during chronic overload. Myosin isoenzyme redistribution 35

SAKS, V. A., G. B. CHERNOUSOVA, N. V. LYULINA, Z. A. KHUCHUA, A. N. PREOBRAZENSKIY and R. VENTURA-CLAPIER (Moscow/Orsay): Role of multienzyme complexes in intracellular compartmentation of adenine nucleotides and in regulation of cardiac energy metabolism . 41

II. Ion movements

HERING, S., A. I. UNDROVINAS and R. BODEWEI (Berlin/Moscow): Frequency- and voltage-dependent block of sodium channels in single rat myocardial cells treated with mexiletine . . 51

NILIUS, B. (Halle): Pacing-dependent properties of the slow inward current in the atrial myocardium 57

SCHOLZ, H. and R. BRÜCKNER (Hamburg): Mechanical and electrophysiological effects of α-adrenoceptor stimulating drugs in the heart 67

III. Ca^{2+} transport and protein phosphorylation

GROSSE, R., E. SPITZER, K. ECKERT and F. BÖHMER (Berlin): Regulation of intracellular Ca^{2+}-concentration in exitable and nonexitable tissues 75

CARAFOLI, E. (Zürich): The regulation of the Ca^{2+} transporting systems of heart plasma membrane 87

KURSKY, M. D. and Z. D. VOROBETZ (Kiev): Effect of cAMP-dependent phosphorylation on passive Ca^{2+} transport in myocardial sarcolemma 95

ZIEGELHÖFFER, A., M. B. ANAND-SRIVASTAVA and N. S. DHALLA (Bratislava/Winnipeg): Possible role of Ca^{2+}-ATPase in mechanism of calcium influx through cardiac sarcolemma . 99

LAMERS, J. M. J. (Rotterdam): Ca^{2+}-calmodulin and cyclic AMP-dependent phosphorylation of cardiac sarcolemma 107

WILL, H., T. LEVCHENKO and C. KEMSIES (Berlin/Moscow): Subunit analysis and cross-linking of phospholamban in cardiac sarcoplasmatic reticulum and sarcolemma 121

IV. Metabolic aspects of myocardial ischaemia

PANAGIA, V., J. A. C. HARROW, G. SINGH, A. GUERIN and N. S. DHALLA (Winnipeg): Myocardial membrane changes due to ischaemia-reperfusion injury in dogs treated with or without acebutolol 133
KAMMERMEIER, H. (Aachen): Free energy of ATP-hydrolysis as a limiting factor of actin-myosin interaction and ion pumping in early failure of the heart 141
KRAUSE, E.-G., P. J. ENGLAND and S. BARTEL (Berlin/Bristol): Isoproterenol-induced protein phosphorylation in the isolated ischaemic rat heart 149
FERRARI, R. and O. VISIOLI (Parma): The functional and metabolical consequence of myocardial ischaemia and reperfusion. Effects of verapamil 157
MOSINGER, B. (Prague): The role of calcium in myocardial ischaemia 169
METSÄ-KETELÄ, T., P. VUORINEN and K. LAUSTIOLA (Tampere): The effect of cyclic GMP-elevating nitrogenous compounds on myocardial glycolysis 177
SZEKERES, L., I. LEPRÁN, I. KRASSOI, J. PATARICZA, E. UDVARY, M. KOLTAI and P. L. VÁGHY (Szeged): Possible pharmacological measures for the prevention of sudden death in acute local myocardial ischaemia 185
MEERSON, F. Z. (Moscow): Stress damages of the heart: Pathogenesis and possibilities of prevention and removing 193
GUDBJARNASON, S., A. EMILSSON and A. GUDMUNDSDOTTIR (Reykjavik): Alterations in fatty acyl chain composition of myocardial phospholipids during stress 203
MONTFOORT, A., C. C. M. RUTTEN-VAN BEYSTERVELD and M. R. WORTELBOER (Rotterdam): Molecular species of phosphatidylethanolamine in rat and mouse heart 207

V. Communication presented as posters

PELOUCH, V., B. OŠTÁDAL and J. PROCHÁZKA (Prag): The effect of hypoxia on the structural and enzymatic properties of cardiac myosin 215
OŠTÁDAL, B., T. JANATOVÁ, V. PELOUCH and E.-G. KRAUSE (Prag): A possible role of cAMP in the cardiotoxicity of catecholamines during embryonic life 217
PORZIG, H., C. BECKER and H. REUTER (Bern): Properties and regulation of β-adrenoceptors in living cardiac cells 221
SCHULZE, W. (Berlin): Ischaemia-induced changes of the cardiac adenylate cyclase system I. Cytochemical studies of adenylate cyclase activity 223
WILL-SHAHAB, L. and I. KÜTTNER (Berlin): Ischaemia-induced changes of the cardiac adenylate cyclase activity. II. Reversible inhibition of adenylate cyclax 227
HYNIE, S. (Prag): Adenylate cyclase activity in the heart and some other tissues treated by α-chymotrypsin 229
WALLUKAT, G., L. WILL-SHAHAB and A. WOLLENBERGER (Berlin): Supersensitivity to isoprenaline in cultured rat myocardial cells exposed to L(+)-lactate and pyruvate 233
BARTEL, S., E.-G. KRAUSE and J. G. REICH (Berlin): Activation of cyclic AMP-dependent protein kinase in the ischaemic myocardium 237
LÖWE, H., I. E. BLASIG, C. HENNIG and B. OCZKO (Berlin): Myocardial protection in vitro by o-(β-hydroxyethyl)-rutoside a flavone derivate and by mannitol 241
BLASIG, I. E., P. MUSCHICK, E. ROHDE, R. RICHTER, D. MODERSOHN and H. LÖWE (Berlin): Can blood flow reduction after isoproterenol overdosage induce myocardial ischaemia? . . . 243
GOOS, H., K.-F. LINDENAU, E.-G. KRAUSE, J. NÖHRING, S. GEHLHAR, J. SCHINKE, C. WAGENKNECHT, H. DAVID, J. LIEBETRUTH, B. JONAS and R. A. PARSI (Berlin): The influence of prostacyclin on experimental myocardial infarction in dogs 247
RABITZSCH, G., H. GOOS, J. NÖHRING, J. LEMBCKE, K.-F. LINDENAU, E.-G. KRAUSE, R.-A.

PARSI and H. HEINE (Berlin): Glycogen phosphorylase b activity in human serum after acute myocardial infarction and coronary bypass surgery 251
FÖRSTER, W., I. HEINROTH, H.-U. BLOCK, P. MENTZ and K. PÖNICKE (Halle): Influence of β-receptor blocking drugs on prostacyclin and thromboxane synthesis 255
SCHIRPKE, B. (Berlin): In vivo experiments on phospholipid metabolism in rat heart. . . . 259
TITLBACH, O., H. MAREK, L. WILL-SHAHAB, P. FEYER, L. BÖLKE and R. FIEBER (Leipzig/Berlin): Influence of drugs, hormones and ischaemia on glucose uptake, CK release and energy potential of rabbit-Langendorff hearts 263
BRASELMANN, H., W. KRAUSE and H. GUSKI (Berlin): Biochemical and electron microscopic findings on the myocardium of trained and untrained rats after infarction 265
POGÁTSA, G. and M. Z. KOLTAI (Budapest): The role of altered diabetic coronary reactivity in myocardial ischaemia 269
LEHMANN, I., R. A. PARSI, B. PAPIES, E. LUDWIG, M. L. KÖNIG, M. NAGI and C. WAGENKNECHT (Berlin): Enzyme pattern in endomyocardial biopsies 275
CAFFIER, G. and R. M. KRÜNES (Berlin): Action of free fatty acids on contractility and action potential of the heart 279
WUSSLING, M. and G. SZYMANSKI (Halle): The influence of Ca^{2+} and passive tension on relaxation phenomena in the mammalian myocardium 281
GÜNTHER, J., E. STORCH, E. KUTSCHERSKIJ and R. VETTER (Berlin): Lipid-diet induced changes of the Ca regulation in the rabbit myocardium 285
HERRMANN, H.-J., V. MORITZ, T. HECHT, C. NORDEN and P. MÜHLIG (Berlin): Appearances of metabolically influenced long-term vasotonus changes in coronary microvessels of rats. . 289
VETTER, R., H. HAASE and H. WILL (Berlin): Potentiating effect of calmodulin and cyclic AMP-dependent protein kinase on the Ca^{2+}-pump of cardiac sarcolemma 293
HOLTZHAUER, M., H. SYDOW and H. WILL (Berlin): Characterization of a phosphorylated protein-lipid complex of heart sarcolemma 297
WETZKER, R., R. KLINGER, I. FLEISCHER and H. FRUNDER (Jena): Activation of (Ca^{2+} + Mg^{2+}) ATPase of erythrocyte membranes by trypsin, fatty acids and Ca^{2+}. A comparison with calmodulin action 301
SCHÖNFELD, P., D. PETZOLD and W. KUNZ (Magdeburg): Simultaneous oxidation of pyruvate and fatty acids by rat heart mitochondria at limiting substrate supply. 305
TAKÁTS, I. and L. SZEKERES (Szeged): Protecting effect of adrenergic β-blocking agents on the energy metabolism of ischaemic myocardium 309
VÁGHY, P. L., M. A. MATLIB and A. SCHWARTZ (Szeged): Diltiazem is a selective inhibitor of the Na^{+}/Ca^{2+} antiporter in heart mitochondria 313
PFEIFFER, C. and Ch. HUCKSTORF (Rostock): Rest versus frequency loaded contractions in the myocardium of rats 319
WUSSLING, M. and G. SZYMANSKI (Halle): Influence of noradrenaline and caffaine on potentiation and staircase phenomena 323
MÖRITZ, K.-U., R. FERMUM and U. TOFELDE (Greifswald): Dissociation of isoproterenol-induced cAMP-increase and vascular relaxation in isolated coronary arteries under the influence of DFP 327
HOFFMANN, P., P. MENTZ and W. FÖRSTER (Halle): Influence of dietary linoleate on the adrenergic response of isolated rat hearts 329
GELLERICH, F. N., and SCHLAME (Magdeburg): Importance of mitochondrial creatine kinase localization for securing the stimulation of mitochondrial ATP-production 333
GOLA, G., K. KOTHE, K.-F. LINDENAU, A. LUN, H. WARNKE and C. WAGENKNECHT (Berlin): Metabolic pattern in the reperfusion period of different cardiovascular operations in the coronary sinus 337
WOLLENBERGER, A.: Closing remarks 341
List of contributors 345

I. Membranes and contractile proteins

USSR Cardiology Research Center, Academy of Medical Sciences, Moscow USSR

Properties of Ca^{2+}-ATPase in Cardiac Sarcoplasmic Reticulum

D. O. Levitsky, M. K. Aliev, D. S. Benevolensky and T. S. Levchenko

In cardiac muscle cells three major events provide periodical changes of contracted and relaxed states of fibers: 1) Ca^{2+} entry into myoplasm from intracellular reservoirs and across sarcolemmal membrane; 2) binding of calcium ions to troponin C resulting in activation of myosin ATPase and contraction of fibers and 3) Ca^{2+} removal from the intracellular fluid leading to heart relaxation [7, 8]. At least half a dozen of Ca^{2+}-channels, pumps and cation exchanges are operating in cardiac cells. These are Ca^{2+}-pumps in sarcoplasmic reticulum (SR) network [10, 12] and mitochondria [2, 4, 6], slow Ca^{2+}-channel [25, 30], Na^+/Ca^{2+} antiporter [30], ATP-dependent Ca^{2+}-pump [3] in sarcolemmal membrane and Ca^{2+}-channels locating in reticular [9] and inner mitochondrial [2, 4] membranes. A quantification of the separate Ca^{2+} transmembrane fluxes is far from complete. This estimate can be achieved using a pure biochemical approach by studying Ca^{2+}-transporting systems on the whole and its main components in purified form.

In this paper the data are summarized on functional and structural properties of cardiac sarcoplasmic reticulum and its calcium pump protein which allowed to determine the place of reticular Ca^{2+}-pump in electrochemical coupling of myocardial cells.

Purification of cardiac SR and reticular Ca^{2+}-ATPase

Microsomal fraction obtained after homogenization of muscle tissue and differential centrifugation of homogenate is enriched by SR fragments. Distinctive feature of cardiac microsomes as compared with microsomes from skeletal muscles is low activity and high lability of the Ca^{2+}-pump and Ca^{2+}-ATPase. This is partly due to the fact that fractions of cardiac SR as a rule are heavily contaminated by mitochondrial membranes, lysosomes, fragments of sarcolemmal and other cellular membranes. One may suggest that major drop in the activity of SR Ca^{2+}-pump occurs already after homogenization of heart muscle when lysosomal enzymes are activated.

For purification of cardiac SR a method of partial Ca^{2+}-oxalate loading of microsomes has been worked out [17]. This procedure allows also to achieve the isolation of less damaged SR vesicles. After centrifugation in sucrose density gradients two supernatant layers are formed containing predominantly sarcolemmal (upper layer) and mitochondrial (lower layer) fragments and a pellet (Ca^{2+}-oxalate preparation), SR-enriched fraction [14, 17, 22, 38]. The major protein component in the Ca^{2+}-oxalate preparation is Ca^{2+}-ATPase with molecular weight of 100000. This enzyme can be purified from membranes of the Ca^{2+}-oxalate preparation by a method of MACLENNAN [21] which is widely used for isolation of Ca^{2+}-ATPase from skeletal muscle SR. The method includes treatment of the membranes with low and high concentrations of sodium deoxycholate. Specific activity of Ca^{2+}-ATPase isolated from pigeon heart SR is 3 times lower than that in the preparation obtained from rabbit skeletal muscle SR [17].

Are these enzymes similar by their structure and functional parameters? The most important characteristics of a Ca^{2+}-pump protein is its sensitivity to calcium ions. As seen from Figure 1, these two Ca^{2+}-ATPases are activated in the same range of concentration of ionized calcium and have identical Ca^{2+}-optima. Dependences of the enzymatic activities on pH are also similar though not identical (Fig. 1b). It is of interest that

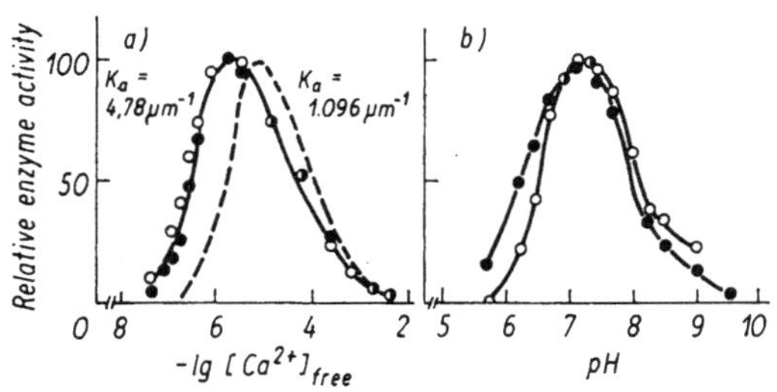

Fig. 1. Calcium ion and pH dependences of Ca^{2+}-ATPase activity. The curves in a were obtained according to the values of association constant of Ca^{2+}-EGTA complex reported by YAMADA et al. [40] (solid line) and OGAWA [26] (dotted line). Incubation medium contained 0.1 M KCl, 30 mM imidazole (pH 7.0), 5 mM sodium azide, 5 mM ATP, 6.5 mM $MgCl_2$, and for b panel 2 mM EGTA and various concentrations of $CaCl_2$. Temperature —37 °C. • — — •, ATPase from pigeon heart SR, ○ — — ○, ATPase from rabbit skeletal muscle SR.

Ca^{2+} sensitivities of the reaction of ATP hydrolysis proceeding in microsomes isolated from heart and skeletal muscle are different [31]. Sensitivity to Ca^{2+} in heart SR appears to be lower in comparison with skeletal muscle SR but it increases after the cAMP-dependent phosphorylation of a regulatory SR protein, phospholamban [11]. One may conclude that a building (Ca^{2+}-pump systems) in muscles of two types is different though major bricks it are formed of (Ca^{2+}-ATPases) are rather similar.

ATP-dependence of Ca^{2+}-ATPase reaction in skeletal muscle SR is complex and does not follow completely Michaelis-Menten kinetics [40]. The second rise in the activity is registered at ATP concentrations higher than 0.1 mM which is taken as an evidence for the existence of the second, regulatory ATP-binding site on the ATPase molecule [24]. The same two-step dependence can be visualized for cardiac Ca^{2+}-ATPase (Fig. 2a). Using double-reciprocal plots, K_m values for ATP, at low concentrations of the substrates, were determined (Fig. 2b). At given experimental conditions, they were found to be close for two enzymes and fell into a range between 12 and 17 µM.

Temperature dependences of ATPase reactions are identical for heart and skeletal muscle enzyme preparations the optima being at 50 °C [17]. That is not surprising since the ratio of unsaturated to saturated fatty acids in phospholipids of the purified SR fractions was found to be the same [18]. Besides, treatment of SR membranes with deoxycholate could modify lipid protein interaction and make the mobility of Ca^{2+}-ATPase molecules identical.

Similarities in functional properties of Ca^{2+}-ATPase from heart and skeletal muscle SR could be explained by similar structures of the enzyme. Comparison of amino acid composition of the Ca^{2+}-ATPases (Table 1, from 20) is an additional evidence for general likeness of the enzymes though this parameter seems to be rough for estimating enzyme structure. Mild treatment of Ca^{2+}-ATPases from skeletal muscle SR by trypsin leads to the splitting of the enzyme into 4 fragments with molecular weights of 55000,

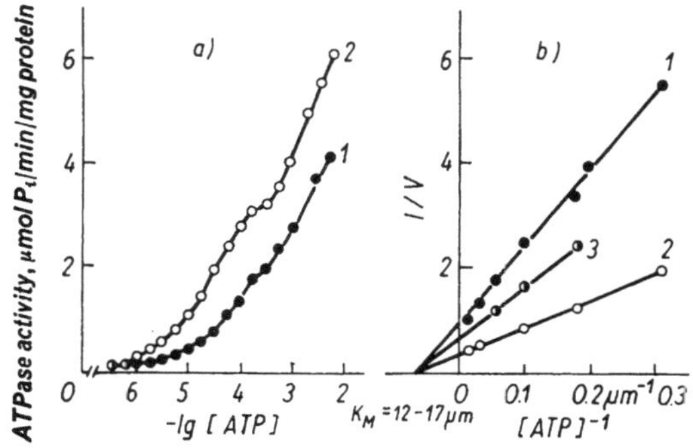

Fig. 2. ATP dependence of ATPase activity. Incubation medium contained 0.1 M KCl, 6.5 mM $MgCl_2$, 15 μM $CaCl_2$, 1 mM phosphoenol pyruvate, 0.2 mM NADH, 6 U/ml lactate dehydrogenase, 1.2 U/ml pyruvate kinase, 15 mM imidazol (pH 7.1, 25 °C).

45000, 30000 and 20000 dalton [34, 36]. Location of the active center in the fragments of the enzyme can be followed by radioactive phosphorus derived from [γ-^{32}P] ATP due to Ca^{2+}-ATPase reaction. It has been found that phosphorylated product becomes localized in 55000 and 30000-fragments [34, 35]. The same distribution of radioactivity is seen in tryptic fragments of Ca^{2+}-ATPase from pigeon heart SR (Fig. 3).

A decisive argument in favour (or against) similarities in the structure of Ca^{2+}-ATPases from heart and skeletal muscles could be obtained after determination of their amino acid sequences. However, one can use a less labour-consuming method and compare antigenic properties of the enzymes. A correlation exists between so-called index of antigenic dissimilarity and variations in primary structure of homologous enzymes [16, 29]. By a complement fixation technique, using sheep antiserum raised to Ca^{2+}-ATPase from rabbit skeletal muscle SR, DeFoor et al. [5] have found different cross-reactivity in Ca^{2+}-ATPases from a number of heart and skeletal muscle SR preparations. The indices of immunological dissimilarity for Ca^{2+}-ATPases increase in a sequence: 1.0 (ATPases from rabbit and rat skeletal muscle SR, immunological identity) < 1.9 (pigeon breast skeletal muscle) < 3.3 (bovine heart) < 5.1 (rabbit heart) < 6.1 (rat heart) < 6.7 (pigeon heart). It follows, therefore, that structures of the polypeptides of the Ca^{2+}-ATPases localized in heart and skeletal muscle SR differ. That might be a basis for lower ATP-hydrolysing and Ca^{2+} accumulating activities in preparations of heart muscle SR.

In favour of this conclusion are the results of our experiment on reconstitution of Ca^{2+}-pumps in a new lipid environment. The vesicles reconstituted by a method of Knowles and Racker [15] after dialysis of a mixture containing cholate, oxalate,

Table 1

Amino acid composition of Ca^{2+}-ATPase isolated from SR of cardiac and skeletal muscles

Amido acid	Pigeon heart muscle	Rabbit skeletal muscle
Lys	47.5	48
His	12.8	12.7
Arg	39.7	37
Asp	85.5	78
Thr	58	55.5
Ser	80	744
Glu	114	114.4
Pro	54.2	64.
Gly	91.5	79
Ala	89.2	84.8
Cys	18.2	21
Val	66.5	75
Met-SO_3	27.5	30
Ile	53.7	53
Leu	91.8	88
Tyr	22.2	20.7
Phe	36.5	33.7
% polar	45	49.4
% nonpolar	55	50.6

The Table shows amount of amino acid residues without tryptophan per 100000 molecule. (From LEVITSKY et al. — 20)

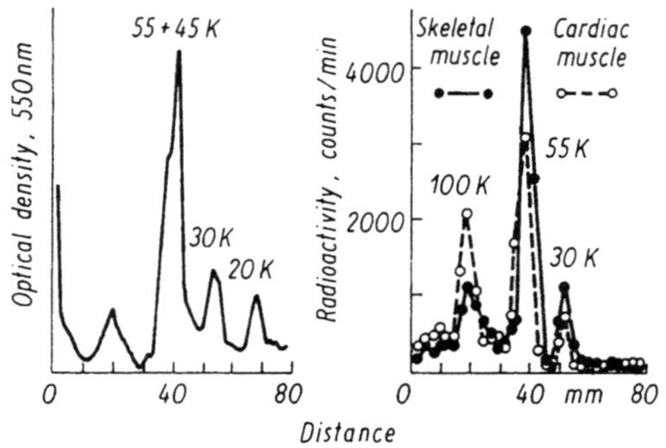

Fig. 3. Splitting of phosphorylated Ca^{2+}-ATPases from heart and skeletal muscle by trypsin. Protein fragments were separated by polyacrylamide gel electrophoresis at pH 2.4.

phospholipids of soy beans and Ca^{2+}-ATPase preparations from either skeletal or cardiac muscles were able to accumulate calcium ions. The proteoliposomes containing Ca^{2+}-ATPase from skeletal muscle transfered Ca^{2+} with a velocity five times higher than proteoliposomes with heart muscle ATPase [18]. Thus, it is the protein but not lipid component of SR membrane that determines higher activity of skeletal muscle Ca^{2+}-pump system.

Ca^{2+}-ATPase and Ca^{2+} consumption by SR of heart muscle

An important problem in excitation-contraction coupling of heart muscle is the contribution of SR network in consuming Ca^{2+} during relaxation period. Molecular activity of reticular Ca^{2+}-ATPase should be high enough to fulfil several turnovers in 100—200 ms. Activity of Ca^{2+}-ATPase in purified cardiac microsomes exceeds at 37 °C 2.6 μmol P_i/min · mg protein [17]. Taking into account a steady state value of the phosphorylated intermediate, 2.45 nmol P_i/mg protein [17], one may estimate that in 100 ms ATPase fulfils about 2 turnovers.

The concentration of the calcium pump protein in a cardiac cell should also be taken into consideration. According to SOLARO and BRIGGS [32] 6.8 mg of microsomal protein are presented in 1 g of the heart. However, since SR fraction isolated by the technique of Solaro and Briggs was not pure, the real amount of SR protein in 1 g of heart should be lower.

To determine concentration of SR in heart muscle, a procedure was devised [19] allowing after a series of short homogenizations and differential centrifugations to extract total fraction of Ca^{2+}-transporting microsomal vesicles (Fig. 4). With each successive cycle of homogenization and centrifugation additional membrane fragments were concentrated in microsomal fraction which consumed Ca^{2+} in the presence and in the absence of oxalate and were phosphorylated by terminal phosphate from [γ-^{32}P] ATP in a calcium--containing medium. After 15th extraction, the curves showing accumulation of active vesicles in the microsomal fraction approached saturation. That indicated termination of SR extraction.

The only component phosphorylated in all fractions extracted from cardiac muscle is a protein which has the same molecular weight as Ca^{2+}-ATPase from skeletal muscle SR (Fig. 5). Values of phosphate incorporation into Ca^{2+}-ATPase localized in micro-

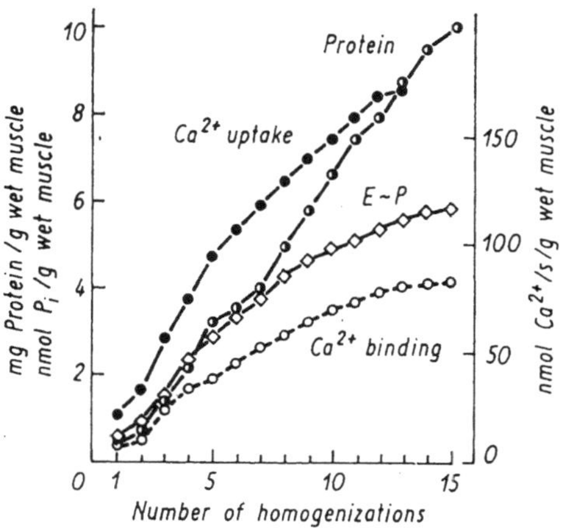

Fig. 4. Yield of SR vesicles after successive cycles of homogenization and differential centrifugation of guinea pig heart. For details see [19]. Ca^{2+} uptake was measured in the presence of 6.5 mM potassium oxalate. "Ca^{2+} binding" was determined in the absence of Ca^{2+}-precipitating anions. Temperature of the incubation medium was 37 °C. Phosphorylation of Ca^{2+}-ATPase was performed at 0 °C.

somal fractions isolated from guinea pig and pigeon hearts are 5.9 and 7.8 nmol/g of wet muscle [19]. Corresponding values for purified SR preparations are 2.8 and 2.45 nmol/mg protein. Thus, in one gram of heart tissue, 2.1 (guinea pig) and 3.2 (pigeon) mg of SR protein are concentrated. Obviously, this estimate concerns only those membranes from reticular network which contain Ca^{2+}-ATPase.

To estimate total Ca^{2+}-pump activity of SR membranes, the measurements of so-called ATP-dependent binding in short time intervals were made [19]. This was done by a technique suggested earlier by WILL et al. [37], using a Durrum mixing apparatus and quenching the process of Ca^{2+} transport by EGTA. At 37 °C and neutral pH,

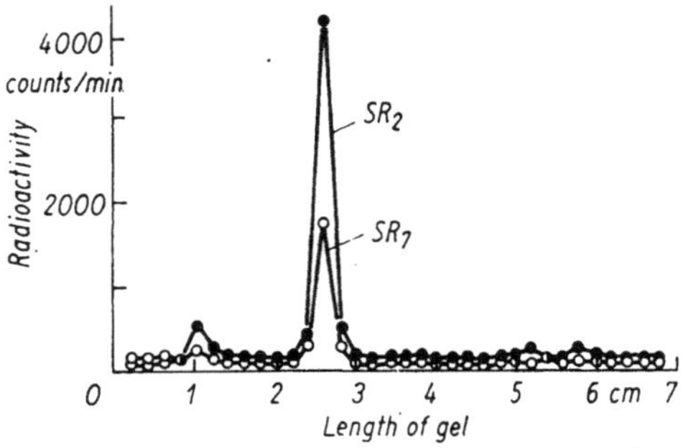

Fig. 5. Phosphorylation of Ca^{2+}-ATPase molecules localized in two different microsomal fractions extracted from guinea pig hearts. Separation of phosphorylated proteins was performed according to a technique described in [17]. Major peak of radioactivity corresponds to the Ca^{2+}-ATPase. Additional small peak represents, most likely, Ca^{2+}-ATPase dimer.

time-course of ATP-dependent Ca^{2+} binding by cardiac microsomes is nonlinear at a range from 0.1 to 1 s (Fig. 6). One-third and a half of Ca^{2+} bound within 1 second was consumed by microsomes in 0.1 and 0.2 s, respectively. Combined fraction of SR extracted from 1 g of guinea pig heart accumulates within 1 second up to 66.5 nmol Ca^{2+} [19]. From the time course of Ca^{2+} accumulation (Fig. 6) it is evident that this fraction is able to bind 22 and 33 nmol Ca^{2+} in 0.1 and 0.2 seconds.

At systole, concentration of ionized Ca^{2+} in myoplasm of a cardiac cell may rise up to 5 μM [1]. According to SOLARO et al. [33], this Ca^{2+} concentration causes 90% activation of cardiac muscle tension. The total amount of Ca^{2+}, free and bound to myofilaments, under these conditions, is about 35 nmol/g muscle [33]. Comparing this value with calculated velocity of Ca^{2+} binding by the fraction of completely extracted SR we may conclude that SR membranes by their Ca^{2+}-pump activity may ensure heart relaxation.

It is of interest to evaluate time-free calcium relationship of the process of Ca^{2+} binding by SR. If the reaction is quenched in 30 seconds the dependence of the amount of bound Ca^{2+} on concentration of ionized Ca^{2+} would be not pronounced at the range between 0.5 to and 20 μM of Ca^{2+} free (Fig. 7, curve a). Decreasing time of the reaction to 1 second one gets a steeper curve with a distinct Ca^{2+}-optimum at about 2 μM (Fig. 7, curve b). Therefore, at short times, Ca^{2+}-pumping activity of cardiac SR is higher at 1 μM of free calcium than at 24 μM (the concentration used in the experiments illustrated by Figs. 3, 5). Troponin C, due to its lower affinity to Ca^{2+} [13, 28], compared to that of reticular Ca^{2+}-ATPase, during relaxation period should behave as a Ca^{2+}-buffer maintaining for tens of milliseconds the myoplasmic concentration of ionized Ca^{2+} above 1 μM. During this period SR pump performs its highest activity. When ionized Ca^{2+} concentration drops down to 0.5 μM the pump would lose only 30% of its efficiency (Fig. 7). At this Ca^{2+} concentration, muscle tension decreases approximately 20 times [33]. It follows that major portion of Ca^{2+} can be removed from the myoplasm of cardiac cell during relaxation by sarcoplasmic reticulum.

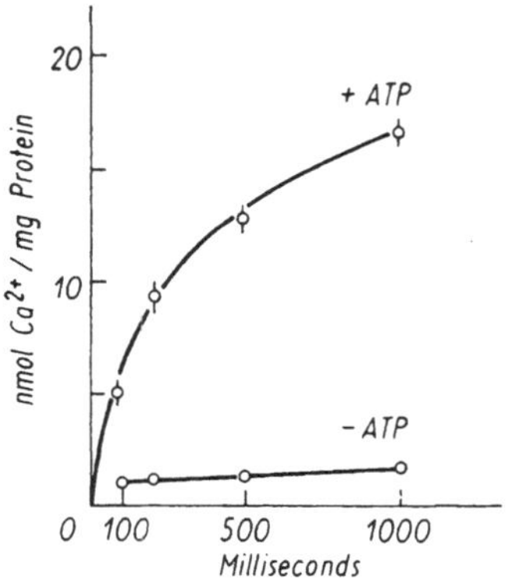

Fig. 6. Accumulation of Ca^{2+} by microsomes from guinea pig heart in short time intervals. For explanations see the text.

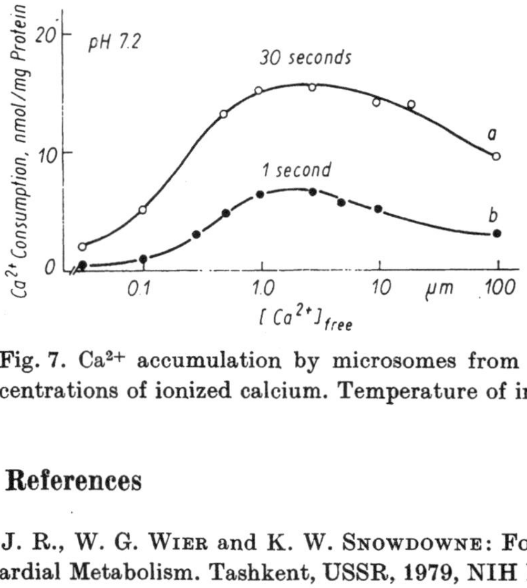

Fig. 7. Ca^{2+} accumulation by microsomes from guinea pig heart at different concentrations of ionized calcium. Temperature of incubation mixture was 37 °C.

References

[1] Blinks, J. R., W. G. Wier and K. W. Snowdowne: Fourth USA-USSR Joint Symposium on Myocardial Metabolism. Tashkent, USSR, 1979, NIH Publication No 80-2017, (1980)

[2] Carafoli, E.: FEBS Letters **104** (1979), 1–5

[3] Caroni, P. and E. Carafoli: J. Biol. Chem. **256** (1981), 3263–3270

[4] Crompton, M., M. Capano and E. Carafoli: Eur. J. Biochem. **69** (1976), 453–462

[5] De Foor, P. H., D. Levitsky, T. Biryukova and S. Fleischer: Arch. Biochem. Biophys. **200** (1980), 196–205

[6] Dhalla, N. S., D. B. McNamara and P. V. Sulakhe: Cardiology **55** (1970), 178–191

[7] Ebashi, S.: Essays Biochem. **10** (1975), 1–36

[8] Ebashi, S. and M. Endo: Progr. Biophys. Mol. Biol. **18** (1968), 123–183

[9] Fabiato, A. and F. Fabiato: Circ. Res. **31** (1972), 293–307

[10] FANBURG, B. and J. GERGELY: J. Biol. Chem. **240** (1965), 2721—2728
[11] HICKS, M. J., M. SHIGEKAWA and A. M. KATZ: Circ. Res. **44** (1979), 384—391
[12] INESI, G., S. EBASHI and S. WATANABE: Am. J. Physiol. **207** (1964), 1339—1344
[13] JOHNSON, J. D., J. H. COLLINS, S. P. ROBERTSON and J. D. POTTER: J. Biol. Chem. **255** (1980), 9635—9640
[14] JONES, L. R., H. R. BESCH, Jr., J. W. FLEMING, M. M. MCCONNAUGHEY and A. M. WATANABE: J. Biol. Chem. **254** (1979), 530—539
[15] KNOWLES, A. F. and E. RACKER: J. Biol. Chem. **250** (1975), 3538—3544
[16] KOPHENHEFFER, T. L., and S. M. GINSBERG: Comp. Biochem. Physiol. **60B** (1978), 163—167.
[17] LEVITSKY, D. O., M. K. ALIEV, A. V. KUZMIN, T. S. LEVCHENKO, V. N. SMIRNOV and E. I. CHAZOV: Biochim. Biophys. Acta, **443** (1976), 468—484
[18] LEVITSKY, D. O., D. S. BENEVOLENSKY, T. S. LEVCHENKO and A. V. KUZMIN: In: Advances in Myocardiology (Ed. by N. S. Dhalla), vol. 3 (1982), 393—405
[19] LEVITSKY, D. O., D. S. BENEVOLENSKY, T. S. LEVCHENKO, V. N. SMIRNOV and E. I. CHAZOV: J. Molec. Cell. Cardiol. **13** (1981), 785—796
[20] LEVITSKY, D. O., E. V. GRISHIN, T. V. BIRYUKOVA, A. V. LEBEDEV and L. N. NIKOLAEVA: Bull. of the All-Union Cardiol. Center. **2** (1981), 7—15
[21] MACLENNAN, D. H.: J. Biol. Chem. **245** (1970), 4508—4518
[22] MISSELWITZ, H.-J., H. WILL, W. SCHULZE, L. WILL-SHAHAB and A. WOLLENBERGER: Biochim. Biophys. Acta **553** (1979), 197—212
[23] MULLINS, L. J.: Am. J. Physiol. **236** (1979), C103—C110
[24] NEET, K. E. and N. M. GREEN: Arch. Biochem. Biophys. **118** (1977), 588—597
[25] NEW, W. and W. TRAUTWEIN: Pflüg. Arch. **334** (1972), 1—23
[26] OGAWA, Y.: J. Biochem. (Tokyo) **64** (1968), 255—257
[27] PATRIARCA, P. and E. CARAFOLI: J. Cell. Physiol. **72** (1978), 29—37
[28] POTTER, J. D. and J. GERGELY: J. Biol. Chem. **250** (1975), 4628—4633
[29] PRAGER, E. M. and A. C. WILSON: J. Biol. Chem. **246** (1971), 7010—7017
[30] REUTER, H.: Circ. Res. **34** (1974), 599—605
[31] SHIGEKAWA, M., J. N. FINEGAN and A. M. KATZ: J. Biol. Chem. **251** (1976), 6894—6900
[32] SOLARO, R. I. and F. N. BRIGGS: Circ. Res. **34** (1974), 531—540
[33] SOLARO, R. I., R. M. WISE, I. S. SHINER and F. N. BRIGGS: Circ. Res. **34** (1974), 525—530
[34] STEWART, P. S. and D. H. MACLENNAN: Ann. N.Y. Acad. Sci. **264** (1975), 326—335
[35] THORLEY-LAWSON, D. A. and N. M. GREEN: Eur. J. Biochem. **40** (1973), 403—413
[36] THORLEY-LAWSON, D. A. and N. M. GREEN: Eur. J. Biochem. **59** (1975), 193—200
[37] WILL, H., J. BLANK, G. SMETTAN and A. WOLLENBERGER: Biochem. Biophys. Acta, **449** (1976), 295—303
[38] WILL, H., T. S. LEVCHENKO, D. O. LEVITSKY, V. N. SMIRNOV and A. WOLLENBERGER: Biochem. Biophys. Acta **543** (1978), 175—193
[39] YAMADA, S., M. SUMIDA and Y. TONOMURA: J. Biochem. **72** (1972), 1537—1548
[40] YAMADA, T. and Y. TONOMURA: J. Biochem. **62** (1967), 558—575

Institute of Pharmacology, University of Vienna, Vienna, AUSTRIA

Calcium Uptake and Phosphorylation in Sarcoplasmic Reticulum: Calmodulin Effect in Cardiac Sarcoplasmic Reticulum and Stopped Flow Fluorescence Measurement of Mg · E* — P in Skeletal Muscle Sarcoplasmic Reticulum

J. Suko, B. Plank, W. Wyskovsky and G. Hellmann

Calmodulin-dependent calcium uptake and phosphorylation in cardiac sarcoplasmic reticulum

The increase in the rate of calcium transport by dog cardiac sarcoplasmic reticulum shown by Katz and Remtula [6] was suggested to be due to phosphorylation of phospholamban by a calcium-, calmodulin-dependent protein kinase [10]. A clear correlation between phosphorylation of phospholamban by a cAMP-dependent protein kinase and increase in the rate of calcium transport has been established [7], but the correlation with the calmodulin-dependent regulatory system has not yet been unequivocally proven.

The effect of calmodulin (CaM) on both calcium uptake and CaM-dependent phosphorylation has been investigated in myocardial sarcoplasmic reticulum (SR) from the dog. It was found that an increase in calcium uptake by CaM was associated with CaM-dependent phosphorylation, whilst experimental conditions which prevent phosphorylation also prevent a CaM-dependent increase in the rate of calcium transport.

Figure 1 shows the effect of 100 nM CaM on the rate of calcium uptake, measured by a filtration method at pH 7.0, 25 °C in the presence of oxalate and a low concentration of free calcium (about 0.5 μM) using 4 different modes of preincubation of SR vesicles: (a) The rate of calcium uptake measured with $^{45}CaCl_2$ following preincubation of SR

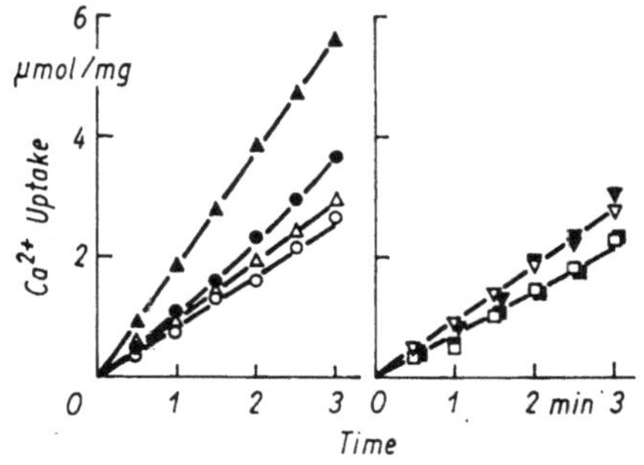

Fig. 1. Effect of CaM on calcium uptake by cardiac SR. Preincubation of SR vesicles (25°C; pH 7.0; 2—5 min; 40 mM histidine-HCl-Tris, 2 mM PEP, 20 μg/ml PK, 5 mM azide, 0.5 mg SR/ml without (open symbols) or with 100 nM CaM (closed symbols) plus (a: ▲, △) 0.1 mM Ca, 1 mM Mg, 1 mM ATP; (b: •, ∘) 0.1 mM Ca, 1 mM Mg; (c: ▼, ▽) zero added Ca, Mg, ATP; (d: ■, □) 0.1 mM EGTA, 1 mM Mg, 1 mM ATP. Calcium uptake: 25°C, pH 7.0; 40 mM histidine-HCl-Tris, 2 mM PEP, 20 μg/ ml PK, 0.2 mM ^{45}Ca, 0.3 mM EGTA, 3.5 mM $MgCl_2$, 5 mM azide, 5 mM oxalate, 0.05 mg/m preincubated SR, with or without 100 nM CaM. Values are means of two experiments.

vesicles with 100 nM CaM in the presence of 0.1 mM $CaCl_2$, 1 mM $MgCl_2$ and 1 mM ATP is markedly greater than the rates obtained with control vesicles preincubated under identical conditions in the absence of CaM. (b) Preincubation of SR vesicles with 100 nM CaM in the presence of 0.1 mM $CaCl_2$, 1 mM $MgCl_2$, but without ATP, results in a delayed and smaller increase in the rate of calcium uptake. On the other hand, preincubation of SR vesicles with 100 nM CaM in the absence of added $CaCl_2$, $MgCl_2$ and ATP (c) or in the presence of 1 mM $MgCl_2$, 1 mM ATP plus 0.1 mM EGTA (d) does not affect the rate of calcium uptake (Fig. 1). The CaM-dependent increase in the rate of calcium uptake following preincubation of SR vesicles with $CaCl_2$, $MgCl_2$ plus ATP (mode a in Fig. 1) was also verified by means of a spectrophotometric method, using arsenazo III as indicator, demonstrating a CaM-dependent increase in calcium net uptake and excluding a CaM-facilitated Ca—Ca exchange.

Half-maximum activation of calcium transport by CaM occurs at about 10 nM CaM (conditions a in Fig. 1). The rate of calcium uptake at about 0.5 μM free calcium and 100 nM CaM using the preincubation conditions with $CaCl_2$, $MgCl_2$ plus ATP (mode a in Fig. 1) was 0.162 ± 0.017 μmol/mg · min, as compared with 0.091 ± 0.009 μmol/mg · min in the absence of CaM (means ± S.E.M. for 10 different SR preparations), whilst the rate of calcium-activated ATP hydrolysis performed with ^{32}P-ATP under otherwise identical conditions was 0.141 ± 0.03 and 0.083 ± 0.010 μmol/mg · min (means ± S.E.M. for 4 different SR preparations) with CaM and control, respectively. The calcium-independent (basic) ATPase was unaffected by CaM.

Figure 2 shows the time course of the CaM-dependent phosphorylation of SR vesicles in the presence of a high free calcium concentration (comparable to the calcium uptake experiments with preincubation of SR vesicles with $CaCl_2$, $MgCl_2$ and ATP; mode a in Fig. 1). 100 nM CaM give rise to the incorporation of about 3 nmol phosphate/mg SR protein which is due to phosphoester bond formation insensitive to hydroxylamine. Half-maximum activation occurs at about 8 nm CaM. More than 90% of this CaM-dependent phosphorylation is due to phosphorylation of phospholamban [10]. The marked increase in the rate of calcium transport (condition a in Fig. 1) and calcium-activated ATP hydrolysis at low free calcium concentrations and low CaM concentrations is thought to be due to the CaM-dependent prephosphorylation of phospholamban.

CaM-dependent phosphorylation of SR vesicles preincubated with 100 nM CaM in the presence of 0.1 mM $CaCl_2$, 1 mM $MgCl_2$, but without ATP, assayed at about 0.5 μM free calcium was 0.967 ± 0.047 nmol/mg, as compared with 0.697 ± 0.065 nmol/mg in the absence of CaM ($n = 6$; 1 min). This CaM-dependent phosphorylation corresponds to the delayed and small increase in the rate of calcium uptake in Figure 1 (mode b).

Preincubation of SR vesicles with 100 nM CaM, 1 mM $MgCl_2$, 1 mM ATP plus 0.1 mM EGTA instead of calcium assayed at about 0.5 μM free calcium does not result in a significant CaM-dependent phosphorylation: 0.528 ± 0.042 and 0.051 ± 0.061 nmol/mg in the presence or absence of CaM, respectively (means ± S.E.M. for 6 different SR preparations; 1 min). This phosphate incorporation represents solely acylphosphate formed by the ATPase protein [12]. CaM has no effect on calcium uptake under these latter conditions i.e. in the absence of CaM-dependent phosphorylation (mode d in Fig. 1).

We confirm the experiments by KIRCHBERGER and ANTONETZ [8] which show that much higher concentrations of CaM, in the μmolar range, are required to stimulate calcium uptake or calcium-dependent ATP splitting at low free calcium concentrations, as used in the present study, when SR vesicles are not prephosphorylated or preincubated with CaM plus a higher free calcium concentration prior to the calcium uptake experiment.

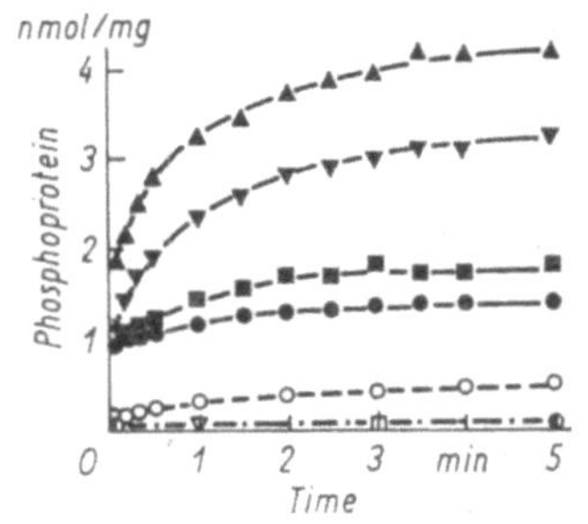

Fig. 2. Time course of CaM-dependent phosphorylation of cardiac SR. Preincubation of SR: 25 °C, pH 7.0, 2–5 min; without CaM (•, ○, ◐) or with CaM (■, □, 2 nM; ▼, ▽, 10 nM; ▲, △, 100 nM), 1 mM Mg, 0.1 mM Ca, 2.5 mg SR/ml. Phosphorylation: 25 °C, pH 7,0, 60 mM histidine-HCl-Tris, 2 mM PEP, 40 µg/ml PK, 10 mM Mg, 0.5 mM Ca, 0.5 mM EGTA, 2–4 mM (^{32}P)-ATP, CaM as above, 0.16 mg preincubated SR/ml. (○) control, zero Ca (5 mM EGTA); control (◐) and CaM (□, ▽, △) zero Ca, zero Mg (1 mM EGTA, 1 mM EDTA, without added Ca and Mg). Values are means of 3 experiments with different SR preparations.

Phosphorylation of sarcoplasmic reticulum ATPase of skeletal muscle by orthophosphate measured by stopped flow fluorescence

Phosphorylation of the calcium transport ATPase by orthophosphate (P_i) characterizes the later steps of the calcium transport cycle and ATP hydrolysis [1, 5]. Phosphorylation by P_i is due to phosphoenzyme formation with the P_i reactive E* form of the transport ATPase (DE MEIS [1]) in both types of phosphorylation, namely dependent on calcium inside [11] and independent of calcium inside [see ref. 1] the sarcoplasmic reticulum. Both phosphoenzymes are magnesium-phosphoenzymes [13]. Phosphorylation of SR ATPase by P_i can be monitored by its alteration of intrinsic tryptophan fluorescence [2, 4, 9] and the $E^* - E \cdot Ca_2$ transition can be followed by the calcium-induced and/or $E^* - E$ induced fluorescence change [3, 4].

Thus stopped flow fluorescence enables the measurement of $Mg \cdot E^* - P$ formation from either E* or $E \cdot Ca_2$, or its decomposition to either E* or $E \cdot Ca_2$ on a single trace. Alterations in tryptophan fluorescence were investigated under these conditions and the mono- or biphasic changes in tryptophan fluorescence following $Mg \cdot E^* - P$ formation or decomposition are shown in Figure 3.

When $Mg \cdot E^* - P$ formation was determined with SR vesicles resuspended in EGTA and Mg, the reaction being started by addition of P_i, the increase in fluorescence appears to be monoexponential and occurs without any lag phase, with apparent half times of 300, 240 and 139 ms with final P_i concentrations of 2.5, 5 and 10 mM, respectively, and a final Mg concentration of 2.5 mM (Fig. 3a).

When $Mg \cdot E^* - P$ formation was carried out with SR vesicles resuspended in 50 µM Ca and the reaction was started by addition of Mg, P_i plus EGTA, the fluorescence chan-

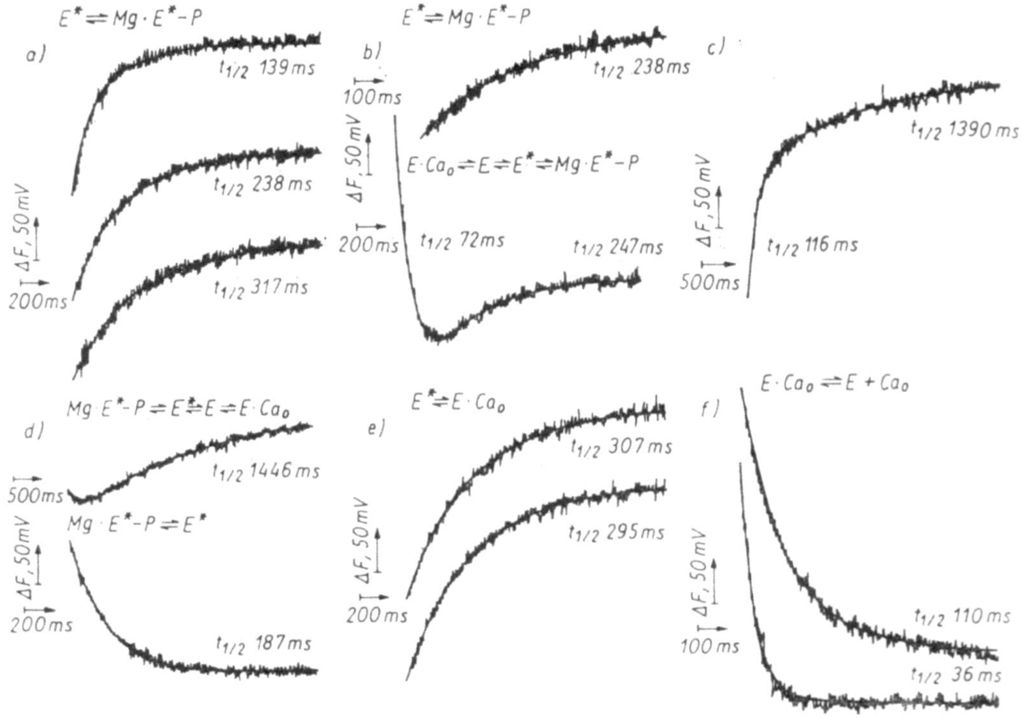

Fig. 3. Mg · E* — P formation and decomposition and E* ⇌ E transition by SR ATPase of rabbit skeletal muscle measured by stopped flow fluorescence. Fluorescence was measured by a Sigma ZWS II spectrophotometer equipped with a stopped flow apparatus (Xenon lamp; ex 280 nm; Schott WG 320 cut-off filter) at pH 6.2, 25 °C with 100 mM Tris-Mes in Syringe I and II and 100 μg SR protein/ml, giving a final concentration of 50 μg/ml after mixing.
a: Syr. I: 1 mM EGTA, 2.5 mM Mg; Syr. II: 1 mM EGTA, 2.5 mM Mg; 5, 10 or 20 mM P_i. b: Syr. I: 0.05 mM Ca; Syr. II: 5 mM Mg, 10 mM P_i, 10 mM EGTA (lower trace), upper trace as in a. c: Syr. I: 2 mM EGTA, 2.5 mM Mg; Syr. II: 2.5 mM Mg, 10 mM P_i, 5 mM Ca. d: Syr. I: 1 mM EGTA, 5 mM Mg, 10 mM P_i; Syr. II: 5 mM Ca (upper trace). Syr. I: 1 mM EGTA, 5 mM Mg, 10 mM, P_i; Syr. II: 20 mM EDTA (lower trace). e: Syr. I: 1 mM EGTA (lower trace) plus 5 mM Mg (upper trace); Syr. II: 5 mM Ca. f: Syr. I: 0.05 mM Ca; Syr. II: 10 mM EGTA (upper trace) or 20 mM EDTA (lower trace). The theoretical curves were obtained by fitting a single exponential (a, b, d, e, f) or two exponential (b, c, d) functions by a least square procedure to the data.

ge was biphasic: A fast decay in fluorescence precedes the increase in fluorescence, due to phosphoenzyme formation (Fig. 3b). This decrease in fluorescence has a similar time course (t 1/2 72 ms) to the fluorescence decrease due to removal of calcium bound to the high-affinity calcium binding sites of the ATPase by EGTA (Fig. 3f; t 1/2 110 ms) [3]. The lag phase in phosphoenzyme formation measured by the fluorescence method corresponds to that observed by quench flow measurements with ^{32}P-orthophosphate (CHALOUB et al. [see ref. 1]).

When phosphoenzyme formation was studied with SR vesicles resuspended in EGTA and the reaction was started by addition of Mg, P_i plus Ca, a biphasic fluorescence change was observed (Fig. 3c), namely a fast increasing phase (t 1/2 116—148 ms), with a time sourse similar to that seen following addition of P_i without Ca (Fig. 3a) and then a slow increasing phase with a similar time course as observed following decomposition of Mg · E* — P by addition of Ca (Fig. 3d, slow phase: t 1/2 1446 ms), showing that phosphorylation under these conditions is faster than E* — E · Ca_2 transition [see ref. 1].

Decomposition of preformed Mg · E* — P by EGTA results in a monophasic fluorescence decay (Fig. 3d; lower trace), whilst decomposition by calcium results in a biphasic fluorescence change, a fast decrease followed by a slow increase in fluorescence (Fig. 3d, upper trace). This biphasic decay of (^{32}P) P_i labelled Mg · E* — P by calcium has been shown by RAUCH et al. [see ref. 5].

On the other hand, the slow calcium-induced fluorescence change (Figs. 3c, 3d: t 1/2 ~ 1400 ms) contrasts markedly with the apparent half time of 300 ms observed on calcium binding to the ATPase (E* → E · Ca_2; Fig. 3e). The reason for this discrepancy is that phosphoenzyme formation and decomposition (E* ⇌ Mg · E* — P) continues following addition of calcium. Since these reactions are faster than the E* → E · Ca_2 formation, the trapping of the enzyme in E · Ca_2 is slowed down. This interpretation is confirmed by the fact that the slow phase of fluorescence change following addition of calcium to the performed phosphoenzyme can be speeded up or slowed down even more when the P_i concentration is decreased or increased, i.e. the apparent rate of Mg · E* — P formation is decreased or increased, respectively.

The data demonstrate that stopped flow measurements of changes in intrinsic fluorescence of the SR ATPase associated with Mg · E — P formation from P_i or its decomposition are a valuable tool in the study of the kinetics of the later steps in the calcium transport cycle of SR membranes [4, 9].

References

[1] DE MEIS, L.: In: Transport in Life Science. **12** (1981), 1–163, J. Wiley & Sons, N.Y.
[2] DUPONT, Y.: Biochem. Biophys. Res. Comm. **82** (1978), 893–900
[3] DUPONT, Y. and J. B. LEIGH: Nature **273** (1978), 396–398
[4] GUILLAN, F., P. CHAMPEIL, J. J. LACAPERE and M. P. GINGOLD: J. Biol. Chem. **256** (1981), 6140–6147
[5] HASSELBACH, W.: In: Topics in Current Chemistry. **78** (1979), 1–56, Springer, Heidelberg
[6] KATZ, S., and M. A. REMTULA: Biochem. Biophys. Res. Comm. **83** (1979), 1373–1379
[7] KIRCHBERGER, M. A., M. TADA and A. KATZ: J. Biol. Chem. **249** (1974), 6166–6173
[8] KIRCHBERGER, M. A. and T. ANTONETZ: J. Biol. Chem. **257** (1982), 5685–5691
[9] LACAPERE, J. J., M. P. GINGOLD, P. CHAMPEIL and F. GUILLAIN: J. Biol. Chem. **256** (1981) 2302–2306
[10] LE PEUCH, C. J., J. HAIECH and J. G. DEMAILLE: Biochemistry 18 (1979), 5150–5157
[11] MAKINOSE, M.: FEBS Letters **25** (1972), 113–115
[12] SUKO, J. and W. HASSELBACH: Eur. J. Biochem. **64** (1976), 123–130
[13] SUKO, J., B. PLANK, P. PREIS, N. KOLASSA, G. HELLMANN and W. CONCA: Eur. J. Biochem. **119** (1981), 225–236

Department of Biochemistry, University of Bristol Medical School,
Bristol BS8 1TD, U.K.

The Phosphorylation of Cardiac Contractile Proteins

P. J. England, D. Mills, H. T. Pask and S. A. Jeacocke

The primary regulation of cardiac contractility by catecholamines is most probably brought about by changes in the intracellular free Ca^{2+} concentration. The mechanisms for this effect, particularly the involvement of phosphorylation of membrane proteins, is discussed at length elsewhere in this volume. However, a number of contractile proteins are phosphorylated in heart in cyclic nucleotide or calcium dependent reactions. In some cases it is clear that the phosphorylation is of considerable importance in the regulation of cardiac contractility, whereas for some proteins the significance of the covalent modification is unclear. Three proteins will be discussed in this article: troponin-I, myosin P-light chain and C-protein. These three proteins represent the major, rapidly phosphorylated contractile proteins in heart. Moreover, because of the large amount of contractile elements present, these proteins are quantitatively the most important of all the phosphorylated proteins in this tissue.

Phosphorylation of troponin-I

Cardiac troponin-I is an excellent substrate for cyclic AMP-dependent protein kinase (cA-PK) [2, 31, 33] either when isolated, or in intact myofibrils. It is phosphorylated rapidly at a specific serine (residue no. 22), and more slowly at a second serine (residue 146). The amino acid sequences around these serines are typical of those found for cA-PK substrates [18].

In intact perfused hearts under control conditions troponin-I is phosphorylated to only a small extent (0.15—0.3 moles phosphate per mole troponin-I), but on perfusion with catecholamine there is a rapid increase in phosphorylation to 1—1.5 moles phosphate per mole [6, 7, 8, 36, 39]. The increase in phosphorylation is predominantly into serine 20 [23], and occurs over a time course similar to the increase in contractile force. However, phosphorylation of troponin-I only occurs with agents which increase cyclic AMP [9, 36], and is not an obligatory event in the inotropic response of the tissue to all stimuli.

The effect of troponin-I phosphorylation is to decrease the Ca^{2+} sensitivity of the contractile system. Thus in experiments with isolated cardiac myofibrils or skinned cardiac fibre preparations, the concentration of Ca^{2+} required for half-maximal activation of ATPase activity or tension is increased 2—3 fold on phosphorylation of troponin-I [1, 11, 13, 20, 27, 31, 32]. As catecholamines in the intact tissue increase contractility, the effect of troponin-I phosphorylation is at first paradoxical. There is apparently a

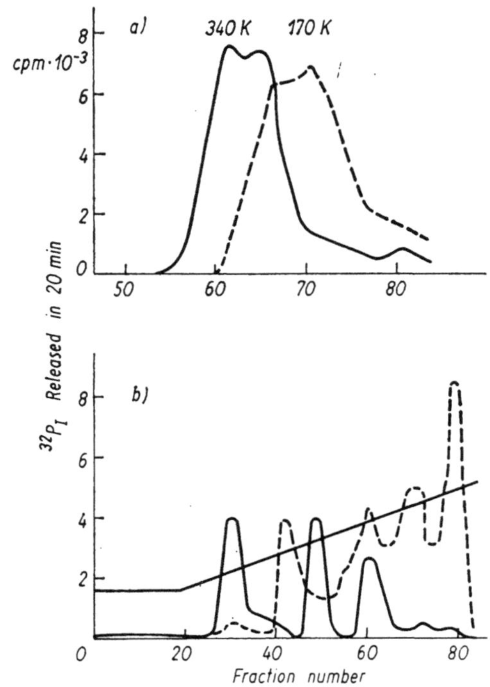

Fig. 1. Separation of phosphoprotein phosphatases from rat heart
a) Rat hearts were homogenised in 1.5 vol. of 25 mM Tris Cl, 10% ethanediol, 50 mM NaCl, 15 mM 2-mercaptoethanol, pH 7.4, centrifuged, and the supernatant chromatographed on a column of Sepharcryl-S300. Fractions were assayed for phosphatase activity by incubation with ^{32}P-labelled histone or troponin (———) or phosphorylase a (– – – –), followed by measurement of $^{32}P_i$ release.
b) The peak fractions from (a) were chromatographed on DEAE-Sepharose in the same buffer, and eluted with a gradient of NaCl from 0—0.3 M NaCl. Activity was measured towards histone (———) or phosphorylase **a** (– – – –).

decreased sensitivity of the myofibrils to Ca^{2+} at a time when the tissue is required to increase contractile force. This implies that catecholamines must cause a large increase in cytoplasmic Ca^{2+} during systole, larger than that which would have been required if troponin-I was not phosphorylated. It is therefore unlikely that phosphorylation of troponin-I is part of the mechanism for the positive inotropic action of catecholamines.

However, the phosphorylation of troponin-I has been implicated in the mechanism whereby catecholamines increase the rate of relaxation of the heart. As discussed elsewhere in this volume, phosphorylation of phospholamban, a protein originally discovered in the sarcoplasmic reticulum but also probably present in the sarcolemma of heart muscle, leads to an increased rate of removal of Ca^{2+} from the cytoplasm. Computer modelling has suggested that in these circumstances the rate of dissociation of Ca^{2+} from troponin could contribute to the overall rate of relaxation of the tissue [34]. It would obviously therefore be advantageous if an increase in the rate of dissociation occurred with catecholamines. The decreased Ca^{2+}-sensitivity of the contractile system discussed above could be brought about either by a decrease in the rate of association of Ca^{2+} with troponin, or an increase in the rate of dissociation. ROBERTSON et al. [35] have measured the rate of dissociation of Ca^{2+} from isolated troponin, and have found that the rate is increased from $14\,s^{-1}$ when troponin-I is dephosphorylated to $21\,s^{-1}$ when it is phosphorylated. Modelling has shown [35] that this increase is sufficient to make a significant contribution to the overall rate of relaxation of the heart.

Certain aspects of troponin phosphorylation in vivo remain unclear, however. In particular, the dephosphorylation of troponin-I (and also C-protein) is slow. Thus if hearts are given a short pulse of catecholamine, there is a transient increase in systolic tension and rate of relaxation. However, troponin-I, which is phosphorylated in response to the catecholamine, remains phosphorylated for several minutes [7, 42]. Phosphorylase, by contrast, shows a transient phosphorylation only. It is clear that the phosphoprotein phosphatases which dephosphorylate troponin-I and phosphorylase are either separate enzymes, or under some form of substrate-directed control. We have recently separated a number of phosphoprotein phosphatases from rat heart, and there are clearly one or more enzymes which are relatively specific for phosphorylase. Figure 1a shows a separation of phosphorylase phosphatase from general, non-specific phosphoprotein phosphatases on the basis of size. The molecular wt. of the general phosphatase is approx. 350,000, while that of phosphorylase phosphatase is 170,000. Figure 1b shows that each peak is composed of several molecular forms. All these forms can be dissociated to monomers of mol. wt. approx. 70,000 which still retain the differences in specificity. The general phosphoprotein phosphatases will dephosphorylate histone H1, troponin-I and C-protein.

While these results give an explanation of how phosphorylase can be rapidly dephosphorylated while the contractile proteins stay phosphorylated, they do not explain why the latter proteins are also not rapidly dephosphorylated. Presumably the general phosphatases are under some form of inhibitory control. Some results in vivo [7, 10, 20], suggest that an increase in cyclic GMP in the heart results in a dephosphorylation of troponin-I. A molecular mechanism for these findings has yet to be discovered, but they open up the possibility of a role for cyclic GMP in protein dephosphorylation.

Phosphorylation of C-protein

C-protein is a component of the thick filament of muscle which is located every 43 nm along the thick filament [4]. In cardiac muscle the protein has a mol · wt. of 150,000, compared to 140,000 for the skeletal muscle enzyme [28, 37, 44]. The exact function of C-protein is not known, although both structural [21, 24, 25] and regulatory [26, 28, 38] roles have been proposed. However, because of the spacing of C-protein not all the myosin molecules will interact with it in an equivalent manner.

When washed cardiac myofibrils were incubated with cA-PK and [γ-^{32}P] ATP, ^{32}P was incorporated into two proteins only, one was troponin-I, the other had a mol. wt. of 150,000 and was later identified as C-protein [16, 31]. C-protein purified from beef heart contains approx. 3 moles phosphate per mole C-protein, and additionally another 1 mole can be incorporated on incubation with cA-PK. This suggests that there are at least 4 phosphorylation sites for cA-PK on cardiac C-protein. C-protein is an excellent substrate for cA-PK. Table 1 shows that C-protein can be phosphorylated probably faster than both troponin-I and lysine-rich histone. As the C-protein already contains conside-

Table 1

Rates of phosphorylation of substrate proteins by the catalytic subunit of cyclic AMP-dependent protein kinase

Substrate	Substrate concentration (mg/ml)	Rate of phosphorylation µmoles/min/mg kinase
Histone H_1	3.0*	6.1
Troponin	5.0*	22.0
C-protein	1.0	16.1

*Approximately V_{max} concentrations

rable phosphate, the rate measured is probably well below the V_{max} value. At least half the endogenous phosphate can be readily removed by the general phosphoprotein phosphatase discussed above. C-protein is not phosphorylated by phosphorylase kinase.

In vivo phosphorylation of C-protein has been demonstrated in perfused rat heart, isolated heart cells and frog atria [10, 16, 29]. In control perfusions, C-protein in rat heart contained approx. 1 mole phosphate per mole C-protein. On perfusion with catecholamine, this was increased to 4—5 moles per mole over a time course parallel to the increase in phosphorylation of troponin-I. C-protein was not phosphorylated following an elevation of extracellular Ca^{2+}. The results in vivo and in vitro all suggest that C-protein phosphorylation is a cyclic AMP-dependent process. As with troponin-I, C-protein dephosphorylation is slow following removal of catecholamine, and is also stimulated by cholinergic agents [10].

At present, no function for C-protein phosphorylation is known. The lack of a clear understanding of C-protein function itself makes speculation difficult. There are probably three C-protein molecules at each 43 nm location on the thick filament, and complete phosphorylation will introduce 15—20 negative charges per C-protein region. Whether this will directly affect thick-filament structure or cross-bridge movement, or will induce conformational changes in nearby proteins, is a matter for speculation at present.

Myosin P-light chain phosphorylation

The P-light chain of myosin (also called the DTNB-light chain or LC2) is phosphorylated in all muscle and non-muscle types by a specific, Ca^{2+}-dependent light chain kinase [39]. Phosphorylation of the P-light chain in fast skeletal muscle causes a change in the kinetics of the actin-myosin interaction, resulting in a slower cross-bridge cycling time [3, 5]. In smooth muscle the effect of P-light chain phosphorylation is generally to considerably increase the actin-activated myosin ATPase [39], although there is considerable disagreement on both this and its role in the control of smooth muscle contraction.

In heart the main interest has been on the state of phosphorylation of the P-light chain in various inotropic states. There are considerable problems in obtaining pure light chains, and in preserving the in vivo phosphorylation levels during isolation [12, 15, 30]. Results from several laboratories show that in control perfusions there is approx. 0.4 to 0.5mole phosphate per mole P-light chain [12, 14, 15, 30]. This value was unchanged following perfusion with adrenaline, increased extracellular Ca^{2+} or K^+. It was also unchanged in short-term ischaemia [17], although long-term perfusion with zero extracellular Ca^{2+} did cause a slow fall in phosphorylation [42]. There was also no change in the level of P-light chain phosphorylation during hormonally-induced changes in myosin isoenzyme content of the heart [19]. In spite of the lack of changes in P-light chain phosphorylation, there is a rapid turnover of the phosphate group in all conditions. Perfusion with $^{32}P_i$ shows a rapid incorporation of ^{32}P into the P-light chain [15]. Although a turnover time cannot be accurately calculated, it is certainly less than 5 min. This indicates a high intracellular activity of the light-chain kinase and phosphatase. STULL et al. [42] have calculated that because of the slow rate of inactivation of myosin light chain kinase when the cytoplasmic Ca^{2+} falls during diastole, in a normally beating heart the kinase remains almost fully active throughout the contraction cycle. As an increase in cytoplasmic Ca^{2+} would therefore cause no further increase in kinase activity, this would explain why various positive inotropic interventions fail to increase the level of P-light chain phosphorylation.

Because of the constant level of P-light chain phosphorylation in various inotropic states, it can have no part in the acute regulation of contraction. There may be long-term changes which affect myosin kinetics or cross-bridge function, but this does not then explain why the kinase/phosphatase couple is so active. The phosphate group is unlikely to be important for the intrinsic activity of myosin, as in skeletal muscle normal contractions can be obtained in the absence of any P-light chain phosphorylation [41].

Acknowledgement

This research was supported by the Medical Research Council of Great Britain.

References

[1] BAILIN, G.: Am. J. Physiol. **236**, (1979), C41–C46
[2] COLE, H. A., and S. V. PERRY: Biochem. J. **149**, (1975), 525–533
[3] COOKE, R., K. FRANKS and J. T. STULL: FEBS Letters **144** (1982), 33–37
[4] CRAIG, R. and G. OFFER: Proc. Roy. Soc. Lond. Ser. B. **192**, (1976), 451–461
[5] CROW, M. and M. J. KUSHMERICK: Biophys. J. **33** (1981), 236a
[6] ENGLAND, P. J.: FEBS Letters **50**, (1975), 57–60
[7] ENGLAND, P. J.: Biochem J. **160**, (1976), 295–304
[8] ENGLAND, P. J.: Biochem J. **168**, (1977), 307–310
[9] EZRAILSON, E. G., J. D. POTTER, L. MICHAEL and A. SCHWARTZ: J. Mol. Cell. Cardiol.
[10] HARTZELL, H. C. and L. TITUS: J. Biol. Chem. **257**, (1982), 2111–2120
[11] HERZIG, J. W., G. KÖHLER, G. PFIZER, J. C. RUEGG and G. WOFFLE: Pflügers. Archiv. **391** (1981), 208–212
[12] HIGH, C. W. and J. T. STULL: Am. J. Physiol. **239**, (1980), H756–H764
[13] HOLROYDE, M. J., E. HOWE and R. J. SOLARO: Biochim. Biophys. Acta. **586**, (1979), 63–69
[14] HOLROYDE, M. J., D. A. P. SMALL, E. HOWE and R. J. SOLARO: Biochim. Biophys. Acta. **587** (1979), 628–637
[15] JEACOCKE, S. A. and P. J. ENGLAND: Biochem. J. **188**, (1980), 763–768
[16] JEACOCKE, S. A. and P. J. ENGLAND: FEBS Lett. **122**, (1980), 129–132
[17] KRAUSE, E.-G., P. J. ENGLAND and S. BARTEL: [This symposium]
[18] KREBS, E. G. and J. A. BEAVO: Ann. Rev. Biochem. **48**, (1979), 923–959

[19] Litten, R. Z., B. J. Martin, E. R. Howe, N. R. Alpert and R. J. Solaro: Circ. Res. **48** (1981), 498–501
[20] McClellan, G. B. and S. Winegard: J. Gen. Physiol. **75**, (1980), 283–296
[21] Miyahara, M. and H. Noda: J. Biochem. **87**, (1980), 1413–1420
[22] Moir, A. J. G. and S. V. Perry: Biochem. J. **167**, (1977), 333–343
[23] Moir, A. J. G., R. J. Solaro and S. V. Perry: Biochem. J. **185**, (1980), 505–513
[24] Moos, C. and I. M. Feng: Biochim. Biophys. Acta. **632**, (1980), 141–149
[25] Moos, C., G. Offer, R. Starr and P. Bennet: J. Mol. Biol. **97**, (1975), 1–9
[26] Moos, C., C. M. Mason, J. M. Besterman, I. M. Feng and J. H. Dublin: J. Mol. Biol. **124**, (1978), 571–586
[27] Mope, L., G. B. McClellan and S. Winegrad: J. Gen. Physiol. **75**, (1980), 271–282
[28] Offer, G., C. Moos and R. Starr: J. Mol. Biol. **74**, (1973), 653–676
[29] Onorato, J. J. and S. A. Rudolph: J. Biol. Chem. **256**, (1981), 10697–10703
[30] Perry, S. V., H. A. Cole, N. Frearson, A. J. G. Moir, A. C. Nairn and R. J. Solaro: Proc. 12th FEBS Meeting **54**, (1979), 147–159
[31] Ray, K. P. and P. J. England: FEBS Lett. **70**, (1976), 11–16
[32] Reddy, Y. S. and L. E. Wyborny: Biochem. Biophys. Res. Commun. **73**, (1976), 703–709
[33] Reddy, Y. S., D. Ballard, N. Y. Giri and A. Schwartz: J. Mol. Cell. Cardiol. **5** (1973), 461–471
[34] Robertson, S. P., J. D. Johnson and J. D. Potter: Biophys. J. **34**, (1981), 559–569
[35] Robertson, S. P., J. D. Johnson, M. J. Holroyde, E. G. Kranias, J. D. Potter and R. J. Solaro: J. Biol. Chem. **257**, (1982), 260–263
[36] Solaro, R. J., A. J. G. Moir and S. V. Perry: Nature **262**, (1976), 615–616
[37] Starr, R. and G. Offer: FEBS Lett. **15**, (1971), 40–44
[38] Starr, R. and G. Offer: Biochem. J. **171**, (1978), 813–816
[39] Stull, J. T.: Adv. Cyclic. Nucleotide Res. **13**, (1980), 39–93
[40] Stull, J. T. and J. E. Buss: J. Biol. Chem. **252**, (1977), 851–857
[41] Stull, J. T. and C. W. High: Biochem. Biophys. Res. Commun. **77**, (1977), 1078–1083
[42] Stull, J. T., C. F. Sanford, D. R. Manning, D. K. Blumenthal and C. W. High: Cold Spring Harbor Conf. Cell. Prolif. **8**, (1981), 823–840
[43] Westwood, S. A. and S. V. Perry: Biochem. J. **197**, (1981), 185–193
[44] Yamamoto, K. and C. Moos: Biophys. J. **33**, (1981), 237a

I.N.S.E.R.M. Unité 127, Hôpital Lariboisière, Paris, FRANCE

Regulation of Cardiac Function During Chronic Overload. Myosin Isoenzyme Redistribution

J. L. Samuel, J. J. Mercadier, Y. Lecarpentier, A. M. Lompré, K. Schwartz and B. Swynghedauw

"It is easier to acquire facts, than to judge what they prove, and how-through the facts we know-to get to those which we want to know". This nice sentence, from John Stuart Mill in 1867, can be specifically applied to studies on cardiac hypertrophy a matter in which data, accumulate with an increasing speed. Usually very few concepts arise from the data and more often attemps to induce confusion around clear features were more than frequent [23].

In response to a chronic overload, both the entire organism and the myocardium itself may adapt to the new situation. As far as the heart is concerned, chronic adaptation involves two different processes: hypertrophy by which the muscle adapts to new requirements by increasing the number of contractile units and the slowing of the shortening speed which is responsible of an improved efficiency [2].

It is necessary to know these factors, and their biological basis in order to estimate the limits of these adaptations and therefore the threshold from which heart failure, at least in term of myocardium, will occur.

This paper is an attempt to summarize the most recent work from our laboratory concerning the biological basis of the slowing of the shortening speed. Most of our data come from the rat a species in which it has been clearly shown that a myosin isoenzymic shift occurs and parallels the shortening velocity. Some data concern the human where the situation is obviously different.

Methods

Male Wistar rats were used except for studies on the spontaneously hypertensive strains (SHR) which have been done with Okamoto rats and, as controls, with the Wistar Kyoto. Animals weighing 200 g were used.

Aortic stenosis, aortic insufficiency, chronic myocardial infarction obtained by coronary ligation, aorto-caval fistulae and the two-step mechanical overload (aortic stenosis + insufficiency) have been created according to procedures described elsewhere [12].

Human hearts were autopsy samples either from traffic injuries or from left ventricular hypertrophy secondary to chronic arterial hypertension. The average heart weight was 302 g for the control and 509 g for the hypertrophic group (N = 7 and 10).

The contractile performances and more specifically the measurements of the maximal contractile velocity by the zero-clamp technique were performed on papillary muscle excised from the left ventricle and analysed according to Brutsaert [4].

Myosin was purified by amonium sulfate precipitation [12]. The early phosphate burst size was measured manually [22] in stoichiometric conditions. Steady state ATPase activities were measured in the presence of either $CaCl_2$ or 1 M KCl and 5 mM EDTA [22]. The pyrophosphate gel were 3.88% in acrylamide and tissue extracts, or myosin, were run 16 h at 2 °C and at 14 Volts per cm according to D'ALBIS [1].

Antibodies against native or SDS-denatured rat hart heavy meromyosin were raised in guinea pigs. The antigen-antibody complex was studied by the microcomplement fixation technique [17—20]. Peptide maping after digestion with chymotrypsin of *Staphylococcus aureus* protease and two-dimensional gels were runs as described elsewhere [20].

Results

Rats

Normal adult rat hearts shorten faster than those from bigger animals, even rabbits. They also contain a myosin whose specific ATPase activity both in the steady state and during the initial fast period ("phosphate burst") is high compared to other mammalians. As can be shown on a pyrophosphate gel electrophoresis in non-dissociating conditions, this is due to the predominancy of a myosin isozyme which has a high ATPase activity (V_1). This isozyme is a minor component in rabbit heart and is absent from dog, pig, human myocardiums. The rat heart does contain two other isozymes called V_2 and V_3, whose ATPase is lower [8]. It has been demonstrated [9] that V_1 and V_3 are two homodimeres αβ and ββ of myosin heavy chains while V_2 is an heterodimere αβ — (Fig. 1). Foetal rat heart contains predominantly V_3 and an abrupt transition occurs after birth from V_3 to V_1 [13] (Fig. 1).

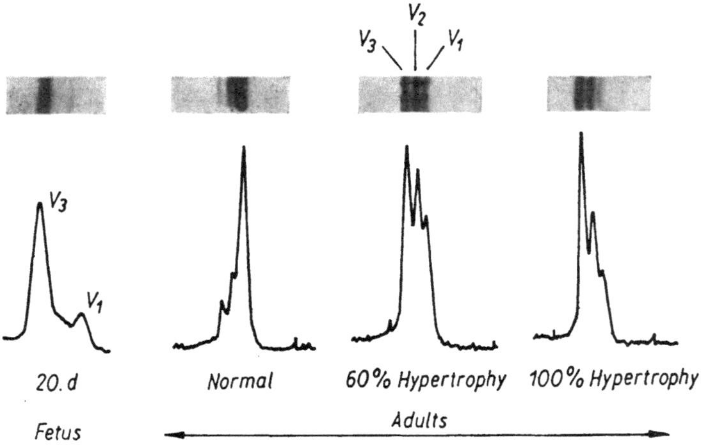

Fig. 1. Myosin isoenzyme redistribution in chronic overload in rat hearts. Pyrophosphate gel electrophoresis (non-dissociating medium) of a tissues extract [12] showing the entire molecule of myosin. Isoenzymic pattern in a foetal heart (a), a normal adult heart (b). and a moderate (c) or a severely overload heart (d) (b, c, d reproduced by permission of Mc MILLAN Cy Ltd from Nature [12].

During chronic overload in rats a transition occurs at the expense of the fast isozyme V_1 to the slow foetal one, V_3. This has been clearly shown on electrophoresis in non-dissociating conditions (Fig. 1) since in advanced hypertrophy, due to a prolonged and severe overload, the normal isoenzyme pattern V_1, $V_2 \gg\gg V_3$ was reversed and since intermediary patterns were observed in moderate overload. This change was seen for all models studied: aortic stenosis or/and insufficiency, chronic arterial hypertension of genetic origin, non infarcted area of myocardium several weeks after a coronary ligation, aorta-caval fistulae. The change involved both endo- and epicardium and occurs earlier in the left than in the right ventricle after a left ventricular overload [14]. It is not due to a contamination by non-muscle cells, whose concentration increases after aortic stenosis [14], since it is also shown in isolated myocytes [6].

All of the above results were based upon pyrophosphate gel electrophoresis. SDS or urea gel electrophoresis did not provide any additional information, since the molecular weight of the myosin heavy remains unchanged This was not unexpected since it has been shown that V_1 and V_3 comigrate in electrophoresis under dissociating conditions. They differ when a two dimensional peptide maping has been performed after proteolytic digestion [unpublished results from our laboratory].

Immunological techniques clearly separate cardiac myosin isolated from different mammalians [17], and also distinguish between myosin extracted from a normal or a hypertrophied heart. (Fig 2) [12, 18]. This was demonstrated using antibodies raised against either native, or SDS-denatured heavy meromyosin, the Ab—Ag reaction was identified by the microcomplement fixation technique. When an Ab raised against normal myosin was made to react against this protein extracted from a hypertrophied heart, a vertical shift of the reaction was observed which indicates a diminution of the common epitopes. Similar results were observed when fetal and adult rat heart myosin were compared [13]. These structural data were also confirmed by using a peptide maping obtained after digestion of myosin with a protease and electrophoresis on one [11] or two dimensions [unpublished from our laboratory].

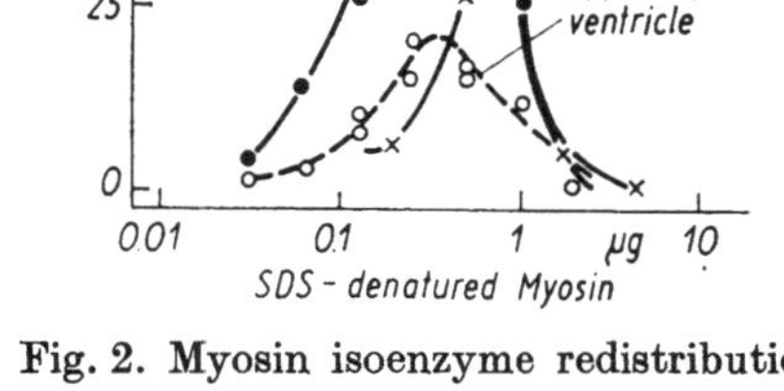

Fig. 2. Myosin isoenzyme redistribution in chronic overload in rat hearts. Microcomplement fixations with an antiserum to normal rat ventricular SDS-denatured heavy meromyosin. Antiserum dilution 1/5,250. The antigens were normal ventricular myosin, normal atrial myosin and myosin from a severely overloaded heart (reproduced by permission of Mc MILLAN Cy Ltd from Nature [12].

Both pressure and volume overload can hypertrophy the heart and modify its myosin isoenzymic pattern, but both phenomena were retarded in volume overload. The stimulation of protein synthesis peaks by the 5th day after aortic stenosis compared to the 15th day after aortic incompetence in rats [15]. Moreover in a pure volume overload model such as aorta-caval fistulae the modification of isozymes of myosin occurs very late, by the 3d to the 4d month, compared to what is observed after aortic stenosis [14].

This isoenzymic change is responsible for a drop in myosin Ca^{2+}-activated ATPase (from 1,200 nmole/$P_i \cdot mg^{-1} \cdot min^{-1}$ in controls to 760 in hypertrophied hearts). This was demonstratedby comparing myosins having the same phosphate burst size (1.6 mole of ATP per mole of myosin), i.e. by comparing myosins preparations having the same amount (about 20%) of denaturated molecules.

It has been shown that this enzymatic activity has a physiological significance since it correlates with the speed of shortening in phylogeny [3]. It does also in chronic overloading. The maximal speed shortening for an unloaded muscle was measured on the papillary muscle which was then homogenized and run on a phyrophosphate gel electrophoresis. The degree of isoenzymic redistribution was quantified by scanning. When hearts of different speed of shortening, i.e. hearts from young or aged, hypophysectomised and overload animals were studied, a linear and positive correlation ($r = 0.90 - p < 0.001$) was found between the percentage of the foetal myosin isoenzyme V_3 and the speed of shortening [19].

Human

The situation in human was different since both adult and foetus have only one isoenzyme in a pyrophosphate gel electrophoresis. Myosin was shown to be resistant, in term of ATPase, to post-mortem proteolysis, and both the ATPase and the initial phosphate burst size were identical in samples taken during surgery and after an autopsy performed less than 24 hours after the death. Myosin from normal and hypertrophied hearts were compared, they both have a burst amplitude of 1.6 mole of ATP per mole of myosin. They also have the same myosin Ca^{2+}-activated ATPase (201 nmole $P_i \cdot min^{-1} \cdot mg^{-1}$ in controls and 124 in hypertrophied hearts) and the same Mg^{2+}-activated myofibrillar ATPase (16 and 18 at pCa 9 and 32 and 33 at pCa 5). Moreover they comigrate both in SDS and pyrophosphate gel electrophoresis. We were unable also to detect any differences between them by routine immunological techniques.

Discussion

There is no doubt that in response to chronic overload a process of adaptation is developed and that this process tends to improve cardiac function in this new situation. Hypertrophy plays that role both by increasing the number of contractile elements and by decreasing the wall stress.

The discovery of a myosin isoenzyme redistribution during chronic overload in rats [12, 14] shows that a process of adaptation does also exist at the molecular level at least in certain conditions and in one animal species. This modification was observed after abrupt overloads, or at least mainly in this conditions, i.e. after a stenosis, an insufficiency rapidly induced by surgery. This correlates nicely with the speed of shortening measured in conditions independent of the load [19]. Several authors have suggested that the change in the speed of shortening may only occur in rapidly induced overloads and was absent when the heart was progressively submitted to an increase in pressure [24]. This could also explain why the slowering of the shortening velocity was not observed after a pure volume overload such as an atrio-septal defect [5]. This distinction was not entirely satisfactory since a striking myosin change was observed in the spontaneously hypertensive rat strain and after an aortocaval fistulae [14]; (see [21].)

Other changes in protein structure have been reported (i) a redistribution in the lactate dehydrogenases isozymes in favor of the M form [16] (ii) recently an increase in the form of creatine kinase isoenzymes; (iii) a slowering of the pumping capacity of the sarcoplasmic reticulum, (iv), an improvement of the mitochondrial function which improves cardiac tolerance to anoxia; references in [21]. The final result was nicely analyzed by N. Alpert's group: both the tension-dependent and the tension independent heat production are lowered for a given tension in a papillary muscle isolated from a hypertrophied heart [2].

In the human the situation is still controversial. It is difficult, if not impossible, to estimate in vivo the unloaded speed of shortening since it is nearly impossible to elevate the wall stress in controls at levels comparable to those observed during overload. The consequence is an increasing number of controversial papers [7, 10]. The few studies on papillary muscle did not solve the problem since it is impossible to have controls and also to make the study on muscles thin enough to guarantee an appropriate oxygenation. Our study was much in favor of a normal contractility in compensatory hypertrophy if we accept the concept according to which the maximal speed of shortening correlates with the myosin ATPase activity. This does not exclude a more subtile change in the sarcomere, for example on the regulatory proteins. Above all it does not explain why the speed of shortening was so much depressed, and this has never been contradicted, at the final stage of the disease.

To date a discrepancy exists between the results obtained in rats, an animal species which undoubtely has the possibility to adapt its contraction speed by modifying its myosin isoenzyme pattern, and those obtained in human which, apparently, does not possess this system. We may find that adaptation to overload in another species is not at the level of the contractile protein, but in another system entirely, for examples at the membrane level.

References

[1] ALBIS (D'), A. and W. B. GRATZER: FEBS Letters **29** (1973), 292—296

[2] ALPERT, N. R. and L. A. MULIERI: Circ. Res. **50** (1982), 491—500

[3] BARANY, M.: J. Gener. Physiol. **50** (1967), 197—216

[4] BRUTSAERT, D. L., N. M. DE CLERCK, M. A. GOETHALS and P. R. HOUSMANS: J. Physiol. (London) **283** (1978), 469—480

[5] COOPER, G. IV, F. J. PUGA, K. J. ZUJKO, C. E. HARRISON and H. N. COLEMAN: III Circ. Res. **32** (1973), 140—148

[6] CUTILLETTA, A. F., M. C. AUMONT, A. C. NAG and R. ZAK: J. Mol. Cell. Cardiol. **9** (1977), 399—407

[7] GROSSMAN, W.: Am. J. Med. **69** (1980), 576—584

[8] HOH, J. F. Y., P. A. MC GRATH and P. T. HALE: J. Molec. Cell. Cardiol. **10** (1977), 1053—1076

[9] HOH, J. F. Y., G. P. S. YEOH, M. A. W. THOMAS and L. HIGGINBOTTOM: FEBS Letters **97** (1979), 330—334

[10] HUBER, D., J. GRIMM, R. KOCH and H. P. KRAYENBUEHL: Circ. **64** (1981), 126—134

[11] KLOTZ, C., B. SWYNGHEDAUW, H. MENDES, F. MAROTTE and J. J. LÉGER: Eur. J. Biochem. **115** (1981), 415—421

[12] LOMPRÉ, A. M., K. SCHWARTZ, A. ALBIS, G. LACOMBE, N. V. THIEM and B. SWYNGHEDAUW: Nature **282** (1979), 105—107

[13] LOMPRÉ, A. M., J. J. MERCADIER, C. WISNEWSKY, P. BOUVERET, C. PANTALONI, A. D'ALBIS and K. SCHWARTZ: Develop. Biol. **84** (1981), 286—290

[14] MERCADIER, J. J., A. M. LOMPRÉ, C. WISNEWSKY, J. L. SAMUEL, J. BERCOVICI, B. SWYNGHEDAUW and K. SCHWARTZ: Circ. Res. **49** (1981), 525—532

[15] MOALIC, J. M., J. BERCOVICI and B. SWYNGHEDAUW: Cardiovasc. Res. **15** (1981), 515—521

[16] REVIS, N. W., R. Y. THOMPSON and A. J. V. CAMERON: Cardiovasc. Res. **11** (1977), 172—176

[17] SCHWARTZ, K., P. BOUVERET, C. SEBAG, J. LÉGER and B. SWYNGHEDAUW: Bioch. Biophys. Acta **425** (1977), 24—36

[18] SCHWARTZ, K., P. BOUVERET, J. BERCOVICI and B. SWYNGHEDAUW: FEBS Letters. **93** (1978), 137—140

[19] SCHWARTZ, K., Y. LECARPENTIER, J. L. MARTIN, A. M. LOMPRÉ, J. J. MERCADIER and B. SWYNGHEDAUW: J. Mol. Cell. Cardiol. **13** (1981), 1071—1075

[20] SCHWARTZ, K., A. M. LOMPRÉ, P. BOUVERET, C. WISNEWSKY and R. G. WHALEN: J. Biol. Chem., **257** (1982), 14412—14418

[21] SWYNGHEDAUW, B. and C. DELCAYRE: In: Patholbiological Annual (edited by H. L. Ioachim), vol. **12** (1982), 137—182

[22] THIEM, N. V., G. LACOMBE and B. SWYNGHEDAUW: Europaen J. Biochem. **91** (1978), 243—248.

[23] WIKMAN-COFFELT, J., W. W. PARMLEY and D. T. MASON: Circ. Res. **45** (1979), 697—707

[24] WILLIAMS, J. F. Jr., and R. D. POTTER: J. Clin. Invest. **54** (1974), 1266—1272

USSR Cardiology Research Center, Moscow, USSR, and Laboratoire de Physiologie Cellulaire Cardiaque, Universite de Paris-Sud, Orsay, FRANCE

Role of Multienzyme Complexes in Intracellular Compartmentation of Adenine Nucleotides and in Regulation of Cardiac Energy Metabolism

V. A. Saks, G. B. Chernousov, N. V. Lyulina, Z. A. Khuchua, A. N. Preobrazenskiy and R. N. Ventura-Clapier

Introduction

For cardiac muscle, a simple concept of intracellular energy channelling by ATP diffusion in cytoplasm [12] has completely failed to explain how the impairment of heart mechanical function may be related to metabolic disturbances when oxygen supply to the heart cells is significantly decreased or ceased at all during hypoxia or ichaemia, or when energy production is otherwise inhibited. Gudbjarnason et al. [6] were first to show clearly that in the absence of oxygen supply to the heart the contractile force quickly decreases to zero within a time interval of several minutes when only small changes in the cellular ATP content are observed. A conclusion made from this observation was that there is a heterogenous distribution of adenine nucleotides, ATP and ADP, in cardiac muscle cells and that only a small pool of ATP localized in myofibrillar compartment is rapidly accessible to the myosin ATPase to support contraction [6]. The data of Gudbjarnason et al. were subsequently confirmed by several groups [3, 11]. Since a fall in the contractile force was observed to be parallel with a decline in phosphocreatine content, the latter compound was suggested to be a high energy phosphate bond carrier between different ATP pools in cardiac muscle cells [6]. During the decade that followed this suggestion has got substantial support both in biochemical and physiological research (see [20, 22]). The phosphocreatine pathway is considered by many authors to be a major way of energy channelling, and its existence is based on heterogenous distribution of creatine kinase isoenzymes inside cardiomyocytes [7, 10, 20, 22]. On the other hand, a unique distribution of creatine kinase isoenzymes and their immediate and efficient interaction with both energy-producing and energy-consuming systems may be a reason for functional compartmentation of adenine nucleotides in the heart cells. The purpose of this report is to describe main features of structurally and functionally coupled systems in which creatine kinase behaves as a part of multienzyme system and thus forms a basis for functional compartmentation of adenine nucleotides.

Mitochondrial creatine kinase: spatial proximity to adenine nucleotide translocase

Because of the strictly aerobic cardiac energy metabolism and the major role of mitochondrial oxidative phosphorylation in biochemically available energy production, mitochondrial creatine kinase connected with the outer side of the inner mitochondrial membrane [7, 21] is one of the key enzymes in the phosphocreatine pathway for the energy transport [7, 20, 22]. The intramitochondrial localization has been found to play an important role in the catalytic activity of this enzyme [17]: under conditions of oxidative phosphorylation the rate of phosphocreatine production is significantly increased due to direct utilization of mitochondrial ATP. It has been suggested on the basis of the kinetic analysis [14] and isotopic studies [24], that the aerobic enhancement of phosphocreatine production is related to the direct channelling of ATP by adenine nucleotide translocase to the creatine kinase active center, that maintaining high steady state level of the central ternary, catalytically active complex E · Mg · ATP · Cr and high rate of aerobic production of phosphocreatine [18]. It has recently been shown in two laboratories that ADP simultaneously formed is immediately transported by translocase back into the matrix to be rephosphorylated into ATP in oxidative phosphorylation [4, 10]. As a result of these coupled reactions, all mitochondrial ATP may be utilized for phosphocreatine production, and adenine nucleotides may be functionally compartmentalized mostly in the intramitochondrial cycle of oxidative phosphorylation the creatine kinase reaction. Such a coupling requires the presence of adenine nucleotide translocase and creatine kinase in equimolar quantities in the mitochondria and their spatial proximity. The first requirement has been shown to be fullfilled in cardiac mitochondria [8]. The second question was investigated in this study. The problem has been approached by using purified antibodies against mitochondrial creatine kinase. Creatine kinase isolated from rat heart mitochondria showed in the SDS-gel electrophoresis the presence of one single protein band with the molecular mass of 42,000 dalton and in the isoenzyme electrophoresis showed only one isoenzyme the mitochondrial form [15]. Antibodies obtained by affinity chromatography by using purified BrCN-Sepharose bound creatine kinase gave only one precipitation band both in the Ouchterlony analysis and immunoelectrophoresis [15], that may be taken to show their purity and monospecifity. These antibodies were used to study intimate environment of the mitochondrial membrane-bound creatine kinase in the mitoplasts obtained from rat heart mitochondrial by a digitonin method [19]. If compared with the intact mitochondria, the mitoplasts are mostly deprived of the outer membrane but the morphological appearance of the inner membrane and matrix system as well as respiratory characteristics are well preserved. The specific activity of creatine kinase of the preparation was not decreased during the removal of the outer membrane, what conforms to the localization of creatine kinase on the inner membrane surface. When antibodies obtained against this creatine kinase were added to the mitoplasts, the creatine kinase was significantly inhibited (Fig. 1a). In the same conditions, the rates of ATP synthesis in the oxidative phosphorylation process from extramitochondrial ADP (0.03 mM) were assessed by a coupled enzyme hexokinase-glucose-6-phosphate dehydrogenase system (Fig. 1b). In this way the rate of mitochondria-produced ATP delivery into the medium via the adenine nucleotide translocation step was determined. As expected, this process was completely inhibited by atractyloside, a translocator inhibitor (Fig. 1b). When mitoplasts were incubated with Ab-CK_{mit}, the rate of ATP production was significantly decreased by a degree similar to that of CK_{mit} inhibition (Fig. 1a and b, traces b). However, when Ab-CK_{mit} were bound into complex with solubilized CK_{mit} prior their mixing with mitoplasts, the rate of ATP production was not changed (Fig. 1b, trace c). Therefore, the step of binding of Ab-CK_{mit} with the antigenic determinant in the creatine kinase molecule is to be necessary for inhibition of oxidative phosphorylation by

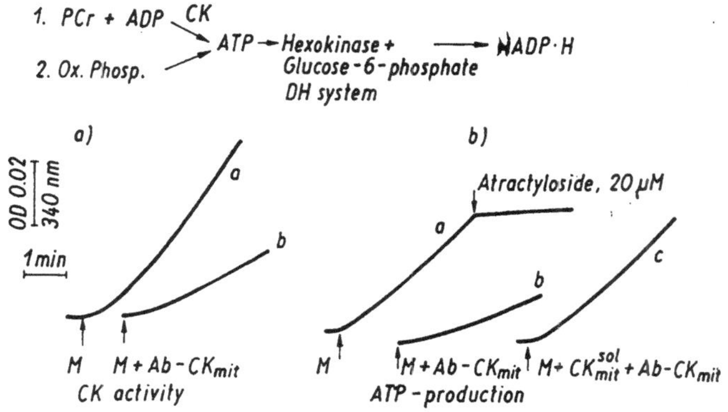

Fig. 1. Inhibition of creatine kinase activity and oxidative phosphorylation by antibodies against mitochondrial creatine kinase, Ab-CK_{mit}, in cardiac mitoplasts, M.
a. Changes in creatine kinase activity.
b. Changes in the rate of ATP production. CK_{mit}^{sol} — solubized mitochondrial creatine kinase, obtained as described in [17], added in 5-fold excess to creatine kinase activity in mitoplasts.

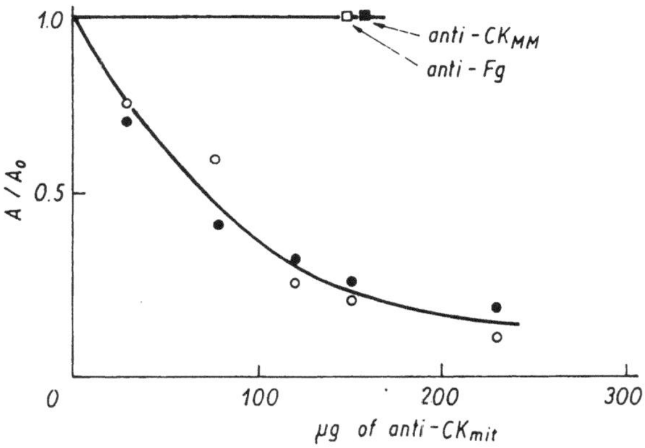

Fig. 2. Titration curves for inhibition of creatine kinase (•) and oxidative phosphorylation (○) reactions by Ab-CK_{mit}. (anti-CK_{mm} and and anti-Fg-antibodies against MM iso-enzyme of creatine kinase and fibrinogen, correspondingly were generous gifts of Dr. Ermolin G. A.).

Ab-CK_{mit}. Further analysis of this inhibition phenomenon is shown in Figure 2. This Figure demonstrates the titration curves for creatine kinase activity (closed circles) and oxidative phosphorylation (open circles) when increasing amount of Ab-CK_{mit} were added to the mitoplasts. A remarkable fitting of both inhibition curves is observed. Both creatine kinase activity and oxidative phosphorylation were inhibited by Ab-CK_{mit} by more than 80%. Antibodies against MM-isoenzyme of creatine kinase, or against fibrinogen (Ab-Fg) did not have any inhibitory action (Fig. 2). The results of these experiments show a specific inhibition of the mitochondrial ATP synthesis by Ab-CK_{mit} after their binding with the mitochondrial creatine kinase at the mitoplasts' membranes. Since the extramitochondrial ADP phosphorylation by mitoplasts is controlled by the adenine nucleotide translocase which connects the matrix space with extramitochondrial medium, the effects described are most probably explained by inhibition of the translocase by Ab-CK_{mit}. This conclusion was directly verified by using ^{3}H-ADP for an assessment of the rate of adenine nucleotide translocation. As it is shown in the Table 2, addition of Ab-CK_{mit} inhibits adenine nucleotide translocation step by 80% — a degree entirely fitting with that for both oxidative phosphorylation and the creatine kinase reaction (see Table 1 and Fig. 2).

The efficient inhibition of oxidative phosphorylation and adenine nucleotide translocation by Ab-CK_{mit} observed in this study is consistent with the concept of the close spatial proximity of the adenine nucleotide translocase and creatine kinase and of their close functional cooperation in heart mitochondria [7, 10, 16, 18]. Schematically, this explanation of the results obtained is given in Figure 3: Ab-CK_{mit} after their binding to the antigenic determinants of the creatine kinase may block simultanously its active center and the nucleotide binding center of the translocator due to the close spatial proximity of these two proteins.

Table 1

Inhibition of ATP-ADP exchange in cardiac mitoplasts by Ab-CK_{mit}

	Rate of ^{3}H-ADP uptake at 2 °C, nmoles $\times$ min^{-1} $\times$ mg^{-1}
1. Control	0.5
2. plus 1.2—1.6 mg per ml Ab-CK_{mit}	0.09
3. % of inhibition	81

Mitoplast were present in concentrations of 0.17—0.22 mg/ml. The rate of ^{3}H-ADP uptake was determined according to [1].

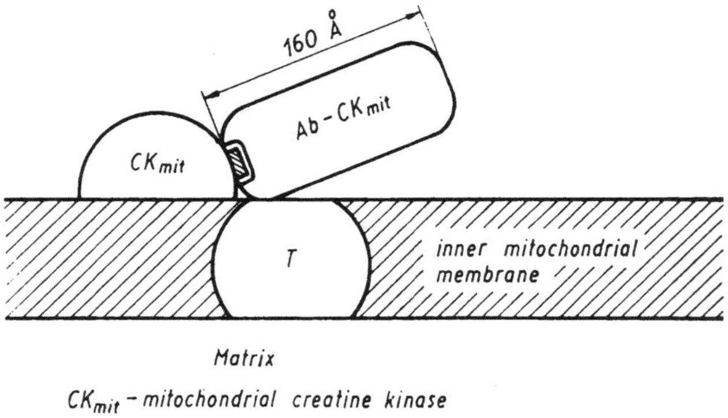

Fig. 3. Schematic explanation of inhibitory action of Ab-CK_{mit} on ATP-ADP translocase (T).

Cardiac myofibrils and sarcolemma: direct channelling of ADP from ATPases to the creatine kinase

Purified preparations of both cardiac myofibrils [16] and sarcolemma [13] have been shown to contain bound MM isoenzyme of creatine kinase (see ref. [20]), functional coupling of which to the actomyosin Mg-ATPase and Na, K-ATPase, correspondingly, has been described in several publications [2, 5]. The molecular mechanisms of this coupling as well as of the control exerted by the creatine kinase system on the contraction of hypodynamic heart [20, 23] are not as yet clear. Therefore, we investigated the fate of ADP, produced in the ATPase reactions. The principle of the approach used is illustrated in Figure 4, and considers the two possibilities of ADP movement. One possible way is a rapid release of ATPase product, ADP, from the enzyme into the medium. In this case ADP will be equally available for all enzymes which utilize it. The second possible way is a direct channelling of ADP to the bound creatine kinase if the latter is localized in the close proximity of ATPase. To differentiate between these two possible

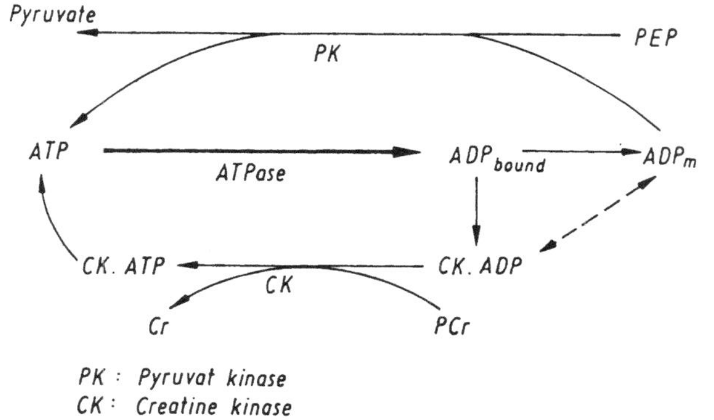

Fig. 4. Principles of investigations of the route of ADP movement in cardiac myofibrils and sarcolemmal preparation. PK-exogenous pyruvate kinase added to remove ADP from the medium. PEP-phosphoenolpyruvate.

ways, we have used a competing enzyme exogenous pyruvate kinase to remove ADP from the medium, and the rates of two competing ADP consuming reactions, creatine release from phosphocreatine and pyruvate release from phosphoenolpyruvate, were determined at saturating concentrations of Mg-ATP for ATPase. As a control system with homogenous distribution of substrates and reaction intermediates, a reconstituted system of soluble hexokinase + glucose (as ATPase) and creatine kinase of equal activity was used and increasing amount of pyruvate kinase was added to enhance the ratio of PK/CK activities up to 100. Figure 5a shows that an increase in PK/CK ratio leads to a rapid drop in the rate of creatine release and causes a symmetrical rise in the rate of pyruvate release, and at PK/CK ratio 20—50 all ADP is trapped by the pyruvate kinase system, ADP concentration in the medium becoming neglectable. In other words, an increase in PK/CK ratio shifts the homogenous system from the creatine kinase to the pyruvate kinase reaction of ADP rephosphorylation, as it should be expected for enzymes with similar affinities for ADP [9] which use the same homogenous pool of substrates.

The effect of enhancing the PK/CK ratio is very different when ADP is used in the myofibrillar creatine kinase reaction. In this case, the rate of creatine release was not decreased more than by 30% and the rate of pyruvate release was not higher than 30% of the value of the ATPase reaction even at very high PK/CK ratio (Fig. 5b). In this structurally organized system the ADP level in the medium was significantly lower than that in the homogenous system, and was not detectable when the PK/CK value exceeded 10—15.

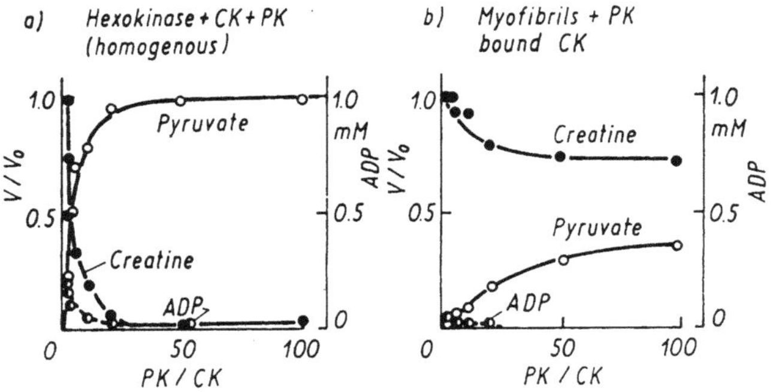

Fig. 5. The effect of elevated ratios of pyruvate kinase/creatine kinase activities, PK/CK, on the rates of creatine and pyruvate release in the myofibrillar + exogenous pyruvate kinase system.
A. Control—homogenous system: 0.6 I U of both hexokinase and creatine kinase were per ml of the reaction medium. The reaction was stopped after 2 min.
B. Cardiac myofibrils. Myofibrils were added to a concentration of 1—2 mg per ml. The ATPase activity was 0.12—0.16 I U/mg, creatine kinase was 0.14—0.15 IU/mg. Reaction was run as indicated in a.

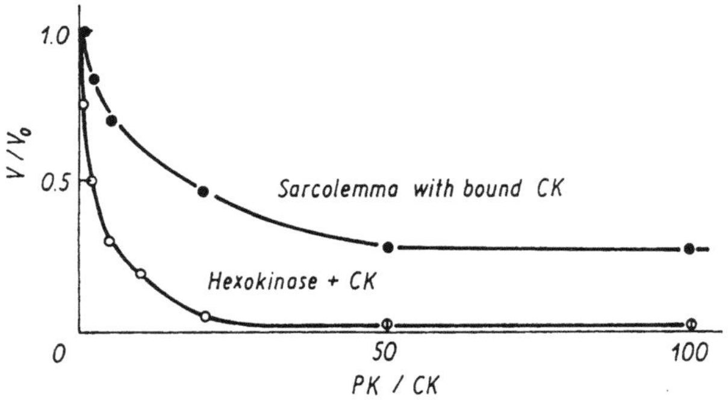

Fig. 6. Investigation of the routes of ADP movement between cardiac sarcolemma. Na, K-ATPase and creatine kinase. Sarcolemmal preparation was added to a concentration of 0.05—0.1 mg/ml. Open circles — control system (see Fig. 5a); closed circles — sarcolemma from rat hearts.

The results of theseseries definitely indicatet hat a major part of ADP produced by the myofibrillar Mg-ATPase is not accessible for the exogenous pyruvate kinase in the medium but seems to be directly channeled to the creatine kinase for rephosphorylation. Figure 6 demonstrates the very similar results obtained for cardiac sarcolemma isolated from rat hearts. As compared to the soluble hexokinase + creatine kinase system, the rate of creatine release decreases much more slowly with the elevation of PK/CK ratio and reaches a plateau at 30% of the original value at PK/CK = 50—100. Somewhat higher sensitivity of the sarcolemmal system to changes in the PK/CK ratio than of myofibrils is probably explained by the presence in membrane preparations of the basal MgATPase activity nonsensitive to inhibition by digitalis and nonrelevant to the NaK-pump system and most probably not coupled to the creatine kinase.

The results reported here are consistent with the concept of the phosphocreatine pathway for energy channelling. This concept is illustrated schematically in Figure 7. Structural closeness of mitochondrial creatine kinase to the adenine nucleotide translocase as well as an aerobic enhancement of phosphocreatine production reported earlier [4, 14, 17, 18, 24] suggests an existence of an enzyme cluster consisting of these two proteins in heart mitochondria. For this cluster, ATP and ADP are internal substrates used for phosphocreatine synthesis coupled with oxidative phosphorylation, and this cluster connects mitochondrial reactions of energy production with cytoplasmic energy consuming reactions via phosphocreatine-creatine shuttle. Very similar clusters consisting of creatine kinase and ATPase, seem to exist in myofibrils and in sarcolemma where phosphocreatine is connected with energy consuming processes via ATP-ADP cycle in the coupled reactions. In both cases, the operation of the whole system of energy supply may include only local turnover of adenine nucleotides, or their functional compartmentation, as it was suggested on a general basis by GUDBJARNASON et al. in 1970 [6].

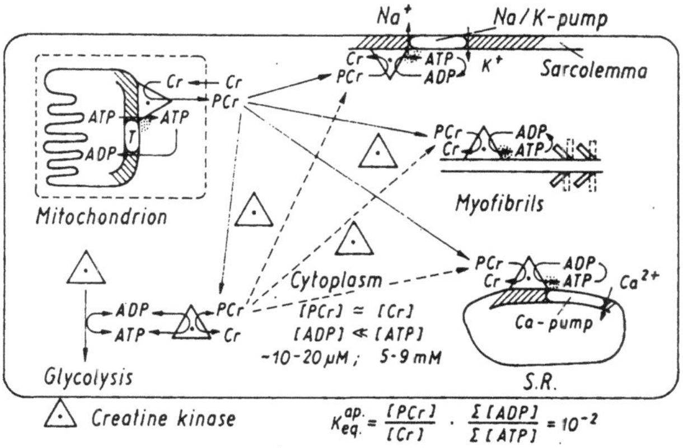

Fig. 7. Compartmentation of the creatine kinase isoenzymes and adenine nucleotides in cardiac cells. Phosphocreatine pathway for intracellular energy chanelling. Reproduced from Advances im Myocardiology, vol. 3, p. 475–497 1982, with permission of Plenum Publishing Corporation.

Acknowledgments

The authors thank Dr. Valery V. KUPRIYANOV for skillful assistance in experiments with the adenine nucleotide translocase determination, and Dr. Victor G. SHAROV for electron microphotographs.

References

[1] BARBOUR, R. L. and S. H. P. CHAN: J. Biol. Chem. **256** (1981), 1940–1948
[2] BESSMAN, S. P., W. C. T. YANG, P. J. GEIGER and S. ERICKSON-VIITANEN: Biochem. Biophys. Res. Comm. **96** (1980), 1414–1420
[3] DHALLA, N. S., Y. C. YATES, D. A. WALZ, V. A. MCDONALD and R. E. OLSON: Can. J. Physiol. Pharmacol. **50** (1972), 333–345
[4] GELLERICH, F., and V. A. SAKS: Biochem. Biophys. Res. Comm. **105** (1982), 1473–1481
[5] GROSSE, R., E. SPITZER, V. V. KUPRIANOV, K. REPKE and V. A. SAKS: Biochim. Biophys. Acta **603** (1980), 142–156

[6] GUDBJARNASON, S., P. MATHES and K. G. RAVENS: J. Molec. Cell. Cardiol. 1 (1970), 325—339
[7] JACOBUS, W. E. and A. L. LEHNINGER: J. Biol. Chem. 248 (1973), 4803—4810
[8] KUPRIANOV, V. V., G. V. ELIZAROVA and V. A. SAKS: Biochimija 46 (1981), 930—941
[9] KUPRIANOV, V. V., E. K. SEPPET, I. V. EMELIN and V. A. SAKS: Biochim. Biophys. Acta 592 (1980), 197—210
[10] MOREADITH, R. W. and W. E. JACOBUS: J. Biol. Chem. 257 (1982), 899—905
[11] NEELY, J. R., M. J. ROVETTO, J. I. WHITMER and H. E. MORGAN: Amer. J. Physiol. 255 (1973), 651—658
[12] OLSON, R. E. and D. A. BARNHORST: In: Recent Advances in Studies on Cardiac Structure and Metabolism (Ed. Dhalla N.S.), University Park Press, Baltimore (1973), 11—30
[13] PREOBRAHENSKIY, A. N. and V. A. SAKS: Biokhimija 46 (1981), 1681 1693
[14] SAKS, V. A., G. B. CHERNOUSOVA, D. E. GUKOYSKY, V. N. SMIRNOV and E. I. CHAZOV: Eur. J. Biochem. 57 (1975), 273—290
[15] SAKS, V. A., B. G. CHERNOUSOVA and N. V. LYULINA: in preparation
[16] SAKS, V. A., G. B. CHERNOUSOVA, R. VETTER, V. N. SMIRNOV and E. I. CHAZOV: FEBS Letters 62 (1976), 293—296
[17] SAKS, V. A., V. V. KUPRIANOV, G. V. ELIZAROVA and W. E. JACOBUS: J. Biol. Chem. 255 (1980), 755—763
[18] SAKS, V. A., V. V. KUPRIANOV, A. N. PREOBRAJENSKY and W. E. JACOBUS: J. Molec. Cell. Cardiol. 14 (1982), Suppl. 3, 1—12
[19] SAKS, V. A., N. V. LIPINA, N. V. LJULINA, G. B. CHERNOUSOVA, R. VETTER, V. N. SMIRNOV and E. I. CHAZOV: Biokhimija 41 (1976), 1460—1470
[20] SAKS, V. A., L. V. ROSENSHTRAUKH, V. N. SMIRNOV and E. I. CHAZOV: Can. J. Physiol. Pharmacol. 56 (1978), 691—706
[21] SCHOLTE, H. R., P. J. WEIJERS and E. M. WIT-PEETERS: Biochim. Biophys. Acta 291 (1973), 764—773
[22] SERAYDARIAN, M. W. and B. ABBOTT: J. Molec. Cell. Cardiol. 8 (1976, 741—746
[23] VENTURA-CLAPIER, R. and G. VASSORT: J. Physiol. (Paris) 76 (1980), 543—561
[24] YANG, W. C. T., P. J. GEIGER, S. P. BESSMAN and B. BORREBACK: Biochem. Biophys. Res. Comm. 76 (1977), 882—887

II. Ion movements

Central Institute of Heart and Circulation Research, Academy of Sciences of the GDR, 1115 Berlin-Buch, GDR, and USSR Cardiology Research Center, Academy of Medical Sciences of the USSR, Moscow, USSR

Frequency- and Voltage-Dependent Block of Sodium Channels in Single Rat Myocardial Cells Treated with Mexiletine[1]

S. HERING, A. I. UNDROVINAS and R. BODEWEI

Introduction

Many aspects of the action of antiarrhythmic drug on the heart may be understood in terms of alterations in cardiac membrane currents [7]. The action of the antiarrhythmic mexiletine on the cardiac membrane currents was studied by several authors with the aid of standard microelectrode technique [5, 6, 17]. In recent studies it could be shown that the "class I agent" mexiletine [18], decreases the upstroke velocity of papillary muscle action potentials in a frequency-dependent fashion [5]. Conflicting findings were reported concerning the effective refractory period [5, 7, 17]. However, according to theoretical considerations and experimental data the upstroke velocity of the action potential is a nonlinear measure of sodium conductance in heart muscle preparations [4]. In view of the difficulties in I_{Na}-measurements in multicellular heart muscle preparations [1] a detailed experimental description of the fast sodium inward current in single mammalian heart muscle cells was a prerequisite for studies of antiarrhythmic drug action on this current [2, 3, 13, 20, 21].

In the present experiments, most of which are reported in greater detail elsewhere [8], the action of mexiletine on some of the properties of the fast Na^+ current was studied in freshly isolated adult rat heart cells, making use of an adaptation of the suction pipette technique for internal perfusion that was introduced by KRISHTAL et al [12]. With the view of recent findings that the antiarythmics attributed to class I [18] might act by different electrophysiological mechanisms special attention was paid to the frequency- and voltage-dependence of the action of mexiletine on the I_{Na} in heart muscle cells [9, 10, 11, 16, 19].

Methods

Single isolated, internally perfused myocardial cells of adult rats were used for voltage clamp analysis of the fast sodium inward current as previously described in detail [2].

Cell isolation: Single ventricular myocytes were obtained according to a modification of the method of RAIS et al. [15] by perfusion of the excised hearts of heparinized adult male Wistar rats with a collagenase-containing solution, followed by disintegration of the minced ventricular tissue during gentle shaking in either "extracellular" solution I (130 mM NaCl, 4 mM KCl, 0.5 mM $MgCl_2$, 0.9 mM $CaCl_2$, 11.1 mM glucose, 10 mM

[1] Material presented at the Young Investigators' Prize Contest during the IX World Congress of Cardiology, Moscow, June 1982

Tris-HCl of pH 7.4) or "extracellular" solution II (100 mM NaCl, 4 mM KCl, 0.5 mM $MgCl_2$, 0.9 mM $CaCl_2$, 11.1 mM glucose, 30 mM Tris-HCl of pH 7.4). Many of the isolated myocytes could be used for as long as 5 to 7 hours for voltage clamping.

Ionic current measurements: The suction pipette technique developed for a voltage clamp study of nervous cells [12] and adapted to the measurement of ionic currents in isolated mammalian heart muscle cells [2, 20, 21] was used.

The series resistance (R_S) was computed from the time constant of the capacitative current flow and amounted to 200—400 kΩ, the leakage resistance (R_L) approximated 10 MΩ. As shown in our earlier work [2], the resulting R_S/R_L ratio guarantees a satisfactory temporal resolution for the measurements to be performed.

Mexiletine hydrochloride was kindly supplied by Boehringer Ingelheim. It was added to the extracellular solutions. The slow inward current was blocked by 0.5 mM $CdCl_2$. All experiments were performed at 18—21 °C.

Results

Effects of mexiletine on the I—V relationship and recovery of I_{Na} at low frequency of stimulation

Figure 1a shows a family of voltage clamp currents from a single internally perfused heart muscle cell sourrounded by extracellular solution I. The test pulses 8 ms applied to this cell with a frequency of 0.1 Hz gave rise to a sodium inward current that reached a maximum value at —30 mV after 1.5 ms. Following a 5-min exposure of the cell to 50 μM mexiletine the current was reduced to about 25 per cent of the control value (Fig. 1b).

The current-voltage relationship of a cell before and during treatment with mexiletine is shown in Figure 2. It is seen that after a 5-min wash following exposure to mexiletine the currents had nearly regained their original strength. The effect of mexiletine on I_{Na} was not associated with changes in the leakage resistance.

In the same experimental series the time course of reactivation of the maximum Na^+ inward current was studied at a holding potential of —100 mV. The reactivation time

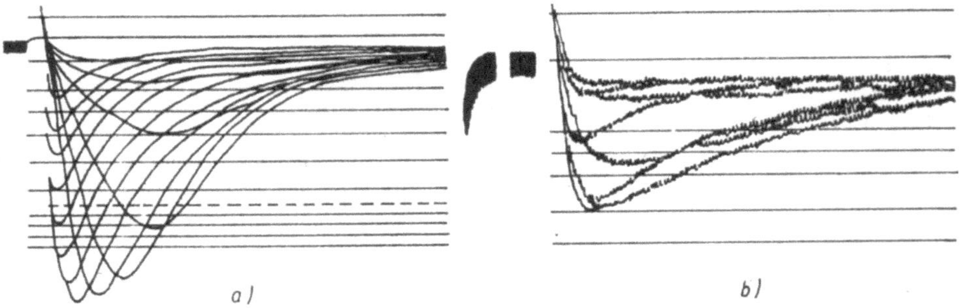

Fig. 1. Families of I_{Na} of a myocardial cell (a) before and (b) during exposure to 50 μM mexilatine. Calibration: Vertical bar, 2 nA for (a) and 1 nA vor (b) 20 mV; horizontal bar, 1 ms. from ref. 21.

constant of the Na^+ current was estimated by a 2-pulse program [2]. A 10-ms depolarieing prepulse of 80-mV amplitude was followed after different time intervals by a 10-ms test pulse of the same amplitude. Mexiletine in a concentration of 40 μM was found to increase the reactivation time constant of the current from 20 ± 7 ms (n = 8) to 190 ± 30 ms (n = 6).

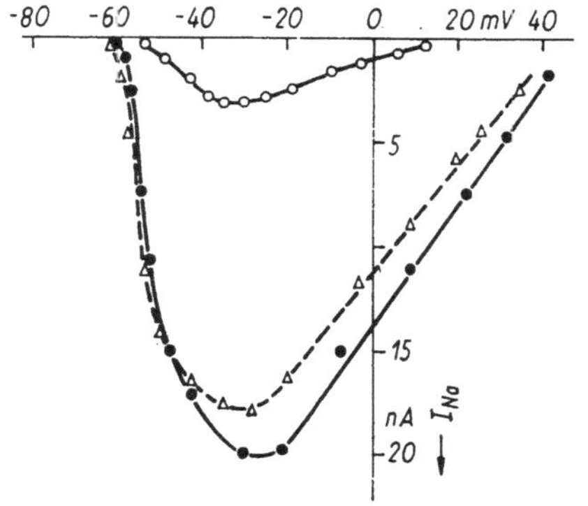

Fig. 2. Current-voltage relationship for the peak I_{Na} of a myocardial cell bathed in solution I. ●: Before mexiletine; ○: 2 min after 60 μM mexiletine in solution I; △ : after a 5-min wash with solution I.

Frequency- and voltage-dependent action of mexiletine on I_{Na}

The possibility of a frequency-dependent Na channel block by mexiletine was examined in cells treated for 5 min with mexiletine in the concentration range of 20 to 30 μM. In this range the drug led on application of 10 ms depolarizing pulses to −20 mV at 0.1 Hz to a "tonic" reduction [19] of I_{Na} by 10 to 20 per cent. Trains of pulses of different duration and spaced at different intervals were then applied. After each train of pulses a rest period of 30 s was interposed during which the current amplitude returned to the initial value.

Figure 3a presents the results of an experiment in which trains of 10-ms test pulses were applied in the presence of 25 μM mexiletine at frequencies ranging 1 to 6 Hz. Peak I_{Na} is plotted here as a function of time. The Figure shows that stimulation at

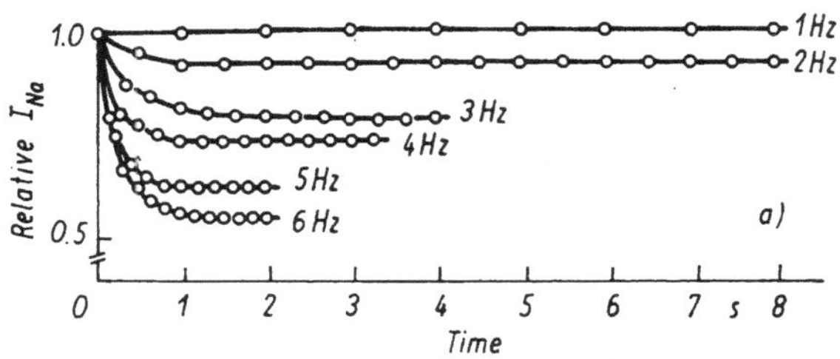

Fig. 3a. Use-dependent block of peak I_{Na} in a single heart cell bathed in solution II containing 25 μM mexiletine. Trains of 10-ms test pulses to −20 mV from V_H of −80 mV were applied at different intervals. Normalized current values, pre-train peak I_{Na} = 1. From ref. 21.

high frequencies enhanced the blocking effect of mexiletine to a greater extent and sooner than did stimulation at low frequencies.

Prior to the addition of mexiletine the peak sodium current was barely reduced even at stimulation frequencies higher than 5 Hz.

The next experiment was concerned with the effect of pulse duration on the frequency-dependent block by mexiletine of peak Na currents. After a 1-min rest period, during which the peak current returned to the pre-train value, the test pulse duration was extended to 100 ms. As seen in Figure 3b, the peak current was reduced by an additional 20 per cent when the 100-ms test pulses were applied at a frequency of 1 Hz.

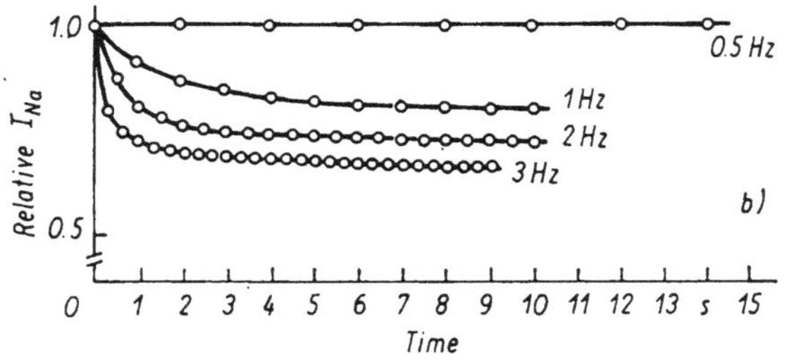

Fig. 3b. Use-dependent block of peak I_{Na} of the cell shown in Fig. 3a, induced by applying 100-ms test pulses to -20 mV from V_H of -80 mV. Normalized values, pre-train peak $I_{Na} = 1$. From ref. 21.

Discussion

Changes of the fast sodium inward current are believed to underlie the therapeutic action of antiarrhythmic drugs of the local anesthetic type on the heart [7, 9]. In recent experiments with isolated myocardial cells of adult rats it was shown that the temporal resolution of voltage clamp measurements can decisively be improved with the aid of the technique of internal perfusion and attention was called to the potential usefulness of this method in the study of the influence of antiarrhythmic and other drugs on the myocardial I_{Na} [2, 13].

The present and related [8] experiments are the first voltage clamp study of the voltage- and frequency-dependent blocking action of one of the newer antiarrhythmic agents, the lidocaine derivative mexiletine, on Na channels of myocardial cells. The drug was applied in concentrations which are of the same order of magnitude as those found in the plasma of patients treated with this drug [14]. It could be shown, first of all, that at a membrane potential of -100 mV the I_{Na} of isolated rat heart muscle cells is severely reduced in the presence of 60 μM mexiletine when short depolarizing pulses were delivered at a frequency of 0.1 Hz. The amplitude of I_{Na} returned to the control value after a 2 to 5-min wash (Fig. 2). This finding and the observation that mexiletine prolongs the reactivation time of I_{Na} confirm the results of studies carried out with the microelectrode technique [5, 6, 17].

It has been reported by several authors [9. 10, 11, 16, 19] that repetitive use of sodium channels caused by short depolarizing voltage pulses progressively reduces the amplitude of sodium currents during exposure to local anesthetics and similarly acting antiarrhythmic drugs. A similar effect of the frequency of depolarization was presently found in single heart cells that were treated with 20—30 μM mexiletine and depolarized by 10-ms and 100-ms pulses (Fig. 3a, b). KHODOROV et al. [11] and HILLE [9] have proposed that local anesthetics interfere with the inactivation mechanism of the Na channel. Our finding that use-dependent block of I_{Na} by mexiletine increases with an increase in pulse duration suggests that this drug, like the just mentioned local anesthetics, interacts preferentially with inactivated Na channels. As could be seen in Figure 3a, b, a rhythmic depolarization of the membrane by 10-ms trains of pulses applied at a frequency of 1 Hz failed to reduce I_{Na}, whereas with 100-ms pulses applied at the same frequency a use-dependent depression of this current was clearly evident. This finding coroborates earlier reports about an interval-dependent inhibition of the upstroke of the cardiac action potential by mexiletine [5, 17]. In agreement with Hille's [9] hypothesis of the mechanism of action of antiarrhythmic agents the pressent results may be interpreted as indicating that binding of mexiletine to the fast sodium channels of rat myocardial cells is facilitated when the cell membrane becomes depolarized.

Acknowledgment

We thank Prof. A. WOLLENBERGER for his encouragement and for helpful discussions and constructive comments on the manuscript.

References

[1] BEELER, G. W. and J. A. S. MC GUIGAN: Progr. Biophys. Molec. Biol. **34** (1978) 219
[2] BODEWEI, R., S. HERING, B. LEMKE, L. V. ROSENSTRAUCH, A. I. UNDROVINAS and A. WOLLENBERGER: J. Physiol. **325** (1982) 301
[3] BROWN, A. M., K. S. LEE and T. POWELL: J. Physiol. **318** (1981) 479
[4] COHEN, C. J., B. P. BEAN, T. J. COLATSKY and R. W. TSIEN: J. Gen. Physiol. **78** (1981) 381
[5] COURTNEY, K.: Europ. J. Pharmacol. **74** (1981) 9
[6] HAAP, K. and H. ANTONI: Klin. Wschr. **56** (1978) 169
[7] HAUSWIRTH, O. and B. N. SINGH: Pharmacol. Rev. **30** (1979) 5
[8] HERING, S., R. BODEWEI and A. WOLLENBERGER: J. Mol. Cell. Cardiol. **15** (1983) 431—444
[9] HILLE, B.: Biophysical Aspect of Cardiac Muscle, M. Morad and M. Tabatabai Eds. New York. Academic Press (1978) 55—74
[10] KHODOROV, B. I., L. D. CHICHKOVA and E. M. PEGANOV: Biochim. Biophys. Acta **433** (1976) 409
[11] KHODOROV, B. I., L. D. SHISHKOVA and E. M. PEGANOV: Bull. Exp. Biol. Med. **3** (1974) 13
[12] KRISHTAL, A. A. and V. J. PIDOPLICHKO: Neirofiziologiya (Kiev) **9** (1977) 644
[13] LEE, K. S., J. R. HUME, W. GIBS and A. M. BROWN: Nature **291** (1981) 325
[14] PODRID, B. J. and B. LOWN: Amer. J. Cardiol. **47** (1981) 895
[15] RAIS, J., M. SUNDBERG, G. V. SUNDBY, N. DONELL, G. TORLING, P. BIEBERFELD and S. JACOBSON: Exp. Cell. Res. **115** (1978) 183
[16] REVENKO, S. V., B. I. KHODOROV and M. YA. AVRUTSKY: Bull. Exp. Biol. Med. **6** (1980) 702
[17] SADA, H., T. BAN and S. OSHITA: Clin. Exp. Pharmacol. Physiol. **7** (1980) 583

[18] SINGH, B. N. and E. M. VAUGHAN WILLIAMS: Brit. J. Pharmacol. **44** (1972) 1
[19] STRICHHARTZ, G. R.: J. Gen. Physiol. **62** (1973) 37
[20] UNDROVINAS, A. I., A. V. YUSHMANOVA, S. HERING and L. V. ROSENSTRAUKH: Physiol. J. USSR **66** (1979) 602
[21] UNDROVINAS, A. I., A. V. YUSHMANOVA, S. HERING and L. V. ROSENSTRAUKH: Experienta **36** (1979) 572

Julius Bernstein Institute of Physiology, Martin-Luther-University Halle—Wittenberg, Halle (Saale), GDR

Pacing-dependent Properties of the Slow Inward Current in the Atrial Myocardium

B. Nilius

Introduction

It is well established that in contrast to the electrical activity in nerve and skeletal muscle the repolarization process in all types of cardiac tissue is highly sensitive to changes in rate and rhythm of pacing (Carmeliet [7], Boyett and Jewell [3]). The changes in repolarization result partly from pacing dependent properties of ionic currents. In the present paper pacing dependent properties of the slow inward current, which is proved to be mainly transported by Ca ions, were examined. It is demonstrated that the Ca influx via the slow inward channel can be controlled by a current (Ca) activated inactivation and that the sensitivity of this channel to variations in the pacing pattern seems to be determined by the inactivation process.
Parts of the experimental findings were published previously [12, 13].

Material and methods

Experiments were performed on single about 2 mm long free running frog atrial trabeculae showing diameters between 40 and 80 μm. A new, improved double sucrose gap chamber was used which consists in three movable parts by which all the gap widthes can be optimized. Seals were made from vaseline (Fig. 1a). The control solution was composed as follows (mmol/l): NaCl 110, KCl 2.5, $CaCl_2$ 4, $NaHCO_3$ 2.38, NaH_2PO_4 0.08, glucose 5.5, pH 7.1—7.2. The depolarizing solution was made from isotonic K aspartat. Fast inward currents were blocked by a depolarizing holding potential at −50 mV or an application of TTX (10^{-5} mol/l). The transgap potential was measured between test node T and one depolarizing compartment K; current was infected into the other peripheral compartment. The transmembrane current was measured in the test node seperately (Fig. 1b). The series resistances R_p could be evaluated supposing the electrical equivalent circuit shown in Figure 1c. It was calculated being between about 3 and 32 kOhm in dependence on the bundle's diameter (for methodical details see Nilius et al. [14]). To demonstrate the realibility of the voltage clamp two examples of an inactivation protocol (Fig. 1d) and a protocol for examining current-voltage "families" (Fig. 1e) of the fast inward current is demonstrated. The records secure a high homogeneity of the used voltage clamp.

To study pacing dependent properties the interval T_0 between the activation pulses was changed from 0.2 to 10 s. A decreases in T_0 always means an increased pacing rate.

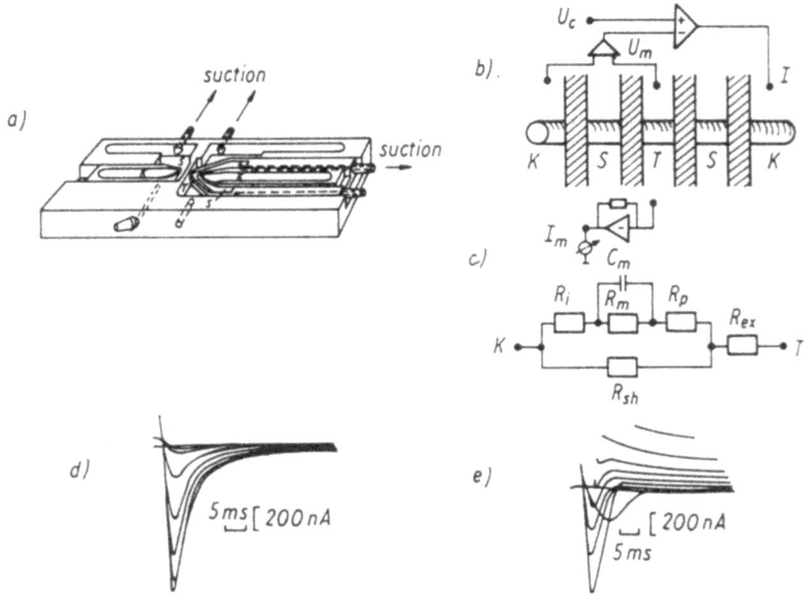

Fig. 1. Scheme of method.
Fig. 1a. perfusion chamber; K, S, T mean the depolarizing (KCl), sucrose, and test compartment, respectively.
Fig. 1b. voltage clamp device; the hatched bars represent the vaseline seals; U_c: command potential, U_m: measured trans-gap potential, I: injected current, I_m: measured membrane current.
Fig. 1c. model of the resistances and membrane capacity C_m between K and T; R_i: internal resistance of the preparation, R_m: membrane resistance of the preparation within the test node, R_p: series resistance due to the preparation (endothelial resistance, cleft resistance), R_{ex}: series resistance due to the solution in the test-node and the electrodes, R_{sh}: shunt resistance (for details see text).
Fig. 1d. experimental protocol for measuring the inactivation of the fast inward current (equidistant conditioning 400 ms lasting voltage steps basic to the holding potential of -15 mV).
Fig. 1e. "family" of currents activated by depolarizing voltage pulses (equidistant depolarizing voltage steps from a holding potential of -80 mV).

Results

Pacing-dependence of current-voltage relationships: The slow inward current was found to be highly sensitive to changes in the activation pattern. Increasing the rate of depolarizing voltage steps the peak inward current (I_{Si}) was decreased (Fig. 2). The current-voltage relationships were shifted upwards to smaller currents due to increasing of the pacing rate. The outward currents taken as current at the end of a 1 s lasting depolarizing step increased in a much smaller extent than the inward current was decreased due to shortening of the pacing interval T_0.

Pacing-dependence of steady-state inactivation: Using a standard double step programme (500 ms conditioning prepulse, 300 ms test pulse to 0 mV) the steady-state inactivation of the slow inward current was examined. If the interval T_0 between the double-

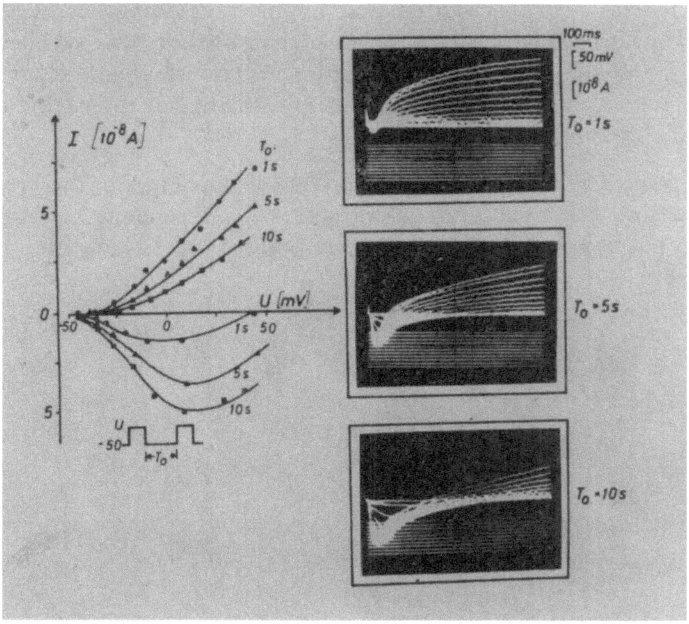

Fig. 2. Membrane currents under steady-state pacing.
Right: families of voltage-current traces at three different pacing intervals T_0. All the single records were taken under steady-state conditions.
Left: current-voltage plots for peak inward current and maximal outward current after 1 s depolarization. Holding potential −50 mV.

step pulses was changed the steady-state inactivation could be studied in its pacing dependence. The inactivation was measured as ratio between test current after the conditioning step and maximal inward current and is described by

$$f_\infty = \left(1 + \exp\,(U - U_S)/S\right)^{-1}$$

(S: slope parameter in mV, U_S: potential for half complete inactivation in mV, f_∞ taken from the ratio between test and maximal inward current). If T_0 was shortened (increase of the pacing rate) U_S was shifted to more negative potentials without a significant change in the slope S (see Fig. 3). Such leftward shift of the steady-state inactivation had been predicted to be mediated by a decrease of the external Ca concentration, a clearing of the external or screening of the internal surface charges (Brown [6]).

Pacing-dependence of recovery from and onset of inactivation: The finding of a pacing-dependent shift in the $f_\infty - U$ relationship referred to an activation-dependent inactivation. Therefore, both recovery from and onset of inactivation were examined. Recovery from inactivation was defined as the increase of the slow inward current due to hyperpolarizing prepulses of successively prolonged duration T. The onset of inactivation was tested by application of depolarizing prepulses of different duration. This double-step pattern could also be delivered at different pacing intervals T_0. Figure 4 demonstrates that the time constant of recovery from inactivation run between 0.35 and 0.40 s independent on the used pacing intervals T_0 between 1 and 10 s. In sharp contrast to it the onset of inactivation was found to be pacing dependent distinctly. If the pacing rate was increased the onset of inactivation was accellerated (Fig. 5). The findings on accelleration of the onset of inactivation favour the hypothesis of the existence of an activation-dependent inactivation: the higher the pacing rate is chosen, the more accellerated inactivation results.

Inactivation studied by a twin-pulse with gap method: Looking for further experimental evidence supporting the hypothesis of an activation-dependent inactivation a twin-pulse with gap method was used: a first conditioning depolarizing step is followed by

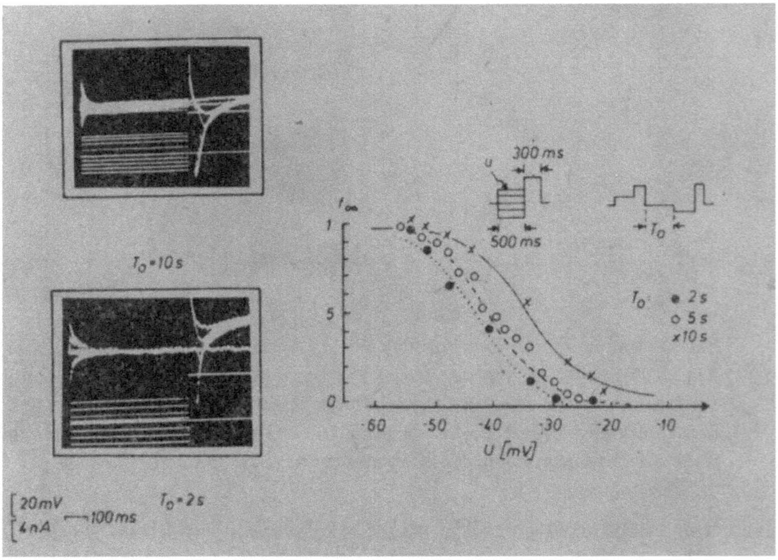

Fig. 3. Pacing dependence of steady state inactivation.
Left: Slow inward current activated by a test pulse to 0 mV, holding potential -40 mV, duration of the test pulse 300 ms. Before each test pulse a 500 ms lasting prepulse had been applied. The double step programme was supplied repetitively with the distance (pacing interval) T_0.
Right: steady state inactivation curve of I_{si}. The measured f_∞-values were fitted by $f_\infty = (1 - \exp((U - U/)S))^{-1}$
The used slope parameter S was calculated to 4.6 mV. • pacing interval $T_0 = 2$ s, $U_s = -40.5$ mV; ∘ $T_0 = 5$ s, $U_s = -43$ mV, × $T_0 = 10$, $U_s = -34$ mV.

a secondary step separated from the first by a 2 s gap. The size of the applied voltage steps was adjusted to activate the slow inward current I_{si} within the overlapping range between steady state activation and inactivation. Prolonging the duration of the twin-pulses the secondary or test current was decreased progressively. At a 50 ms conditioning pulse the test current was nearly unchanged but at a 900 ms prepulse the test current disappeared. If during the conditioning step inward transported charge was considered a monotonous decrease of both the normalized inward transported charge and peak I_{si} during the test step was observed as the inward transported, conditioning charge was increased (Fig. 6).

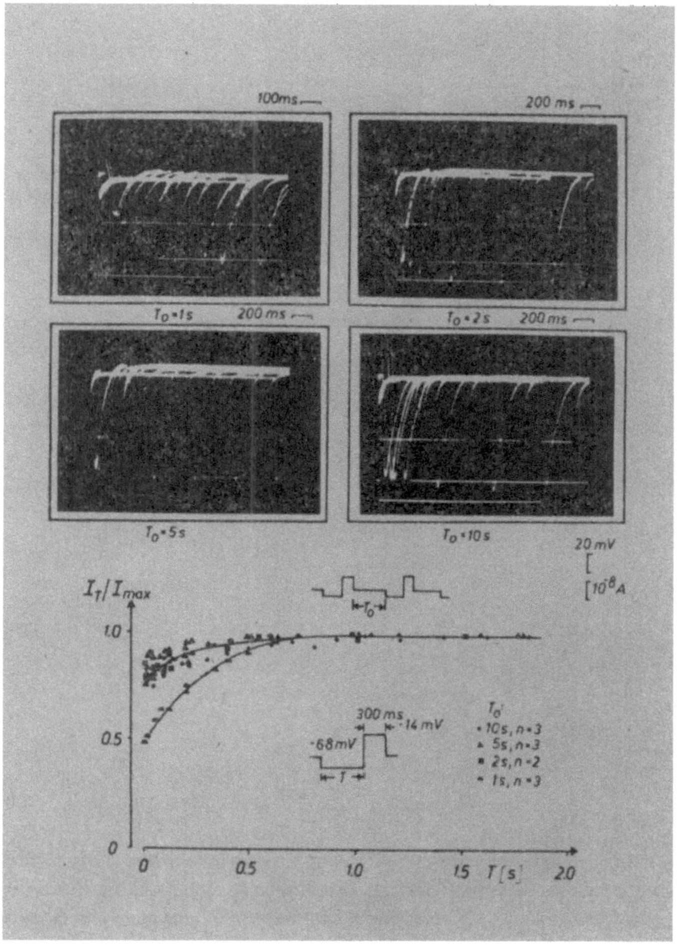

Fig. 4. Recovery from inactivation at different pacing intervals. top: families of current-voltage records at different durations of the hyperpolarizing prepulse (double step programme, see inset). T_0: interval between the voltage clamp double steps during repetitive activation. Bottom: abscissa-duration of the hyperpolarizing prepulse before a 300 ms lasting test step to −14 mV. Ordinate-normalized peak slow inward current. n: number of measurements.

Currents activated by voltage steps different in size showed an U-shaped dependence of the normalized secondary test inward current on the depolarizing voltage (Fig. 7). From the same finding comes the main evidence for a Ca-dependent inactivation in other tissues [1, 4, 5, 15, 16].

Discussion

It is evident from the experimental findings that the slow inward current is highly sensitive to changes in the activation pattern. The results showed a decrease of the peak inward current due to an increase of the pacing rate. It is unlikely that the pacing-

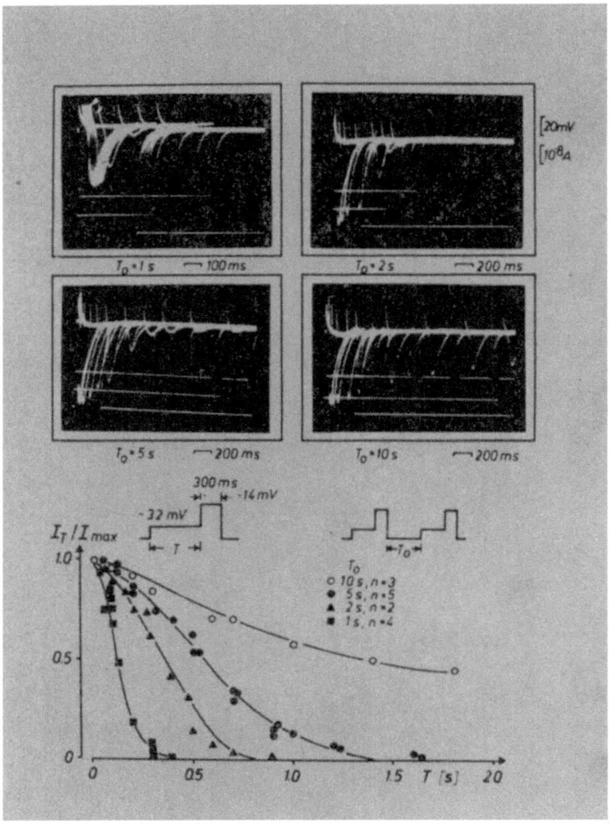

Fig. 5. Onset of inactivation at different pacing intervals. Top: families of current-voltage traces at different pacing intervals. A depolarizing prepulse precedes the test pulse (see inset). T_0 represents the interval between the double step voltage clamp pulses.
Bottom: abscissa-duration of the depolarizing prepulse before a 300 ms lasting test step to −14 mV. Ordinate-normalized peak slow inward current.
n: number of measurements

dependent decrease of I_{si} is provoked by a decrease of the maximal conductance g_{si} for being the positive slope conductance taken from the peak I_{si}-voltage relationships pacing-independent. A pacing-induced increase of outward currents is also ruled out because the findings were also obtained under 4-aminopyridine. Figure 2 demonstrates that the pacing-induced decrease in the peak inward current is much larger than the shift in the outward currents. Also, a Ca depletion or accumulation changing the driving force is unlikely. A change in the inward current by about 80% of the control level (see also Fig. 2 and 6) would need a drastic variation in the Ca gradient through the sarcolemma. Using a constant field model a Ca depletion from 4 to about 10^{-4} mmol/l or an internal Ca accumulation from about 100 nmol/l to 0.1 mmol/l would be necessary to explain changes in current. From the inward transported charge (Fig. 6) it seems quite unlikely that such a distinct alteration in the Ca concentration on either side of the membrane can take place. The most plausible explanation of the pacing-dependence

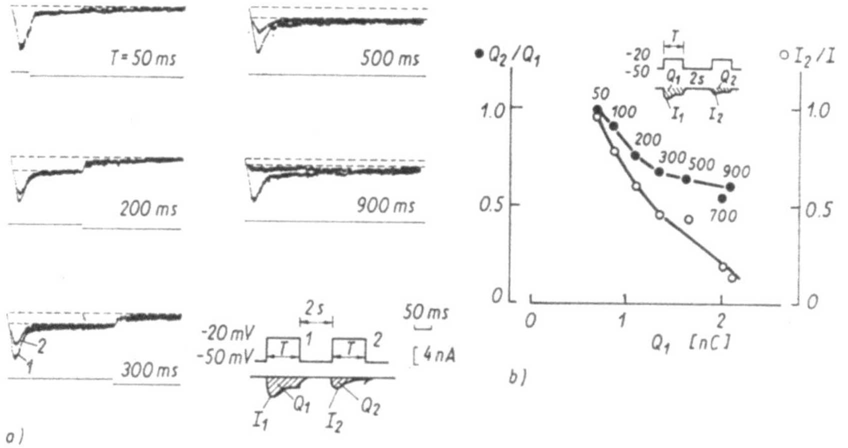

Fig. 6a. Slow inward currents recorded using a twin-pulse with gap programme. The pulse duration T was varied. The gap was kept constant at 2 s (see inset). All currents were activated by depolarizing voltage steps from a holding potential of −50 mV to −20 mV. The smaller current always coincides with the secondary test current. The duration T of the depolarizing steps is indicated at each trace (upper trace: current, lower trace: voltage).

Fig. 6b. Dependence of the relative sizes of both the inward transported charge and the peak inward current during the test pulse on the inward transported charge during the conditioning pre-pulse. ○ : test peak inward current relative to the conditioning inward current, • : relative charge during the test pulse (note the different ordinates). The numbers mark the duration T of the conditioning pulse. All the measurements were taken from depolarizing steps of different duration from −50 to −20 mV (see inset). Abscissa: inward transported charge during the conditioning pulse in nC.

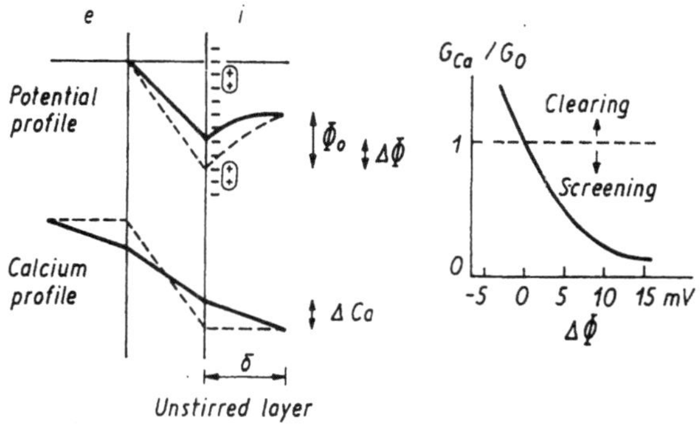

Fig. 7. Dependence of the test current on the depolarizing voltage step.

Fig. 7a. Slow inward currents recorded by a twin-pulse with gap programme. The duration of the twin-pulses was 400 ms. From a holding potential of −50 mV currents were activated by clamping the membrane potential to various depolarizing voltages U. The duration of the gap was chosen to 2 s (see inset right).

Fig. 7b. Effect of the conditioning pulse size on the inactivation. Ordinate: peak current at the test pulse relative to the peak current at the conditioning pulse. Abscissa: potential of the depolarizing twin-pulses. For twin-pulse programme see inset (duration of the gap between the pulses was 2 s). The different symbols mark diverse experiments. The dotted line was drawn by hand.

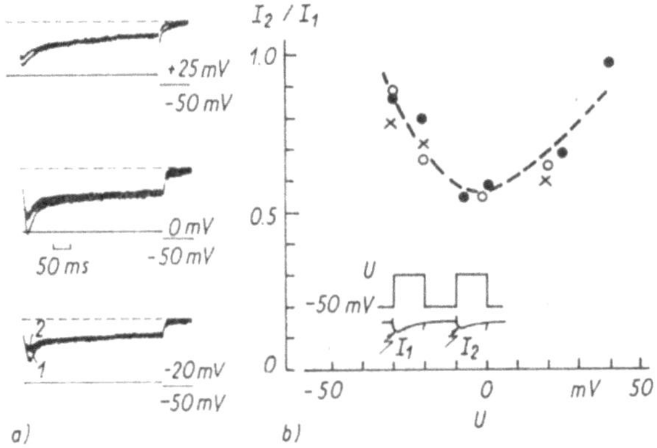

Fig. 8. Supposed mechanism of current-induced inactivation (see also HALL, and CAHALAN [10]).
Left: Potential profile and calcium concentration profile through the membrane before (- - - -) and after (———) the conditioning voltage step. Inward transported Ca would screen the internal surface charges resulting in a drop of the surface potential $\Delta\Phi$ (initial surface potential Φ_0) and a flattening of the Ca concentration profile (rise in the internal Ca concentration ΔCa near the inner side of the membrane). δ marks an unstirred layer's thickness. Stirring or convection might mix completely the solutions up to a distance $\delta \cdot \delta$ was chosen being about ten times the Debye-length.
Right: Effects of changes in the surface potential $\Delta\Phi$ on the relative membrane conductance G_{Ca}/G_0. In the used context G_{Ca}, G_0 mean the maximum conductance during the test step, conditioning step, respectively. Clearing of surface charges would increase the relative conductance, screening of surface charges diminished the conductance. The smooth line was obtained from a graph defined by formulae

$$\Delta\Phi = (4RT/F) \tan h \, (F\Phi_0/RT) \cdot \frac{K_M \cdot Ca}{1 + K_M \cdot Ca}$$

and

$$\frac{G_{Ca}}{G_0} = \exp(-\Delta\Phi/U_0)$$

(K_M: binding constant for Ca to the sarcolemm, Ca: Ca concentration in the undirect layer, R, F, T with usual meaning; Ca is related to Q and Vδ, see Figure 6 and text by Ca $= Q/(F \cdot V\delta)$).

of I_{si} seems to be an activation-dependent inactivation. Figure 8 presents a possible mechanism by which a activation-dependent inactivation or pacing-dependent inactivation could be mediated similar to that proposed by HALL and CAHALAN [10].

The sarcolemmal membrane may be occupied by fixed charges. For sake of simplicity all the outer negative are regarded as screened. The dotted lines on the left-hand side demonstrate both the potential profile and the profile of the calcium concentration if no internal Ca accumulation takes place, the smooth line if Ca has been accumulated internally in a unstirred layer of thickness. Increasing the Ca influx (that means an increased pacing rate or an increased conditioning current) would screen the internal negative sides resulting in a drop of the negative surface potential. Such a change in surface potential might decrease a Ca conductance. From the Gouy-Chapman-theory the effect of changes in the surface potential on the conductance can be expressed quantitatively [10].

Mark Q the during the conditioning step inward transported charge in the twin-pulse with gap method (Fig. 6, 7), G_{Ca} the maximum conductance during the test pulse (obtained from both activating voltage and peak inward current) and G_0 during the conditioning pulse than it can derived that

$$\frac{G_{Ca}}{G_0} = \exp\left((-4RT/FU_0) \cdot \tan(F\Phi_0/RT) \cdot \frac{Q}{F \cdot V_\delta K_M + Q}\right)$$

(Φ_0: internal surface potential before activating the Ca current, U_0: voltage for an e-fold increase in the membrane conductance for Ca, K_M the binding constant of Ca to internal binding sites). U_0 can be easily obtained from the steady-state activation of I_{si}, V_δ is the volume of the unstirred layer supposing a thickness of ten DEBYE-lengthes (about 100 Å) and is calculated by

$$V_\delta = \frac{R^2}{\left(a + (b/2)\right)^2} \cdot \pi \cdot L \cdot \delta \cdot (2a - \delta)$$

(R: bundle radius, a: mean fibre radius chosen to 2.5 µm, b: mean cleft width set to 0.2 µm, L: length of the test-gap, see ATTWELL and COHEN [2]). From best approximation of the experimental data obtained from twin-pulse with gap experiments as shown in Figure 6 Φ_0, K_M, V_δ and U_0 values were calculated between −10.5 and −36.7 mV, 1.02 and 3.12 mol/l^{-1}, $3.15 \cdot 10^{-10}$ and $1.28 \cdot 10^{-9}$ cm^3, 8 and 13 mV, respectively.

Such mechanism would explain the pacing induced accelleration of inactivation (Fig. 5) and the pacing-induced shift of the steady-state inactivation (Fig. 3). Pacing dependent inactivation can be explained by lowering of the density of internal surface charges as a screening effect mediated by the inward transported calcium. The existence of a Ca-induced inactivation, a special case of it might be the pacing dependent inactivation, is proved in several tissues: Paramecium: [4, 5]; Aplysia neurons: [16]; Helix neurones: [15]; embryonic chick sensory neurons: [8]; skeletal muscle: [1] and also supposed in heart muscle [9, 11]. In the present experiments a consequence of such a mechanism is demonstrated: the slow Ca inward current can be modulated by the pacing rate. The importance of such a mechanism would be evident: The sarcolemma would be able to control the slow channel inward transported calcium acting against a cellular Ca overload.

Acknowledgment

Most of the experiments were practised during a study stay of B.N. in the Centre of Physiology, Slovak Academy of Sciences Bratislava, CSSR (head: Academic J. Zachar). I am much obliged to Ing. M. HENCEK for helpful advice in performing the experiments.

References

[1] ASHCROFT, F. M. and P. R. STANFIELD: Science **213** (1981), 224–226
[2] ATTWELL, D. and I. COHEN: Prog. Biophys. Mol. Biol. **31** (1977), 201–245
[3] BOYETT, M. R., and B. R. JEWELL: Prog. Biophys. Mol. Biol. **36** (1980), 1–52
[4] BREHM, P. and P. ECKERT: Science **202** (1978), 1203–1206
[5] BREHM, P., P. ECKERT and D. TILLOTSON: J. Physiol. (Lond.) **306** (1980), 193–203
[6] BROWN, R. H. Jr.: Prog. Biophys. Mol. Biol. **28** (1974), 343–370
[7] CARMELIET, E.: J. Physiol. (Paris) **73** (1977), 903–923
[8] DUNLAP, K. and G. D. FISCHBACH: J. Physiol. (Lond.) **317** (1981), 519–535
[9] FISCHMEISTER, R., D. MENTRARD and G. VASSORT: J. Physiol. (Lond.) **320** (1981), 27P–28P
[10] HALL, J. E. and M. D. CAHALAN: J. Gen. Physiol. **79** (1982), 387–409
[11] MARBAN, E. and R. W. TSIEN: Biophys. J. **33** (1981), 143a
[12] NILIUS, B. and M. HENCEK: Ref. 5. Gem. Tagung Ges. exp. Med. DDR, Teil 1, P 91 (1981)
[13] NILIUS, B., and M. HENCEK: Gen. Physiol. Biophys. **1** (1982), 307–318
[14] NILIUS, B., K. BENNDORF and W. SCHENK: Biomed. Biochim. Acta **42** (1983), 203–213
[15] PLANT, T. D. and N. B. STANDEN: J. Physiol. (Lond.) **321** (1981), 273–285
[16] TILLOTSON, D.: Proc. nat. Acad. Sci U.S.A. **76** (1979), 1497–1500

Abteilung Allgemeine Pharmakologie, Universitäts-Krankenhaus Eppendorf, Martinistraße 5b, D-2000 Hamburg 20, FRG

Mechanical and Electrophysiological Effects of α-Adrenoceptor Stimulating Drugs in the Heart

H. Scholz and R. Brückner

The present paper summarizes briefly the mechanism of the positive inotropic effect of β-adrenoceptor stimulation. The main part, however, is concerned with the increase in myocardial force of contraction mediated by alpha-adrenoceptors.

It is widely accepted [11, 13] that the positive inotropic effect of β-adrenoceptor stimulating agents, e.g. isoprenaline, in mammalian cardiac muscle results from an increase in slow inward current (I_{si}), which is primarily carried by Ca ions, and from a stimulation of Ca uptake by the sarcoplasmic reticulum (SR). Both actions are probably due to an elevation of intracellular cAMP levels with subsequent activation of cAMP-dependent protein kinases and phosphorylation of sarcolemmal and SR proteins, respectively. The increase in I_{si} supposedly leads to a greater release of Ca from intracellular stores (and hence to an increase in force of contraction), either because it enhances Ca-dependent Ca release and/or because it produces a greater filling of these stores with releasable Ca. A greater filling with Ca is also brought about by the cAMP dependent stimulation of Ca uptake by the SR. This explains probably also the so-called relaxant effects of the β-adrenoceptor stimulating catecholamines, namely the abbreviation of the contraction and the depression of potassium-induced contractures.

There is no doubt that the mechanical effects of the catecholamines on the heart are mainly due to stimulation of β-adrenoceptors. However, there is an increasing evidence that α-adrenoceptors exist in the myocardium and that a positive inotropic effect is produced by stimulation of these sites [1, 2, 11]. The positive inotropic effects of β- and α-adrenoceptor stimulating agents are qualitatively different from each other in several points. For instance, the positive inotropic effect (PIE) of α-adrenoceptor stimulation develops relatively slowly (Fig. 1a). This might suggest an intracellular localization, but kinetic studies with labelled α-adrenergic agonists or iontophoretic injections are still lacking. Moreover, the α-adrenoceptor mediated increase in force of contraction is not accompanied by a decrease in the duration of contraction (Fig. 1b), and potassium contractures are not suppressed. This indicates that α-adrenoceptor stimulation does not produce relaxant effects which is consistent with the failure to increase cAMP levels as mentioned below. Furthermore, the positive inotropic response to α-adrenoceptor stimulation is greatly dependent on the frequency of stimulation. It is barely detectable at frequencies below 0.1 Hz and higher than 4 Hz. There is as yet no convincing explanation for this phenomenon. Finally, both the β- and α-adrenergic positive inotropic effects are dependent on thyroid hormone. However, in contrast to the β-adrenergic effect, the α-adrenergic response is increased in hypothyroidism and decreased in hyperthyroidism. These effects are also largely unexplained at present.

The mechanism by which α-adrenoceptor stimulation increases the force of contraction is not known. Most importantly, cAMP is unlikely to be involved as a mediator. There is no convincing evidence for an increase in cAMP during the α-adrenergic PIE which, in addition, is not increased in the presence of phosphodiesterase inhibitors. Moreover, there is no detectable change in cGMP levels and in $(Na^+ + K^+)$-ATPase activity [10].

It appears reasonable to assume that the α-adrenoceptor-mediated PIE results primarily from an increase in the intracellular Ca concentration. In order to obtain information on the question whether an increase in slow inward current is involved in this

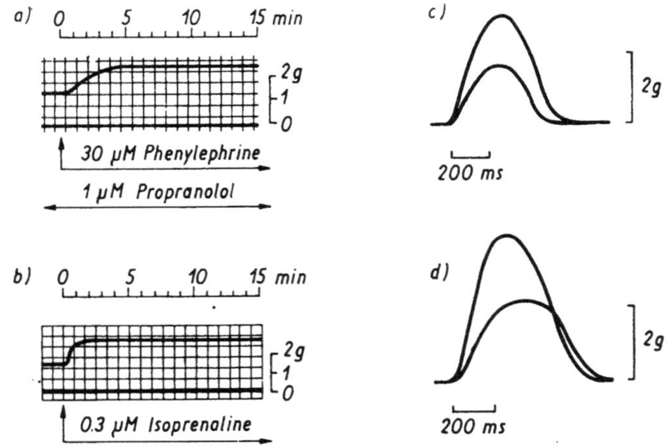

Fig. 1. Effects of 30 µM phenylephrine in the presence of 1 µM propanolol (a and c) and of 0.3 µM isoprenaline (b and d) on force of contraction in electrically driven papillary muscles from cats. a and b: time course of the positive inotropic effects. C and D: Isometric contraction curves in the absence (lower traces) and in the presence (upper traces) of phenylephrine (c; incubation time 15 min) or isoprenaline (d; incubation time 1 min). Note that the positive inotropic effect of phenylephrine developed relatively slowly and that it was accompanied by a prolongation of the contraction. From ([3]; a—c), ([5]; d).

PIE, we studied the effects of phenylephrine on normal transmembrane action potentials and on calcium-dependent slow action potentials in electrically driven trabeculae isolated from the right ventricles of cow hearts. Voltage-clamp experiments with the single sucrose-gap method [9] were also performed, and all experiments were done in the presence of 1—5 µM (±)-propranolol in order to avoid interference from β-adrenoceptor stimulation.

Figure 2 shows that the positive inotropic effect of phenylephrine in the presence of propranolol was accompanied by an increase in the duration of the normal action potential. Figure 3 shows that the duration of calcium-dependent slow action potentials was also prolonged by phenylephrine and that there was a marked increase in the maximal rate of depolarisation (Fig. 3, upper panels). Mechanical and electrophysiological effects of phenylephrine followed a similar time course and were maximal after about 10 min. All effects were not altered by increasing the concentration of propranolol from 1 µM

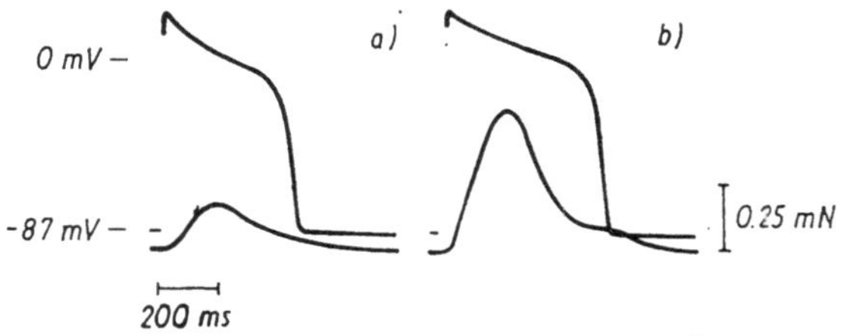

Fig. 2. Transmembrane action potentials (upper traces) and force of concentration (lower traces) in an electrically driven (0.3 Hz) cow right ventricular trabecula mounted in a single sucrose-gap chamber in bathing solution with 5.4 mM K^+ and 1.8 mM Ca^{2+} at 35 °C as described by [9]. a, control. b, 15 min after the addition of 10 μM phenylephrine in the presence of 1 μM propranolol.

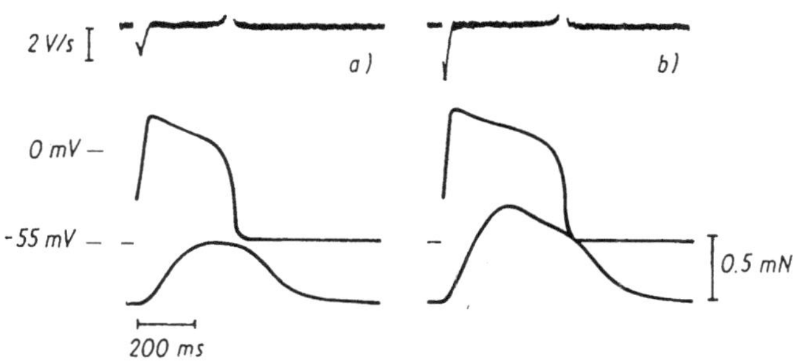

Fig. 3. Maximal rate of depolarisation (upper traces), transmembrane calcium-dependent slow action potentials (middle traces) and force of conctraction (lower traces) in an electrically driven (0.3 Hz) cow right ventricular trabecula mounted in a single sucrose-gap chamber [9]. Bathing solution with 22 mM K^+ and 1.8 mM Ca^{2+} at 35 °C. A, control. B, 15 min after the addition of 10 μM phenylephrine in the presence of 5 μM propranolol.

to 5 μM, were completely reversible on washing within 30 min and were surmountably blocked by 5 μM of the α-adrenoceptor blocking agent phentolamine.

An increase in the maximal rate of depolarisation of calcium-dependent slow action potentials may theoretically be caused by an increase in I_{si} and/or a decrease in K outward current. However, a direct determination of the effects of phenylephrine in the presence of propranolol on I_{si} with the single sucrose-gap voltage-clamp method revealed that the drug increased I_{si} without any detectable change in outward current (Fig. 4). This indicates that the phentolamine-sensitive and hence presumably α-adrenoceptor-mediated effects of phenylephrine on normal and slow action potentials, at least in bovine ventricular muscle, are mainly, if not entirely, due to an increase in I_{si}. In the light of the failure of α-adrenoceptor stimulation to increase myocardial cAMP levels, this effect appears somewhat surprising. One might have expected that a sympathomimetic agent which fails to increase cAMP also would not enhance I_{si}.

The present results are in accord with those of [7] who found that phenylephrine in the presence of the β-adrenoceptor blocking agent bufetolol induced phentolamine-sensitive slow action potentials in *rabbit* papillary muscles. Handa et al. [6] also obtained prazosin-sensitive slow action potentials with phenylephrine in the rabbit heart, although this was at least partially attributed to a suppression of a time-dependent outward current. However, our results are in contrast to those of [8] who reported that the phenylephrine-produced effects on calcium-dependent action potentials in guinea-pig papillary muscles were completely abolished by β-adrenoceptor blocking agents, and were thus apparently due to β-adrenoceptor and not to α-adrenoceptor stimulation. The discrepancies mentioned are probably due to species differences. Obviously, α-adrenoceptors are of minor importance or only poorly developed in guinea-pig ventricular tissue, as has been pointed out by [12].

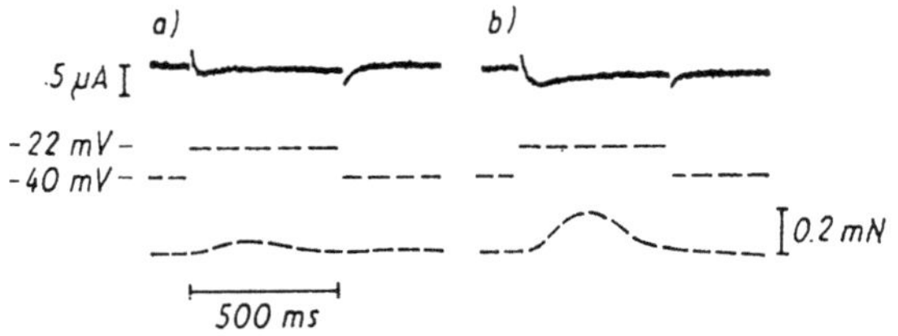

a) 1 µM Propranolol (control , 30 min)
b) 1 µM Propranolol + 10 µM Phenylephrine (10 min)

Fig. 4. Voltage-clamp steps (middle traces; depolarization from a holding potenia of —40 mV to —22 mV for 500 ms), corresponding membrane currents (upper traces) and contractions (lower traces) under control conditions (a, 1 µM propanolol) and, 10 min after addition of 10 µM phenylephrine (b). Cow right ventricular trabecula frequency of stimulation 0.3 Hz, 35 °C, 1.8 mM Ca. Single sucrose-gap voltage-clamp method [9]. Note that the positive inotropic effect of phenylephrine was accompanied by a small increase in I_{si} (downward deflection in the upper traces) whereas the current at the end of the 500 ms voltageclamp step remained unaltered.

It was mentioned above that the phentolamine sensitive electrophysiological and mechanical effects of phenylephrine in the presence of propranolol developed with a similar time course. Hence, it is quite conceivable an increase in I_{si} contributes to the positive inotropic effect of α-adrenoceptor stimulation. However, the phenylephrine-produced increase in I_{si}, as judged from the effect on the rate of depolarisation of slow action potentials, was smaller than that of an equieffective (with respect to the PIE) concentration of isoprenaline [3, 6]. This indicates that other (still unknown) mechanisms are very likely to be also involved in the positive inotropic response to α-adrenoceptor stimulation.

Acknowledgment

This work is supported by the Deutsche Forschungsgemeinschaft (grant Scho 15/8).

References

[1] BENFEY, B. G.: Can. J. Physiol. Pharmacol. **58** (1980), 1145—1157
[2] BENFEY, B. G.: Life Sci. **31** (1982), 101—112
[3] BRÜCHNER, R., I. HACKBARTH, T. MEINERTZ, B. SCHMELZLE, and H. SCHOLZ: Naunyn-Schmiedebergs Arch. Pharmacol. **303** (1978), 205—211

[4] Brückner, R. and H. Scholz: Naunyn-Schmiedeberg's Arch. Pharmacol. 311 (Suppl.) (1980), R 37
[5] Hackbarth, I., W. Schmitz, H. Scholz, E. Erdmann, W. Krawietz, and G. Philipp: Biochem. Pharmacol. **29** (1980), 1429—1432
[6] Handa, Y., J. Wagner, J. Inui, H. Averesch and H. J. Schümann: Naunyn-Schmiedeberg's Arch. Pharmacol. **318** (1982), 330—335
[7] Miura, Y., J. Inui and H. Imamura: Naunyn-Schmiedeberg's Arch. Pharmacol. **301** (1978), 201—205
[8] Ledda, F., L. Mantelli and A. Mugelli: Br. J. Pharmacol. **69** (1980), 565—571
[9] Reuter, H. and H. Scholz: J. Physiol. (Lond.) **264** (1977), 17—47
[10] Schmitz, W., H. Scholz, E. Erdmann and K. Werdan: Experientia **36** (1980), 1313—1315
[11] Scholz, H.: In: Heffter-Heubner's Handbook of Experimental Pharmacology, Adrenergic activators and inhibitors, Part I (L. Szekeres, ed.) Berlin, Heidelberg, New York; Springer, (1980), 651—733
[12] Shibata, S., D. G. Seriguchi, S. Iwadare, Y. Ishida and T. Shibata: Gen. Pharmac. **11** (1980), 173—180
[13] Tsien, R. W.: Adv. Cycl. Nucleot. Res. 8 (1977), 363—420

III. Ca^{2+} transport and protein phosphorylation

Biomembrane Section, Central Institute of Molecular Biology, Academy of Sciences of GDR, 1115 Berlin, GDR

Regulation of Intracellular Ca^{2+}-Concentration in Excitable and Nonexcitable Tissues

R. GROSSE, E. SPITZER, K. ECKERT and F. BÖHMER

Introduction

In cardiac muscle, synaptosomal and kidney preparations as well as in dialyzed squid axons two mechanisms for extrusion of Ca^{2+} from cytoplasm, a $Na^{+}—Ca^{2+}$ exchange and an ATP-driven Ca^{2+} transport, have been reported to reside in the plasma membrane [4, 28, 29, 31, 37, 38, 40]. The presence of Ca^{2+}-stimulated ATPase and Ca^{2+}-transport activity has been reported for plasma membrane preparations of several cell types [15, 16, 19, 21, 22]. To relate the (Ca^{2+}, Mg^{2+})-ATPase and Ca^{2+}-transport activities to a plasma membrane bound Ca^{2+}-pump it is necessary to differentiate the presumed enzyme from the well characterized Ca^{2+}-pump of endoplasmatic reticulum. The latter was shown to consist of a catalytic subunit with a molecular mass of 100 kD [18, 39].

Using calmodulin affinity chromatography for the first time CARONI and CARAFOLI [5] succeeded in demonstration of the phosphoprotein of heart sarcolemma (Ca^{2+}, Mg^{2+})-ATPase of 150 kD. We were not succesful in demonstrating this phosphoprotein when using native sarcolemmal vesicles [37]. However, we could demonstrate a Ca^{2+}-dependent phosphoprotein (molecular mass 135 kD) in native plasma membranes from Ehrlich ascites carcinoma cells which is unambigously different from the catalytic subunits of the (Na^{+}, K^{+})-ATPase of the plasma membrane and of the reticular (Ca^{2+}, Mg^{2+})-ATPase.

$Na^{+}—Ca^{2+}$ exchange activity has been found in cardiac plasma membrane [4, 28, 40]. However, the protein nature of the $Na^{+}—Ca^{2+}$ antiporter has not been clarified. For answering the question, we compared liposomes in which we had incorporated brain or kidney (Na^{+}, K^{+})-ATPase preparations by means of the cholate dialysis method [25] or the octylglucoside dilution technique [26], respectively. Various pieces of circumstantial evidence pointed to the eventual involvement of (Na^{+}, K^{+})-ATPase. First, both systems are found to coexist or to copurify with (Na^{+}, K^{+})-ATPase [23, 28, 32, 37]. Second, both show an absolute specificity for sodium [3, 6]. Third, (Na^{+}, K^{+})-ATPase after incorporation into liposomes appears to act as ionophore for Na^{+} [9] or K^{+} [1]. Fourth, Ca^{2+} can substitute for Na^{+} in eliciting transphosphorylation from ATP to enzymeprotein [34]. Fifth, Ca^{2+} may also substitute for Na^{+} in inducing ouabain binding conformation of phosphoenzyme formed [35]. In the present paper, we used the reconstitution technique to answer the question whether (Na^{+}, K^{+})-ATPase is a molecular machine involved in promoting Ca^{2+}-movements across the membrane of proteoliposomes.

Materials and Methods

All details concerning studies with sarcolemmal preparations are given in [37], with plasma membranes of Ehrlich ascites carcinoma cells the corresponding data are given in [38] and the reconstitution technique has been described in [8].

Results

Demonstration of plasma membrane-bound Ca-$^{2+}$pump

Figure 1 presents the results of Ca^{2+}-transport measurements using different ATP-regenerating systems.

Ca^{2+}-accumulation in vesicles was obtained with both the endogenous and the external ATP-regenerating systems, but they remarkably differed in the MgATP-concentration needed to drive Ca^{2+}-accumulation. At ATP-concentrations of 0.3 mM, the initial rates of Ca^{2+}-accumulation were higher in the presence of phosphocreatine than in the presence of pyruvate kinase and phosphoenolpyruvate. In vesicle preparations from guinea-pig heart muscle cells addition of creatine phosphokinase caused only a small further increase of Ca^{2+}-accumulation. However, in vesicle preparations from rat heart muscle cells maximal accumulation was obtained in some experiments in presence of added

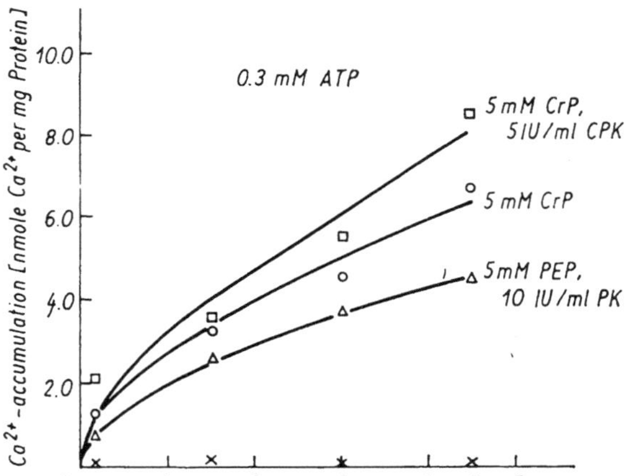

Fig. 1. MgATP- or MgATP plus phosphocreatine-effected change of intravesicular Ca^{2+}-content. The intravesicular Ca^{2+}-content present in cation equilibrium with the extravesicular space was set to be zero in this and the other Figures. It remained unchanged in the presence of Mg^{2+}, ATP, PCr or PEP when added separately. It became increased in presence of 0.3 mM MgATP plus 5 mM PCr (○), 0.3 mM MgATP, 5 mM PCr plus 5 IU per ml added creatine phosphokinase (□), or 0.3 mM MgATP, 5 mM PEP plus 10 IU per ml pyruvate kinase (△). Addition of 2 μg/ml of the Ca^{2+}-ionophore A 23187 to the incubation medium prevents the Ca^{2+}-accumulation in presence of ATP or ATP plus PCr (×). Guinea-pig heart plasma membrane vesicles were used. Initial uncomplexed calcium concentration amounted to 0.45 μM.

creatine kinase. As shown in Figure 1 the Ca^{2+}-specific ionophore A23187 completely inhibited the ATP-driven accumulation of Ca^{2+}, indicating that a Ca^{2+}-gradient was formed. The Ca^{2+}-accumulation is not inhibited by oligomycin, ruthenium red or Cl-CCP (not shown). Ca^{2+}-accumulation in sarcolemmal vesicles was not promoted by 2 mM MgCTP or 2 mM MgITP. By contrast, the Ca^{2+}-uptake into the sarcoplasmic reticulum is stimulated by MgCTP and MgITP [11]. The dependence of ATP-driven Ca^{2+}-transport on Ca^{2+} concentration yielded an apparent K_m-value of 0.2 μM (not shown). The concentrations of ATP required for half-maximal Ca^{2+}-uptake were found to be dependent on the nature of the ATP-regenerating system, being 7 μM with the endogenous and 170 μM with the external ATP-regenerating system (not shown). The remarkable reduction of the ATP-concentration required for half-maximal Ca^{2+}-accumulation can be explained by spatial clustering of the endogenous ATP-regenerating system and the transport enzyme [10].

We have shown that the normalized Ca^{2+}-accumulation rates strongly correlated with the specific (Na^+, K^+)-ATPase activities of the different preparations used [37]. Further evidence for localization of the Ca^{2+}-pump in the plasma membrane has been provided by our finding that, in accordance with the presence of a Na^+—Ca^{2+} exchange system in cardiac sarcolemma [3, 6, 32], externally added Na^+ was found to release about 45% of the intravesicularly trapped Ca^{2+}. Li^- in the same concentration caused a release of only 7% (not shown).

As demonstrated in Figure 2 phosphorylation of proteins in intact sarcolemmal preparations with [^{32}P]-ATP was stimulated by Ca^{2+}. Polyacrylamide gel electrophoresis revealed only one radioactive peak which corresponded to a phosphoprotein with a molecular weight of 100000. When analyzed in parallel tracks of polyacrylamide gels this phosphoprotein could not be separated from the phosphorylated intermediate of (Na^+, K^+)-ATPase and from the phosphoprotein of sarcoplasmic reticulum showing like-

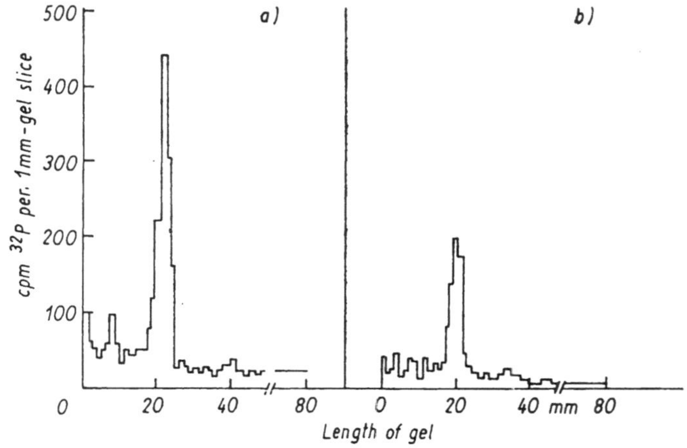

Fig. 2. Electrophoretic demonstration of the Ca^{2+}-dependent phosphoprotein formation. Panel a shows the distribution of radioactivity in the gel after phosphorylation of the sarcolemmal vesicle preparation (1 mg/ml) in the presence of 0.6 μM γ-[^{32}P]-ATP, 0.45 μM Ca^{2+}, 10 mM Mg-acetate, 10 mM K-acetate and 10 μM Cl-CCP. The results shown in Panel b were obtained by omitting Ca^{2+} in the incubation medium and adding EGTA (final concentration 5 mM).

wise a molecular weight of 100000 [11]. To avoid contaminations of sarcoplasmic reticulum in the vesicular preparation we isolated plasma membranes from Ehrlich ascites tumour cells known to consist of much less reticular membranes. As described in a previous paper [38] these membranes are entirely free of mitochondrial and reticular membranes, show high (Na^+, K^+)-ATPase activity and accumulate Ca^{2+} in presence of ATP.

Plasma membranes were phosphorylated with [γ^{32}P]-ATP at 0 °C and undergone an SDS-electrophoresis under acidic conditions.

A typical result of electrophoretic separation (the same principal patterns were obtained with 5 independent membrane preparations) is shown in Figure 3b—d as an autoradiograph. The corresponding plasma membrane proteins have been visualized by

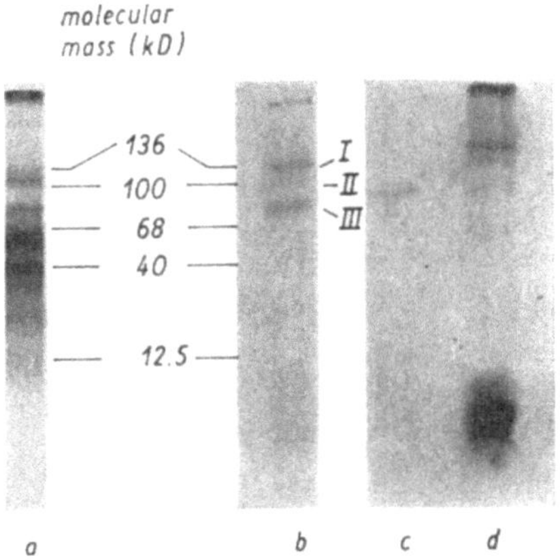

Fig. 3. Autoradiographic demonstration of the Ca^{2+}-dependent phosphoproteins in plasma membrane of Ehrlich ascites carcinoma cells. Plasma membrane proteins were separated on SDS-polyacrylamide gels and visualized by autoradiography after phosphorylation (lane b—d, about 90 µg protein were applied per lane) or staining with Coomassie blue (lane a, about 40 µg protein were applied to the gel). Phosphorylation was performed with 2 µM [γ^{32}P]-ATP in the presence of 160 mM KCl, 12.5 µM $MgCl_2$ and 20 µM Ca^{2+} (lane b) or 160 mM KCl, 12.5 µM $MgCl_2$ and 500 µM EGTA (lane c) or 160 mM KCl, 5 mM $MgCl_2$ and 20 µM Ca^{2+} (lane d).

staining with Coomassie blue (Fig. 3, lane a). In the presence of Ca^{2+} and micromolar Mg^{2+} (Fig. 3, lane b) three distinct bands are visualized migrating with molecular masses of 135 kD (I), 100 kD (II) and about 90 kD (III).

Bands I and II disappear completely upon addition of EGTA into the phosphorylation medium (Fig. 3, lane c). Both bands are sensitive to hydroxylamine.

Band III was independent on the presence of EGTA in the phosphorylation medium and insensitive to hydroxylamine treatment. Therefore the identity of this band was not further investigated.

Phosphorylation in the presence of millimolar Mg^{2+} revealed the same pattern of phosphoproteins in the high molecular mass range as found with the low Mg^{2+}-concentration (Fig. 3, lane d). A number of additional phosphoproteins became detectable presumably because of the activation of protein kinases by Mg^{2+} as described for instance for erythrocyte membranes [30]. A further increase of protein kinase dependent background phosphorylation made a clear demonstration of the EGTA effect on the 135 kD band in the presence of millimolar Mg^{2+} difficult. The acyl-phosphate character of phosphorylation of the 100 kD and the 135 kD band was proven under these conditions as well (not shown).

The presence of millimolar Mg^{2+} permitted the clear identification of the 100 kD protein as the catalytic subunit of the (Na^+, K^+)-ATPase. As shown in Figure 4 in the presence of Na^+, the ^{32}P-incorporation into the 100 kD-peak is remarkably increased (Figs. 4a and b).

The stimulation of the Mg^{2+}-dependent phosphorylation by sodium [24] is demonstrated with a highly purified preparation of (Na^+, K^+)-ATPase from pig kidney in Figure 4c and d.

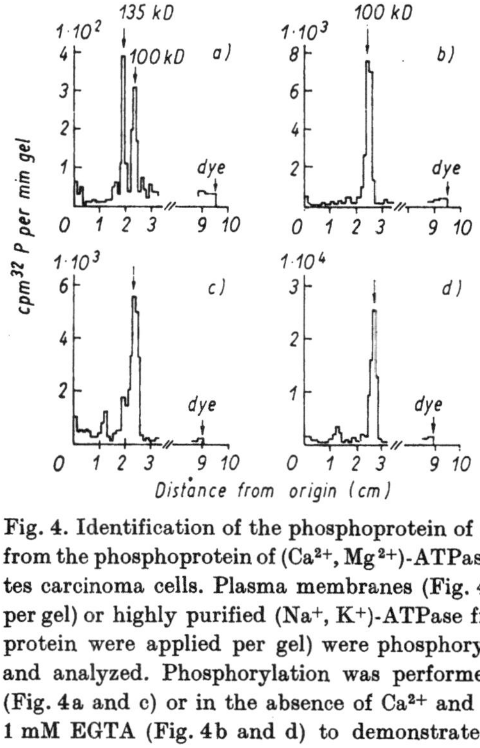

Fig. 4. Identification of the phosphoprotein of (Na^+, K^+)-ATPase and differentiation from the phosphoprotein of (Ca^{2+}, Mg^{2+})-ATPase in plasma membranes of Ehrlich ascites carcinoma cells. Plasma membranes (Fig. 4a and b, 60 μg protein were applied per gel) or highly purified (Na^+, K^+)-ATPase from pig kidney (Fig. 4c and d, 40 μg protein were applied per gel) were phosphorylated in the presence of 5 mM $MgCl_2$ and analyzed. Phosphorylation was performed either in presence of 20 μM Ca^{2+} (Fig. 4a and c) or in the absence of Ca^{2+} and in the presence of 140 mM NaCl and 1 mM EGTA (Fig. 4b and d) to demonstrate the effects of Ca^{2+} and Na^+ on ^{32}P-incorporation into the different proteins.

Demonstration of plasma membrane-bound Na^+—Ca^{2+} antiporter

The freeze fracture electron micrographs of the proteoliposomes characterized in detail in a previous paper [8] showed a uniform population of fractured membrane faces which appeared either concave or convex. The diameters of most vesicles lay in the range of 100—130 nm. The presence of ATP in the extravesicular space accelerated Na^+-transport into the intravesicular space of both PC and dioleoyl phosphatidylcholine (DOPC) proteoliposomes (not shown). Ouabain known as specific inhibitor of (Na^+, K^+)-ATPase suppressed the Na^+-transport into PC proteoliposomes only when intravesicularly applied. The Ca^{2+}-influx into the proteoliposomes occurred slowly when high NaCl, LiCl or KCl concentrations were present on both sides of the membrane (Figs. 5 and 6), and was not changed when a K^+- or Li^+-concentration gradient was present (Fig. 6). Contrary to the K^+- and Li^+-gradient, the Na^+-gradient strongly enhanced the Ca^{2+}-influx (Fig. 5). The Na^+ gradient-driven Ca^{2+}-accumulation ceased essentially within 15 min apparently due to the exhaustion of the Na^+-gradient (inset to Fig. 5). In the presence of the Ca^{2+} ionophore A 23187, all Ca^{2+} was removed from the proteoliposomes during their separation from the incubation medium (Fig. 5). This suggests that Ca^{2+} binding to the vesicle constituents was not involved in the Ca^{2+}-uptake data.

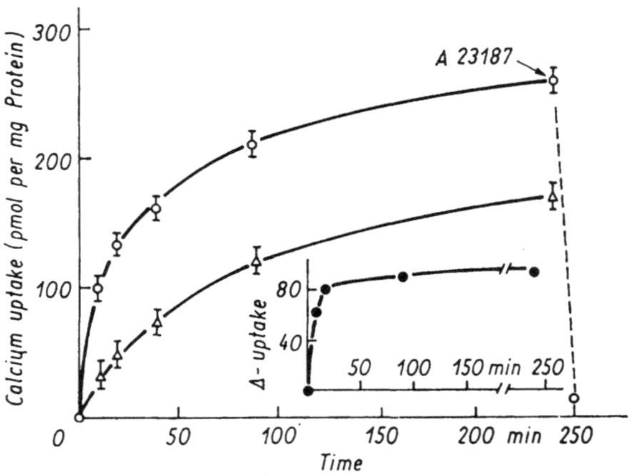

Fig. 5. Ca^{2+} influx at 28 °C into proteoliposomes from brain (Na^+, K^+)-ATPase preparation and DOPC in presence (○ — ○) or absence (△ — △) of a Na^+-concentration gradient over the liposome membrane directed from the intra- to the extravesicular space. The proteoliposomes were loaded with 160 mM NaCl during the vesiculation procedure. Aliquots of the proteoliposome suspension were added to buffer solutions containing besides 25 μM $^{45}CaCl_2$ either 160 mM LiCl (Na^+-gradient) or 160 mM NaCl (no Na^+-gradient). — INSET. Na^+-gradient dependent Ca^{2+}-accumulation in the vesicles.

In presence of extravesicular Ca^{2+}-concentration far below the $K_{0.5}$ (Ca^{2+}) value lying near 40 μM [3] the Na^+-efflux along its concentration gradient occurred slowly. At Ca^{2+}-concentration surpassing the $K_{0.5}$ (Ca^{2+}) value the Na^+-efflux became increased (Fig. 7). The Ca^{2+}-dependent fraction of Na^+-efflux ceased essentially within 15 min apparently due to the dissipation of the gradient (inset to Fig. 7). A similar time parameter was found for the Na^+-gradient dependent Ca^{2+}-uptake (inset to Fig. 5). The observations lead to the conclusion that a Na^+—Ca^{2+} antiporter sensitive to sodium and calcium ions has been incorporated into the liposomes. 0.2 μM tetrodotoxin, intravesicularly trapped during vesiculation did not inhibit Na^+-efflux (not shown). The following experiments have been carried out to prove the question whether the (Na^+, K^+)-ATPase can operate as Na^+—Ca^{2+} antiporter. To this end we measured in parallel the ATP promoted Na^+-transport and the Na^+-gradient dependent Ca^{2+}-uptake with liposomes containing (Na^+, K^+)-ATPase preparations of different specific activities. As expected the proteoliposomes from kidney (Na^+, K^+)-ATPase preparation with high specific activity

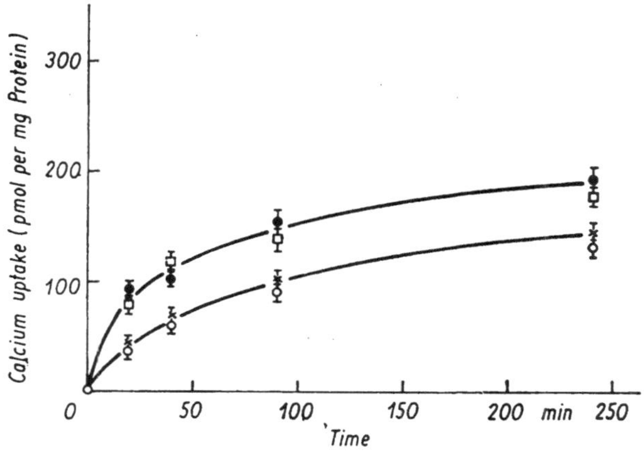

Fig. 6. Ca^{2+}-influx at 28 °C into proteoliposomes from brain (Na^+, K^+)-ATPase preparation and DOPC in presence [□ — □) or absence (• — •) of a K^+ concentration gradient, and in presence (○ — ○) or absence (× — ×) of a Li^+-concentration gradient. The proteoliposomes were loaded with 160 mM KCl or LiCl during the vesiculation procedure. Aliquots of the proteoliposome suspension were added to buffer solutions containing besides 25 μM $^{45}CaCl_2$ either 160 mM NaCl or 160 mM KCl, and 160 mM NaCl (Li^+-gradient) or 160 mM LiCl (no Li^+-gradient), respectively.

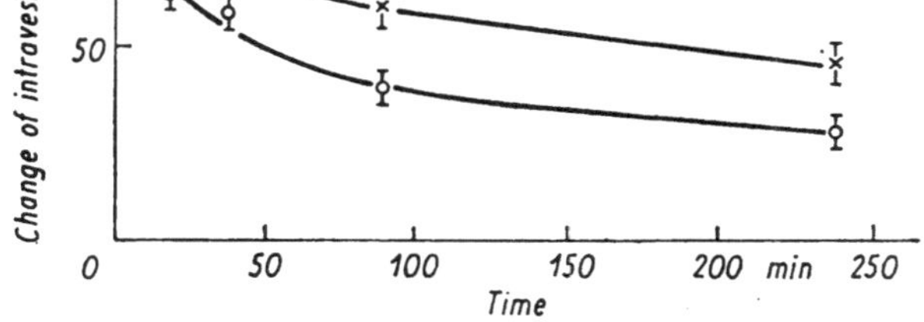

Fig. 7. Na^+-efflux at 28 °C from proteoliposomes, formed from brain (Na^+, K^+)-ATPase preparation and DOPC, in absence (× — ×) or presence (○ — ○) of a Ca^{2+}-gradient. The proteoliposomes were loaded with 160 mM NaCl containing 0.3 mCi/l $^{22}NaCl$ and 0.9 mM EGTA during the vesiculation procedure. Aliquots of the proteoliposome suspension were tenfold diluted with buffer solutions containing 160 mM LiCl, 1.0 mM $CaCl_2$ and EGTA concentrations to get 0.23 μM Ca^{2+} or 160 μM Ca^{2+} (steep Ca^{2+}-gradient). The Ca^{2+} concentrations were calculated from $K_{(Ca.EGTA)} = 0.15$ μM [38]. — INSET. Ca^{2+}-dependent fraction of Na^+-efflux from the vesicles.

(300 μMol P_i mg^{-1} h^{-1}) accumulated in presence of ATP by about one order of magnitude more Na^+ than the less active (42 μMol P_i mg^{-1} h^{-1}) liposomes containing (Na^+, K^+)-ATPase from brain (Fig. 8).

In contrast to this finding the proteoliposomes from kidney did not accumulate significant higher amounts of Ca^{2+} in presence of an outwardly directed Na^+-gradient (Fig. 9). The passive cation permeabilities were similar in all preparations. The liposomes containing higly purified kidney (Na^+, K^+)-ATPase did not catalyze a Na^+-efflux sensitive to extravesicular Ca^{2+}-ions (not shown).

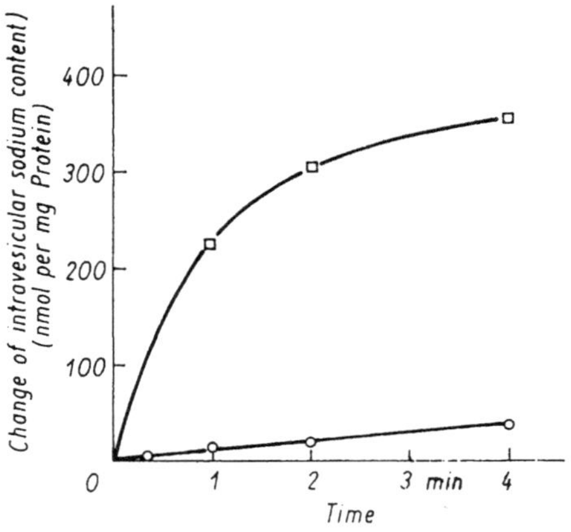

Fig. 8. ATP-promoted Na^+-transport into proteoliposomes from kidney (Na^+, K^+)-ATPase (□ — □) or into proteoliposomes from brain (Na^+, K^+)-ATPase preparations (○ — ●).

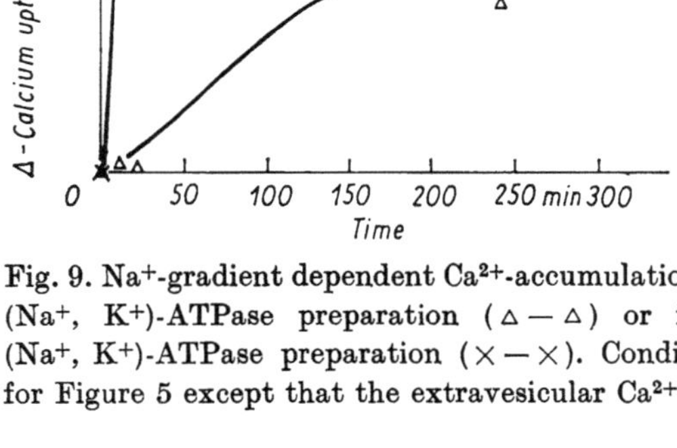

Fig. 9. Na^+-gradient dependent Ca^{2+}-accumulation into proteoliposomes from kidney (Na^+, K^+)-ATPase preparation (△ — △) or into proteoliposomes from brain (Na^+, K^+)-ATPase preparation (× — ×). Conditions were the same as described for Figure 5 except that the extravesicular Ca^{2+}-concentration amounted to 55 μM.

Discussion

Plasma membrane-bound Ca^{2+}-pump

In the present paper we could demonstrate Ca^{2+}-dependent ATP-splitting, ATP-dependent Ca^{2+}-transport and the Ca^{2+}-dependent hydroxylamine-sensitive phosphorylation of a 135 kD protein in highly purified plasma membranes from Ehrlich ascites carcinoma cells. For the following reasons we would like to suggest that the three phenomena are attributed to the plasma membrane bound Ca^{2+}-transporting ATPase. Firstly, the molecular mass of the Ca^{2+}-dependent phosphorylated intermediate is clearly different from the known molecular mass of the very well investigated catalytic subunit of (Ca^{2+}, Mg^{2+})-ATPase of endoplasmic reticulum with a molecular mass of 100 kD [18, 39]. Secondly, the formation of a phosphorylated intermediate in dependence on the transported ion has been shown to be characteristic for all cation transporting ATPases [14, 18, 24].

Finally, the characteristics of the enzyme described in the present paper are remarkably similar to those of the (Ca^{2+}, Mg^{2+})-ATPase of human erythrocyte membranes. The K_m-values for ATP and Ca^{2+} were equal to 44 ± 9 μM or 0.25 ± 0.10 μM, respectively. The corresponding values for the (Ca^{2+}, Mg^{2+})-ATPase of erythrocyte were found to be in the range of 25—60 μM [17, 42] and 0.3—0.6 μM [20, 42]. The molecular mass of the (Ca^{2+}, Mg^{2+})-ATPase of erythrocyte was estimated in the range of 140—150 kD [20] while we have determined about 135 kD for the Ca^{2+}-pump of Ehrlich ascites carcinoma cells.

Hinnen et al. [12] have analyzed the Ca^{2+}-fluxes in Ehrlich ascites tumour cells.

Treating the plasma membranes of these cells with phospholipids by the freeze-thaw sonication technique they obtained vesicles which exhibited an ATP-dependent Ca^{2+}-accumulation. The identity of the (Ca^{2+}, Mg^{2+})-ATPase was not further investigated.

Several authors dealt with attempts to identify phosphorylated intermediates of a putative plasma membrane bound (Ca^{2+}, Mg^{2+})-ATPase:

DeJonge et al. [7] and Schneider et al. [33] have published results of phosphorylation experiments with plasma membrane preparations from rat duodenal epithelium and macrophages, respectively. With macrophage plasma membranes [33] the authors suggested Ca^{2+}-dependent phosphorylation of a 132 kD protein. In the case of membranes from rat duodenal epithelium [7] a Ca^{2+}-dependent phosphoprotein is demonstrated as a poorly resolved shoulder of 115 kD of a major Ca^{2+}-insensitive peak of 84 kD. In native sarcolemmal membranes, which are presumably any time slightly contaminated by sarcoplasmic reticulum, we [37] and others [17] however, could not exclude that Ca^{2+}-dependent phosphorylation is due to the Ca^{2+}-pump of sarcoplasmic reticulum.

Evidence for a Ca^{2+}-dependent phosphoprotein in sarcolemmal membranes with a molecular mass (150 kD) which is clearly different from that of the sarcoplasmic Ca^{2+}-pump has been presented hitherto only by Caroni and Carafoli [5].

Plasma membrane-bound Na^{+}—Ca^{2+} antiporter

The analysis of a Na^{+}—Ca^{2+} exchange mechanism in cells of excitable tissues have been attempted hitherto by the use of purified membrane fractions from heart muscle [2, 4, 28, 23] or brain synaptosomes [27, 32]. The results suggest that vesicular membranes derived from heart muscle or from synaptosomes contain both reversible Na^+—Ca^{2+}-exchange and ATP-dependent Ca^{2+}-uptake processes.

No serious attempts are known to identify the supposed carrier which presumably is an integral plasma membrane protein. Using sarcolemmal vesicles this seems to be extremely difficult as even the best characterized preparations consist of at least 20 proteins of different molecular weights [17].

For demonstration of a Na^+—Ca^{2+}-exchange activity in (Na^+, K^+)-ATPase preparations from brain we prepared proteoliposomes. The cholate-dialysis reconstitution procedure described by GOLDIN [27] has been improved in this work. The majority of Mg^{2+}-ATPase activity could be removed during the incorporation procedure consisting finally of no more than 5% of the (Na^+, K^+)-ATPase activity [8]. The following pieces of evidence support our conclusion, that a Na^+—Ca^{2+} antiporter of brain plasma membranes has been incorporated into proteoliposomes. First, a Na^+-concentration gradient was required to accelerate Ca^{2+}-movement across vesicle membrane. The gradient-promoted Ca^{2+}-transport was specific for Na^+; K^+- or Li^+-gradients were ineffective. Second, the antiporter was specific for Ca^{2+}; a high Mg^{2+} excess did not inhibit Ca^{2+}-antiport.

Third, the Na^+-efflux depends on the Ca^{2+}-concentration at the other side of the membrane as it was shown by BLAUSTEIN and RUSSEL [3] for Na^+—Ca^{2+}-exchange in squid giant axons. Fourth, the Na^+-efflux was not inhibited by tetrodotoxin known as inhibitor of Na^+ conductance channels. However, the demonstrated Na^+—Ca^{2+} antiporter activity could not be related to (Na^+, K^+)-ATPase protein, since it was absent from proteoliposomes with incorporated kidney (Na^+, K^+)-ATPase devoid of contaminating proteins. The exclusion of (Na^+, K^+)-ATPase involvement in Na^+ gradient-promoted Ca^{2+}-antiport or in ATP-driven Ca^{2+}-transport coincides with the demonstration that proteoliposomes with incorporated kidney (Na^+, K^+)-ATPase showed neither Ca^{2+}-activated K^+-transport nor bumetanide-inhibited Na^+, K^+ cotransport [13]. Besides kidney plasma membrane we have looked for a Na^+—Ca^{2+} antiporter in plasma membrane of Ehrlich ascites tumour cells (K. ECKERT, unpublished results) and of hepatocytes (R. GROSSE, K. KOCH and H. LEFFERT, in preparation). Both cell types do not possess Na^+—Ca^{2+} exchange activity in the plasma membrane. Therefore, in these cells the only driving force for Ca^{2+} extrusion across the plasma membrane seems to be the ATP-dependent Ca^{2+}-pump. One could speculate that the need for a Na^+—Ca^{2+} antiporter is related to the cell function. Because of the relative small changes of free intracellular Ca^{2+}-concentrations in cells of non excitable tissues a Ca^{2+}-pump alone is sufficient for uphill Ca^{2+}-transport.

Acknowledgments

We are indebted to Dr. H. MEYER for performance of the electron-microscopic investigations, to Mrs. R. FRANKE for expert technical assistance, to Dr. R. LACHMANN for delivery of the phospholipids.

References

[1] ANNER, M. B.: Biochem. Intern. 2 (1981), 365—371

[2] BERS, D. M., K. D. PHILIPSON, and A. Y. NISHIMOTO: Biochim. Biophys. Acta 601 (1980), 358—371

[3] Blaustein, M. P. and J. M. Russel: J. Membrane Biol. **22** (1975), 285—312
[4] Caroni, P. and E. Carafoli: Nature **283** (1980), 765—767
[5] Caroni, P. and E. Carafoli: J. Biol. Chem. **256** (1981), 3263—3270
[6] Dahl, J. L. and E. L. Hokin: Ann. Rev. Biochem. **43** (1974), 327—356
[7] DeJonge, H. R., W. E. J. M. Ghijsen, and C. H. Vanos: Biochim. Biophys. Acta **647** (1981), 140—149
[8] Eckert, K. and R. Grosse: Biochim. Biophys. Acta **692** (1982), 69—80
[9] Goldin, S. M. and S. W. Tong: J. Biol. Chem. **249** (1974), 5907—5915
[10] Grosse, R., E. Spitzer, V. Kuprianov, V. Saks, and K. R. H. Repke: Biochim. Biophys. Acta **603** (1980), 142—156
[11] Hasselbach, W.: Biochim. Biophys. Acta **515** (1978), 23—53
[12] Hinnen, R., H. Miyamoto, and E. Racker: J. Membrane Biol. **49** (1979), 309—327
[13] Karlish, S. J. D., J. C. Ellory, and V. L. Lew: Biochim. Biophys. Acta **646** (1981), 353—355
[14] Knauf, P. A., F. Proverbio, and I. F. Hoffman: J. Gen. Physiol. **43** (1974), 324—336
[15] Lichtman, A. H., G. B. Segel, and M. A. Lichtman: J. Biol. Chem. **256** (1981), 6148—6154
[16] Lotersztajn, S., J. Hanounce, and F. Pecker: J. Biol. Chem. **256** (1981), 11209—11215
[17] Louis, St. P. J. and P. V. Sulakhe: Biochemistry **17** (1978), 4540—4550
[18] Martonosi, A. and R. A. Halpin: Arch. Biochem. Biophys **144** (1971), 66—77
[19] Morcos, N. C.: Biochim. Biophys. Acta **643** (1981), 55—62
[20] Niggli, V., E. S. Adunyah, J. T. Penniston, and E. Carafoli: J. Biol. Chem. **256** (1981), 395—401
[21] Niggli, V., J. I. Penniston and, E. Carafoli: J. Biol. Chem. **254** (1979), 9955—9958
[22] Pershadsingh, H. A. and J. M. McDonald: J. Biol. Chem. **255** (1980), 4087—4093
[23] Pitts, B. J. R.: J. Biol. Chem. **254** (1979), 6232—6235
[24] Post, R. L. and S. Kume: J. Biol. Chem. **248** (1973), 6993—7000
[25] Racker, E.: J. Biol. Chem. **247** (1972), 8198—8200
[26] Racker, E., B. Violand, S. O'Neal, M. Alfonso, and J. Telford: Arch. Biochem. Biophys. **198** (1979), 470—477
[27] Rahamimoff, H. and R. Spanier: FEBS-Lett. **104** (1979), 111—114
[28] Reeves, J. P. and J. L. Sutko: Proc. Natl. Acad. Sci. U.S.A. **76** (1979), 590—594
[29] Requena, J., R. Dipolo, F. Brinley, and L. J. Mullins: J. Gen. Physiol. **70** (1977), 329—353
[30] Sarkadi, B.: Biochim. Biophys. Acta **604** (1980), 159—190
[31] Schatzmann, H. J.: Experientia **22** (1966), 364—368
[32] Schellenberg, G. D. and P. D. Swanson: Biochim. Biophys. Acta **648** (1981), 13—27
[33] Schneider, C., C. Mottola, and D. Romeo: J. Supramol. Struct. **10** (1979), 433—441
[34] Schön, R., W. Schönfeld, K. H. Menke, and K. R. H. Repke: Acta Biol. Med. Germ. **29** (1972), 643—659
[35] Schönfeld, W. R., Schön, K. H. Menke, and K. R. H. Repke: Acta Biol. Med Germ. **28** (1972), 935—956
[36] Skriver, E., A. B. Maunsbach, and P. L. Jørgensen: J. Cell. Biol. **86** (1980), 746—754
[37] Spitzer, E., R. Grosse, V. Kupriyanov, and A. Preobrazhensky: Acta Biol. Med. Germ. **40** (1981), 1111—1121
[38] Spitzer, E. F. D. Böhmer, and R. Grosse: Biochim. Biophys. Acta. 728 (1983), 50—58
[39] Tada M., T. Yamamoto, and Y. Tonomura: Physiol. Rev. **58** (1978), 1—79
[40] Trumble, W. R., I. Sutko, and J. P. Reeves: Life Sci. **27** (1980), 207—215
[41] Vogel, F., H. W. Meyer, R. Grosse, and K. R. H. Repke: Biochim. Biophys. Acta **470** (1977), 497—501
[42] Waisman, D. M., J. M. Gimble, D. B. P. Goddman, and H. Rasmussen: J. Biol. Chem. **256** (1981), 409—414

Laboratory of Biochemistry, Swiss Federal Institute of Technology (ETH), 8092 Zürich, Switzerland

The Regulation of the Ca^{2+} Transporting Systems of Heart Plasma Membrane

E. Carafoli

The penetration of Ca^{2+} into heart cells occurs through a specific channel, which is sensitive to the level of polarization of the plasma membrane. The Ca^{2+} that has entered into the cell must eventually be ejected again to avoid intracellular Ca^{2+} overload. Ejection has been shown to occur through 2 systems, a specific ATPase, and a Na^+—Ca^{2+} exchanger. The existence of the first system has been documented conclusively only recently (Caroni and Carafoli [7]) the second system has been demonstrated more than 10 years ago (Reuter and Seitz [30]). The 2 transport systems are under the control of complex regulatory processes, which will be discussed in this article. A synthetic survey of the most important properties of the 2 systems will also be presented.

The Ca^{2+}-pumping ATPase

In 1966, Schatzmann [32] demonstrated that erythrocytes extrude Ca^{2+} through a specific ATPase. Subsequent studies, carried out essentially in erythrocytes, characterized the enzyme in the membrane (see Schatzmann [33], for a recent review), and established it as the system responsible for the ejection of Ca^{2+} from non-excitable cells. Later work, summarized in a recent review by Penniston [24] showed that Ca^{2+}-pumping ATPases are present in most, and probably all, plasma membranes. Of particular interest are the findings by Di Polo and Beaugé [15] and Caroni and Carafoli [9] that a Ca^{2+}-specific ATPase, having characteristics very similar to those of the erythrocyte enzyme, is present in excitable plasma membranes (the giant axon of the squid and the sarcolemma of heart). These findings on neurons and heart plasma membranes have been instrumental in disposing of the generally accepted view that the only Ca^{2+} ejecting system of excitable plasma membranes is the Na^+/Ca^{2+} exchanger.

Table 1 summarizes the most important properties of the Ca^{2+}-pumping ATPase in situ. The enzyme is a high-affinity, low-capacity system, ideally qualified for ejecting Ca^{2+} from cells in which the level of free Ca^{2+} in the cytosol is not expected to undergo substantial variations above the normal μM or sub-μM level In excitable cells, where periodic increases of free Ca^{2+} above the resting level are normally occurring, the ATPase is probably the enzyme responsible for the Ca^{2+} homeostasis at rest, when the low levels of Ca^{2+} in the cytosol would be sufficient to activate the high affinity ATPase, but presumably not the other Ca^{2+}-ejecting system, the Na^+/Ca^{2+} exchanger (see below).

Interestingly, for the case of erythrocytes it has been calculated that the ATPase is in large excess with respect to the Ca^{2+}-pumping requirements dictated by the pene-

Table 1

The Ca^{2+}-pumping ATPase of plasma membranes

Ca^{2+} affinity (K_m)	$< 0.5\ \mu M$
V_{max} (nmol Ca^{2+} × mg^{-1} prot. × sec^{-1})	0.5–1.0 nmol × mg^{-1} prot. × sec^{-1}
Ca^{2+}/ATP stoichiometry	1–2*
Inhibition	vanadate ($K_{1/2} < 1\ \mu M$)
Calmodulin sensitivity	present**
Enzyme cycle	$E_1 - E_2$, acyl phosphate
Concentration	~ 0.1% of total membrane protein
Acidic phospholipids	activate
Controlled proteolysis	activates

* opinions on this point diverge (see SCHATZMANN [33] for a discussion).
** there maybe exceptions (see PENNISTON [2, 4], for a discussion)

tration of Ca^{2+} into the cell through the specific channel (LEW and FERREIRA [18], VARECKA and CARAFOLI [35]). It is possible, however, that the permeability of the erythrocyte membrane to Ca^{2+}, which is normally very low, increases substantially when the cells are forced to pass through narrow capillaries. As a result, the cytoplasm of the cells would become inundated with Ca^{2+} and the large excess of Ca^{2+}-pumping ATPase would at this point be particularly convenient to rapidly return the situation to normal.

Of interest among the properties listed in Table 1 is the sensitivity of the ATPase to calmodulin. Although exceptions may exist (for example liver, see legend for Table 1) this can be considered as a distinctive property of the plasma membrane Ca^{2+} ATPase. The stimulation by calmodulin was first observed by GOPINATH and VINCENZI and JARRETT and PENNISTON [16, 17] and was later shown by NIGGLI et al [23] and LYNCH and CHEUNG [19] to be due to the direct interaction of the activator with the ATPase. The last finding has provided the rationale for the successful attempt (NIGGLI et al. [22]) to purify the ATPase on calmodulin affinity chromatography columns. The large body of data now collected on the purified enzyme, has been summarized in a recent review (CARAFOLI and ZURINI [6]) and will be briefly discussed here.

As Table 2 shows, the purified ATPase is a polypeptide of M_r 138,000, which repeats

Table 2

The isolated Ca^{2+}-pumping ATPase of plasma membranes

M_r	138,000
Ca^{2+}-affinity (K_m)	$< 0.5\ \mu M$
V_{max} (nmol × mg^{-1} prot × sec^{-1})	up to 500
Ca^{2+}/ATP stoichiometry (liposomes)	1
Inhibition	vanadate ($K_{1/2} < 1\ \mu M$)
Calmodulin sensitivity	present*
Enzyme cycle	forms acyl-phosphate
Acidic phospholipids	activate
Controlled proteolysis	activates

* There may be exceptions (see CARAFOLI and ZURINI [6] for a discussion)

the functional properties of the enzyme in situ. It forms an acyl-phosphate during the reaction cycle, it is inhibited by vanadate, and has high affinity for Ca^{2+}. Its V_{max} of Ca^{2+} transport in reconstituted systems may be as high as 500 nmoles per mg per sec, and its Ca^{2+}/ATP stoichiometry, which studies on the enzyme in situ have left undecided between 1 and 2, seems to be consistently 1 (CLARK and CARAFOLI [13]). The stimulation of the enzyme by fatty acids and acidic phospholipids (see Table 1) is alternative to that produced by calmodulin, and is essentially expressed by the transition of the enzyme to a higher Ca^{2+} affinity. The mechanism of the activation by calmodulin, fatty acids-phospholipids, and controlled proteolysis is obscure, but it has been suggested that the 3 treatments lead to increased substrate (Ca^{2+} and/or ATP) accessibility of the active site (CARAFOLI and ZURINI [6]). Of interest is the fact that a number of so-called antical-modulin drugs remove the stimulation of the enzyme by calmodulin **and** by the alternative activating treatments mentioned (ADUNYAH et al. [1]). This shows unequivocally that these drugs (e.g., phenothiazines) interact directly with the ATPase molecule, and not only with calmodulin.

The interest of the activating effects of acidic phospholipids resides in the fact that they are present in plasma membranes, and are concentrated in the inner layer of the bilayer leaflet, where the active site of the Ca^{2+} ATPase is presumably located. Assuming homogeneous distribution in the horizontal plane of the membrane, acidic phospholipids are present in sufficient amounts to produce about 50% activation of the Ca^{2+} ATPase [21]). It is thus possible to think of them as physiological modulators of the enzyme. Changes in the phospholipids composition in the ambient surrounding the Ca^{2-} ATPase, e.g., by lateral diffusion, would determine its modulation. Of potential interest is also the activation of the Ca^{2+} transporting ATPase by di- and triphosphoinositides [5, 20] metabolites that are known to be produced in plasma membranes. Of no physiological interest, by contrast, is probably the activation of the enzyme by limited proteolysis. As a tool, however, it has now become important for the molecular study of the purified ATPase. Recent studies on the purified erythrocyte enzyme with trypsin as a proteolytic agent (see CARAFOLI and ZURINI [6], for a review of the topic) have now permitted the mapping of some regions of functional interest in the ATPase molecule. The acyl-phosphate is formed on a polypeptide of M_r 76,000—81.000, whereas the minimal size for the calmodulin receptor seems to be a fragment of M_r 8,000. It has also been possible to show that the trypsin attack produces a polypeptide of M_r about 33,000 which is particularly hydrophobic, and might thus contain (most of) the membrane-spanning regions of the molecule.

The Ca^{2+} pumping ATPase of erythrocytes seems thus to be regulated by calmoduliu and by the composition of the lipid ambient surrounding it. One additional regulatory mechanism which is apparently not present in erythrocytes has recently been documented in heart sarcolemma. The Ca^{2+}-pumping ATPase of the latter plasma membrane is modulated by a phosphorylation-dephosphorylation cycle [10]. The demonstration of the phenomenon required the previous dephosphorylation of the sarcolemmal membranes by an exogenous protein phosphatase: only after this treatment could the activating effect of ATP be demonstrated. The latter depends on a cAMP-dependent, membrane-bound protein kinase, since it is inhibited by a protein-kinase inhibitor, cAMP-dependent. However, Ca^{2+} also plays a role, since the activation of the Ca^{2+} pumping by ATP is decreased in the presence of Ca^{2+} chelators. The target of the membrane-bound activating kinase is not the ATPase enzyme, but must evidently be some other accessory protein of the sarcolemmal membrane. This is a neccessary conclusion, since the purified Ca^{2+} pumping ATPase of sarcolemma is not influenced by the phosphorylation/dephosphorylation cycle described.

The Na^+/Ca^{2+} exchanger

Recent reviews on the Na^+/Ca^{2+} exchange have appeared (BAKER [2], REUTER [31], BLAUSTEIN and NELSON [4]), and the reader is referred to them for detailed information. A concise survey of the most important properties of the system will be presented here, followed by a somewhat more detailed discussion of some recent developments pertaining to its regulation.

The system, originally described in excitable plasma membranes, has now been recognized also in a number of non-excitable cells (see BLAUSTEIN and NELSON [4], for a review). It normally operates in the direction of Ca^{2+} efflux, but it is very likely that under given in vivo conditions it may become reversed, and mediate the influx of Ca^{2+} into cells. Under *in vitro* conditions, the system is indeed perfectly reversible, and mediates both the influx and efflux of Ca^{2+}, and Na^+, in preparations like the giant axon of the squid or the vesicles of heart sarcolemma.

One important point, in connection with the suggestion that the Na^+/Ca^{2+} exchanger is the system responsible for the bulk of Ca^{2+} ejection from cells, is whether the energy content of the inwardly directed Na^+ gradient is adequate. A neutral exchange ($2Na^+$ per $1Ca^{2+}$) would not be sufficient for the maintenance of the very low Ca^{2+} concentration normally found inside cells, but an electrogenic exchange (e.g., $3Na^+$ per $1Ca^{2+}$), in which an electrical term is added to the total Ca^{2+}-pulling force, would be. Clear-cut evidence for the electrogenicity of the exchanger has now been provided by several lines of investigation on isolated sarcolemmal vesicles: direct isotopic measurements of Na^+ and Ca^{2+} fluxes (PITTS [27]) movement of lipophilic cations in the direction of Ca^{2+} during Na^+ efflux (REEVES and SUTKO [29], CARONI et al. [8]) stimulation of the exchanger by the establishment of a positive potential inside the vesicles, and inhibition by the establishment of a negative potential (PHILIPSON and NISHIMOTO [25], BERS et al. [3]).

Work on heart sarcolemmal vesicles has established that the affinity of the exchanger for Na^+ is expressed by a K_m of about 20 mM (REEVES and SUTKO [28]). When measured under non-limiting conditions, the $K_{m(Ca)}$ is of the order of 2 μM (CARONI et al. [8], however, see below). The maximal rate of Ca^{2+} transport through the exchanger is very high (in heart, up to 15–20 nmoles per mg of protein per sec). These findings characterize the exchanger as a (relatively) low-affinity, high-capacity system, suited for rapidly ejecting Ca^{2+} during the physiological phases of cell life in which substantial increases of cytosolic Ca^{2+} may be expected. In the case of heart, an integrated view (see Table 3)

Table 3

A comparison of the Ca^{2+}-pumping ATPase and the Na^+/Ca^{2+} exchanger of heart plasma membrane

	ATPase	Exchanger
K_m (μM)	~ 0.5	~ 2
V_{max} (nmol × mg prot^{-1} × sec^{-1})	~ 0.5	15–20
Functional role	diastolic	peak activation

would have the exchanger functioning optimally at peak activation, when the cytosolic concentration of Ca^{2+} presumably rises past the levels necessary to activate the exchanger. As indicated above, the Ca^{2+} pumping ATPase would on the other hand already function optimally during diastole.

The Na^+/Ca^{2+} exchanger has been reported to be inhibited by amiloride, albeit at rather high concentrations (SMITH et al. [34] and by doxorubicin and other anthracyclines (CARONI et al. [11]). The inhibition by the latter compounds correlates, at least partially, with their cardiotoxicity, and seems to be competitive with Ca^{2+}.

One interesting aspect of the Na^+/Ca^{2+} exchanger is its sensitivity to ATP. In the giant axon of the squid the latter increases the affinity of the exchanger for Ca^{2+} and Na^+ (reviewed by BLAUSTEIN and NELSON [4]). Evidently, the effect of ATP requires its hydrolysis, since only hydrolyzable analogues stimulate (DI POLO [14]). This observation, which suggests the involvement of a phosphorylation reaction, has now been extended in experiments with heart sarcolemma vesicles (CARONI et al. [12]). The affinity of the exchanger for Ca^{2+} is enhanced (to a K_m of about 0.8 μm) by a kinase-mediated phosphorylation step, and decreased by a phosphatase-mediated dephosphorylation reaction. The kinase is membrane-bound, and requires, in addition to ATP, Ca^{2+} and calmodulin, but not cAMP (Table 4). In order to make the stimulating effect of protein phosphorylation more evident, it has been found convenient to previously dephosphory-

Table 4

Inhibition of the Na^+/Ca^{2+} exchange activity by preincubation of the heart sarcolemma vesicles with phosphorylase phosphatase. Reactivation by an endogenous mechanism requiring Ca^{2+}, endogenous calmodulin, and ATP

The sarcolemmal vesicles (for details on their and on the testing of the Na^+/Ca^{2+} exchange activity see [12]). were incubated for 20 min in 160 mM NaCl, 20 mM Hepes, pH 7.4 to load them with Na^+. Then, they were incubated in the same medium for 5 min at 37° in the presence of the compounds listed in the column labeled (first preincubation) and then treated with 100 mM EDTA to arrest the reaction. After washing, the vesicles were submitted to the second preincubation under the condition of the first, and then washed and suspended (5 mg protein per ml in NaCl-Hepes). Concentrations in the preincubation media were: phosphorylase phosphatase, 20 μg/ml; protein kinase (cAMP-dependent) inhibitor, 20 μg/ml; R 24571 (an anticalmodulin compound), 0.5 μM-$MgCl_2$, 1 mM, $CaCl_2$, 20 μM; EGTA, 0.2 mM. When ATP (1 mM) was present in the preincubation medium, 10 μM vanadate and 10 μM digitoxigenin were included to prevent the comsumption of ATP and the loading of the (inside-out) vesicles with Na^+ by the Na, K-ATPase. The Na^+/Ca^{2+} exchange activity was measured with the arsenazo III technique, in the presence of 10 μM Ca^{2+}.

Additions to the first preincubation medium	Additions to the second preincubation medium	Na^+/Ca^{2+} exchange activity (nmol Ca^{2+} × mg protein × sec^{-1})
Phosphorylase Phosphatase,	none	9.7
Mg^{2+}	Ca^{2+}, Mg^{2+}, ATP	28.1
Mg^{2+}	Ca^{2+}, Mg^{2+}	9.5
Mg^{2+}	Ca^{2+}, ATP	10.7
Mg^{2+}	EGTA, Mg^{2+}	9.9
Mg^{2+}	Ca^{2+}, Mg^{2+}, ATP, R 24571	10.6
Mg^{2+}	Ca^{2+}, Mg^{2+}, ATP, protein kinase inhibitor	28.4

late the sarcolemmal vesicles with an exogenous phosphatase, in this case phosphorylase phosphatase. The latter is most probably not the enzyme physiologically active in dephosphorylating the exchanger or the sarcolemmal substrate that is responsible for its activation. However, the exchanger can be inactivated by a treatment with Ca^{2+} and calmodulin (Table 5). Since appropriate controls have excluded that the latter treatment artificially damages the sarcolemmal vesicle membrane, thus making it leakier to Ca^{2+} and Na^+, it must be concluded that a Ca^{2+} and calmodulin-sensitive protein phosphatase is present in the sarcolemmal membrane, and inactivates the exchanger.

One last recent finding on the Na^+/Ca^{2+} exchanger deserves to be mentioned, i.e., its stimulation by a controlled treatment of heart sarcolemmal vesicles with trypsin (PHILIPSON and NISHIMOTO [26]). The activating effect, which is reminescent of the activation of the plasma membrane Ca^{2+} pumping ATPase by protolysis, is apparently additive with that induced by the kinase-mediated phosphorylation (CARONI et al. (12]).

Table 5

Inactivation of the Na^+/Ca^{2+} exchange process by an endogenous Ca^{2+} and calmodulin-dependent mechanism

The first and the second preincubation of the sarcolemmal vesicles were carried out as described in the legend for Table 4. When added, R 24571 was incubated for 1 min at 37 °C with the calmodulin-containing preincubation medium to allow full interaction of the drug with calmonulin. Concentrations in the preincubation medium to allow full interaction of the drug with calmodulin. Concentrations in the preincubation media were: phosphorylase phosphatase, 20 μg ml; calmonulin 5 μg/ml;, R 24571, 0.5 μM; ATP, 1 mM; $MgCl_2$, 1 mM; EGTA, 0.2 mM; $CaCl_2$, 20 μM. When ATP was present in the preincubation medium, 10 μM vadanate and 10 μM digitoxigenin were included to prevent ATP consumption by the sarcolemmal. The Na^+/Ca^{2+} exchange activity was measured with the arsenazo III technique in the presence of 10 μM $CaCl_2$.

Additions to the first preincubation menium	Additions to the second preincubation medium	Na^+/Ca^{2+} exchange activity nmol Ca^{2+} × mg protein × sec^{-1}
none	none	19.8
Ca^{2+}, Mg^{2+}, calmodulin	none	9.6
Ca^{2+}, Mg^{2+}, R 24571, calmodulin	none	19.0
EGTA, Mg^{2+}, calmodulin	none	19.7

References

[1] ADUNYAH, E. S., V. NIGGLI and E. CARAFOLI: FEBS Letters **143** (1982), 65–68
[2] BAKER, P. F.: In: Calcium Movement in Excitable Cells, P. F. Baker and H. Reuter, eds., Pergamon Press, Oxford (1975), pp. 6–54
[3] BERS, D. M., K. D. PHILIPSON and Y. NISHIMOTO: Biochim. Biophys. Acta **601** (1980), 358 to 371
[4] BLAUSTEIN, M. P. and M. J. NELSON: In: Membrane Transport of Calcium, E. Carafoli, ed. Acad. Press, London (1982), pp. 217
[5] BUCKLEY, J. T. and J. N. HAWTHORNE: J. Biol. Chem. **247** (1972) 7218–7223
[6] CARAFOLI, E. and M. ZURINI: Biochim. Biophys. Acta **683** (1982), 279–301

[7] CARONI, P. and E. CARAFOLI: Nature **283** (1980), 765–767
[8] CARONI, P., L. REINLIB and E. CARAFOLI: Proc. Nat. Acad. Sci., U.S.A. **77** (1980), 6354–6358
[9] CARONI, P. and E. CARAFOLI: J. Biol. Chem. **256** (1981), 3263–3270
[10] CARONI, P. and E. CARAFOLI: J. Biol. Chem., **256** (1981), 8371–9373
[11] CARONI, P., F. VILLANI and E. CARAFOLI: FEBS letters, **130** (1981), 184–186
[12] CARONI, P., L. SOLDATI and E. CARAFOLI: In: Electrogenic Transport, M. P. Blaustein and M. Liebermann, Eds., Raven Press, New York, in press
[13] CLARK, A. and E. CARAFOLI: Cell Calcium, **4** (1983), 83–88
[14] DI POLO, R.: J. Gen. Physiol. **64** (1974), 503–517
[15] DI POLO, R. and L. BEAUGÉ: Nature, **278** (1979), 271–273
[16] GOPINATH, R. M. and F. F. VINCENZI: Biochem. Biophys. Res. Commun. 77
[17] JARETT, H. W. and J. T. PENNISTON: Biochem. Biophys., Res. Commun. **77** (1977), 1210 to 1216
[18] LEW, V. and H. G. FERREIRA: Current Topics Membr. Transp. **10** (1978), 218–279
[19] LYNCH, Th. J. and W. Y. CHEUNG: Arch. Biochem. Biophys. **194** (1979), 165–170
[20] MICHELL, R. H., C. J. KIRK, L. M. JONES, C. P. DOWNES and J. A. CREBA: Phil. Trans. R. Soc. Lond. B. **299** (1981), 123–137
[21] NIGGLI, V., E. S. ADUNYAH and E. CARAFOLI: J. Biol. Chem. **256** (1981), 8588–8592
[22] NIGGLI, V., J. T. PENNISTON and E. CARAFOLI: J. Biol. Chem., **254** (1979), 9955–9958
[23] NIGGLI, V., P. RONNER, E. CARAFOLI and J. T. PENNISTON: Arch. Biochem. Biophys. **198** (1979), 124–130
[24] PENNISTON, J. T.: In: Calcium and Cell Function, W. Y. Cheung, ed., Vol. 4, Acad. Press, New York, in press
[25] PHILIPSON, K. D. and A. Y. NISHIMOTO: J. Biol. Chem. **255** (1980), 6880–6882
[26] PHILIPSON, K. D. and A. Y. NISHIMOTO: Am. J. Physiol. **243** (1982), C 191–C 195
[27] PITTS, B. J. R.: J. Biol. Chem., **254** (1979), 6232–6235
[28] REEVES, J. P. and J. L. SUTKO: Proc. Nat. Acad. Sci., **76** (1979), 590–594
[29] REEVES, J. P. and J. L. SUTKO: Science, 208 (1980), **1461–1464**
[30] REUTER, H. and N. SEITZ: J. Physiol. (London) **195** (1968), 451–470
[31] REUTER, H.: In: Calcium Movement in Escitable Cells, P. F. Baker and H. REUTER, eds., Pergamon Press, Oxford (1975), pp. 55–98
[32] SCHATZMANN, H. J.: Experientia **22** (1966), 364–265
[33] SCHATZMANN, H. J.: In: Membrane Transport of Calcium, E. Caraboli, ed., Acad. Press, London (1982) pp. 41–108
[34] SMITH, R. L., I. G. MACARA, R. LEVENSON, D. HANSMAN and L. CANTLEY: J. Biol. Chem. **257** (1982), 773–780
[35] VARECKA, L. and E. CARAFOLI: J. Biol. Chem. **257** (1982), 7414–7421

A. V. Palladin Institute of Biochemistry, Academy of Sciences of the Ukrainian SSR, Kiev

Effect of cAMP-Dependent Phosphorylation on Passive Ca^{2+} Transport in Myocardial Sarcolemma

M. D. KURSKY and Z. D. VOROBETZ

Concentrations of intracellular Ca^{2+} which are necessary for normal function of myocardial cells are maintained by systems of passive and active Ca^{2+} transport. These systems are located in sarcolemma, sarcoplasmic reticulum and possibly mitochondria which implies that the study of nervous and humoral regulation of Ca^{2+} transport in these subcellular structures is very important.

The effects of β-adrenergic agonists on strength and velocity of contractions are mediated by cAMP-dependent phosphorylation of proteins which are constituents of sarcolemma and sarcoplasmic reticulum [2, 7]. cAMP-dependent phosphorylation of the sarcolemma effects both the passive flux of Ca^{2+} into the cell [10, 15] and its active extrusion out of the cell [4, 13]. It is suggested that increase in passive Ca^{2+} influx into the cell is correlated with activation of both Ca^{2+}- and Mg^{2+}-ATPase which are thought to regulate opening of Ca^{2+} channels [16]. cAMP-dependent phosphorylation increases the Ca^{2+} influx into inside-out orientated sarcolemmal vesicles which posses Ca^{2+}, Mg^{2+}-ATPase activity. According to theses data it is difficult to understand how cAMP-dependent phosphorylation can simultaneously influence these two opposite processes.

The purpose of the present paper is to show the results of the effect of cAMP-dependent phosphorylation on passive Ca^{2+} transport in vesiculated preparations of cardiac sarcolemma prepared by the method of JONES et al. [5]. The obtained vesicles exhibit high activities of Na^+, K^+-ATPase, adenylate cyclase and cAMP-dependent protein kinase but had no Ca^{2+}, Mg^{2+}-ATPase activity. Approximately 80% of the vesicles were inside-out orientated.

Under these conditions Ca^{2+} release from vesicles was taken as an equivalent of passive Ca^{2+} influx into the cell. Vesicles (3 mg of protein/ml) were preloaded with Ca^{2+} over night at 2 °C in a medium containing 500 μM $^{45}CaCl_2$, 140 mM KCl and 20 mM Tris-HCl buffer of pH 7.4 with subsequent preincubation at 37 °C for 10 minutes. To investigate the influence of phosphorylation on Ca^{2+} release from vesicles 2.5 mM $MgCl_2$, 25 μM ATP, 0.01—1.0 μM cAMP, 10 mM NaF and/or 100 μg of protein kinase have been added to the loading medium during preincubation. At the same time and under same conditions phosphorylation level was determined using ^{32}P ATP. Ca^{2+} release from vesicles was initiated by 30-fold dilution of Ca^{2+}-loaded vesicles with a medium containing 20 mM Tris-HCl, pH 7.4, 0.2 mM EGTA and 140 mM NaCl. The reaction was stopped at different time intervals by addition of a solution composed of 280 mM sucrose and 0.5 mM $LaCl_3$, pH 7.4 Samples were filtered through Millipore filters (0.45 μm) and rinsed with 5 ml of the same solution to remove adsorbed Ca^{2+}.

Figure 1 shows that the major portion of Ca^{2+} (more than 50%) has been released during the first minute of incubation. It is clearly shown that Ca^{2+} release is decreasing with time due to dissipation of Ca^{2+} gradient. About 80% of accumulated Ca^{2+} has been released from vesicles at the sixth minute. Ca^{2+} ionophore A 23187 (5 μM) and sodium dodecylsulfate (SDS, 0.3 mg/ml) caused leakage of vesicles and fast release of accumulated Ca^{2+}. It may indicate that the passive Ca^{2+} transport from inside-out vesicles does not relate to their leakage due to the mechanical damage but is caused by transmembra-

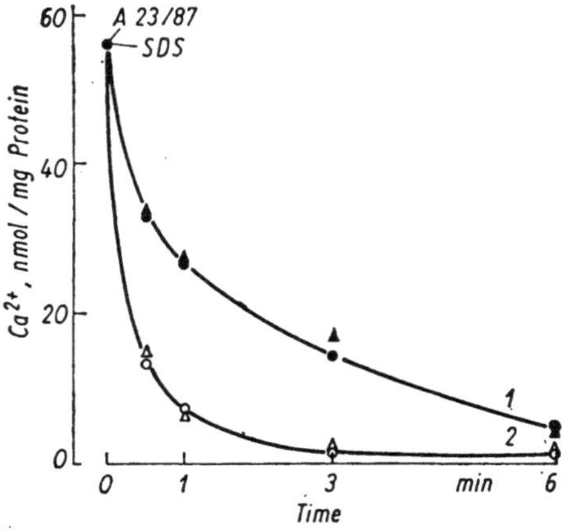

Fig. 1. Kinetics of Ca^{2+} release from sarcolemmal vesicles.
1 — Vesicles were loaded with 500 μM $^{45}CaCl_2$, 140 mM KCl and 20 mM Tris-HCl, pH 7.4 and then 30-fold diluted in medium containing: • — • — • 20 mM Tris-HCl, pH 7.4, 02 mM EGTA and 140 mM NaCl; ▲ — ▲ — ▲ 20 mM Tris-HCl, pH 7.4, 02 mM EGTA and 140 mM KCl.
2 — ○ — ○ — ○ Ca^{2+}-ionophore A 23187 was added to loading medium and to solution which has been used for dilution
▽ — ▽ — ▽ Instead of A 23187 sodium dedecylsulfate was added

ne ionic movement from a certain volume through the corresponding ion channels which are inherent in cardiac sarcolemma. Ca^{2+} binding at the inner surface of vesicles does not affect Ca^{2+} release.

Both the endogenous and the exogenous cAMP-dependent phosphorylation of sarcolemmal protein components lower the rate of Ca^{2+} release from vesicles (Fig. 2) Moreover, the rate of Ca^{2+} release was inversely proportional to the level of membrane phosphorylation.

Table 1 shows that the level of phosphorylation of sarcolemmal vesicles is elevated by the increase in cAMP concentration and addition of exogenous protein kinase. In the presence of cAMP (10^{-6} M) and exogenous protein kinase a small incorporation of ^{32}P into sarcolemmal proteins occured. Under these conditions the Ca^{2+} release was minimal. To proof these data the effect of specific inhibitor of cAMP-dependent protein kinase, tolbutamide, on both the cAMP-dependent phosphorylation and the Ca^{2+} flux has been studied in vesicular preparation of sarcolemma [6]. Tolbutamide (10^{-4} M) inhibited cAMP-dependent sarcolemmal phosphorylation. The inhibitory effect of protein phosphorylation on Ca^{2+} release was markedly reduced by tolbutamide.

The presented data are in good agreement with literature [7, 14]. The results of Ca^{2+}

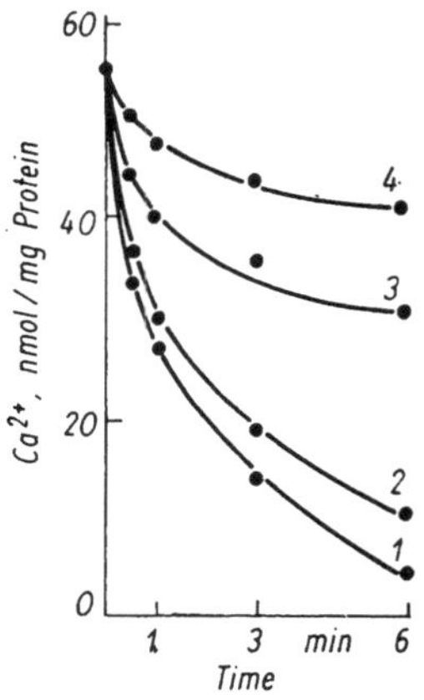

Fig. 2. Effect of cAMP-dependent phosphorylation on Ca^{2+} release from sarcolemmal vesicles.
1 — Control, nonphosphorylated vesicles
2 — Enogenous phosphorylation in presence of 10^{-8} M cAMP
3 — Endogenous phosphorylation in presence of 10^{-6} M cAMP
4 — Phosphorylation by exogenous protein kinase in presence of 10^{-6} M cAMP.

Table 1

Phosphorylation of myocardium sarcolemmal vesicles

Additiods	pmol ^{32}P/mg Protein/5 min
Mg + ATP	260 ± 41
Mg + ATP + 10^{-8} M cAMP	376 ± 35
Mg + ATP + 10^{-6} M cAMP	457 ± 44
Mg + ATP + 10^{-6} M cAMP + Protein kinase	547 ± 56
Mg + ATP + 10^{-6} M cAMP + tolbutamide 10^{-4} M	2,8

flux experiments fit with those of electrophysiological investigations of Kostyuk et al. [8] who have shown that introduction of cAMP into snail neuron decreased the magnitude of Ca^{2+} current which was inversely proportional to the concentration of cAMP. Phosphorylation of microvilli membranes of the intestine mucosa brush border caused also a decrease in the membrane Ca^{2+} permeability. The results obtained with presynaptic neurons [12] and pancreatic β-cells [3] also showed an inhibitory effect of cAMP on Ca^{2+} current through plasma membranes.

The Ca^{2+} channel blocker D 600 which inhibits predominantly slow potential-dependent Ca^{2+} inward current [11] was also shown to diminish Ca^{2+} release from vesicles. This effect was similar to Figure 4 that observed by phosphorylation. D 600 (0.1 mM) incort-

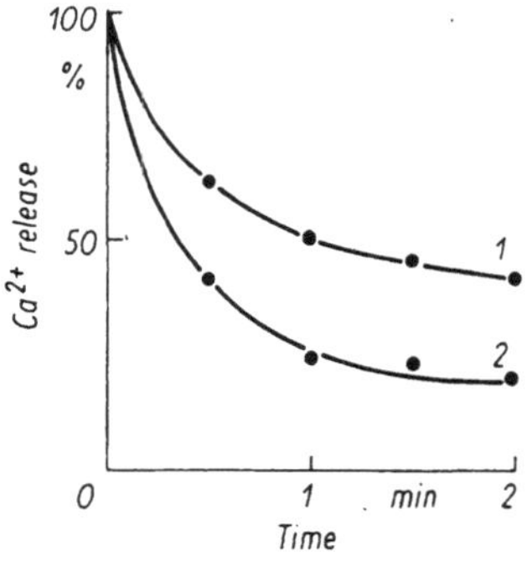

Fig. 3. Effect of tolbutamide on Ca^{2+} release from sarcolemmal vesicles.
1 — Vesicles which has been phosphorylated by endogenous protein kinase in presence of 10^{-6} cAMP
2 — Vesicles which has been phosphorylated by endogenous protein kinase in the presence of 10^{-6} M cAMP and of 10^{-4} M tolbutamide.

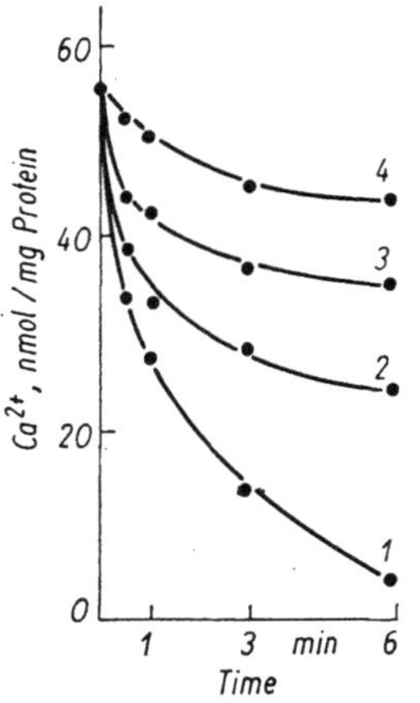

Fig. 4. Effect of D 600 enclosed in sarcolemmal vesicles on Ca^{2+} release.
1 — Control, nonphosphorylated vesicles
2 — Effect of D 600 on nonphosphorylated vesicles
3 — Effect of D 600 on vesicles phosphorylated by endogenous protein kinase in presence of 10^{-6} M cAMP
4 — Effect of D 600 on vesicles phosphorylated by exogenous protein kinase in presence of 10^{-6} M cAMP.

porated into nonphosphorylated sarcolemmal vesicles during homogenization lowered twofold the rate of Ca^{2+} release at sixth minute. Certain potentiation of the inhibitory effect of D 600 on passive Ca^{2+} release by phosphorylation has been observed. It is suggested that D 600 and phosphorylation affect different types of Ca^{2+} channels.

Thus, the obtained data show that Ca^{2+} transport into myocardial cells is a complicated process in which cAMP-dependent phosphorylation is involved.

References

[1] DRUMMOND, J. I.: Texas Report on Biol. Med. **39** (1979), 37—52
[2] DUPIS, Y., G. GROUZOULON and P. FOURNIER: Int. J. Biochem. **13** (1981), 1163—1170
[3] GYLFE, E. and B. HELLMAN: Biochem. Med. **26** (1981), 365—376
[4] HUI, C. W., G. J. DRUMMOND and M. DRUMMOND: Arch. Biochem. Biophys. **173** (1976), 415—427
[5] JONES, L. R., H. R. BESCH, Jr., J. W. F. FLEMING, M. M. MC CONNAUGHEY and A. M. WATANABE: J. Biol. Chem. **254** (1979), 530—539
[6] KANAMORI, T., T. HAYAKOVA and T. NAGATSU: Biochim. Biophys. Acta **429** (1976), 147—162
[7] KATZ, A. M.: In: Adv. Cycl. Nucl. Res. **11** (1979) edited by P. Greengard and G. A. Robison, Raven Press, New York, 303—343
[8] KONONENKO, N. Í. and P. G. KOSTJUK: Njeurofisiologija **14** (1982), 291—299
[9] KURSKY, M. D., Z. D. VOROBETZ and C. N. MARTSCHENKO: Ukrainskij Biochim. J. **54** (1982), 643—649
[10] LASAREW, A. W., W. I. POROTIKOW and T. S. KSCHUTASCHWILI: Dokl. Akad. Nauk **244** (1979), 747—750
[11] RASMUSSEN, H. and D. B. P. GUDMAN: Physiol. Rev. **57** (1977), 422—509
[12] SHAPIRO, E., V. F. CASTELLUCH and E. R. KANDEL: Proc. Nat. Acad. Sci. USA **77** (1980), 1185—1189
[13] SULAKHE, V. and P. J. St. LOUIS: Gen. Pharmacol. **7** (1976), 313—319
[14] TADA, M. and A. M. KATZ: Ann. Rev. Physiol **44** (1982) 401—423
[15] WOLLENBERGER, A., and H. WILL: Life Sci. **22** (1978), 1159—1178
[16] ZIEGELHÖFER, A., M. B. ANNAND-SRIVASTAVA, R. L. KHANDELWAL and N. S. DHALLA: Biochem. Biophys. Res. Commun. **89** (1979), 1073—1081

Experimental Cardiology Section, Department of Physiology, Faculty of Medicine, University of Manitoba, Winnipeg, Canada R3E OW3

Possible Role of Ca^{2+}-ATPase in the Mechanism of Calcium Influx through Cardiac Sarcolemma

A. ZIEGELHÖFFER, M. B. ANAND-SRIVASTAVA and N. S. DHALLA

Heart sarcolemma has been shown to possess ATP hydrolyzing activities in the presence of Ca^{2+} or Mg^{2+} [1, 4, 15, 20]. Earlier studies have revealed that Ca^{2+}/Mg^{2+} ATPase in heart sarcolemma was depressed by divalent cations such as Ni^{2+}, Mn^{2+} and Co^{2+}, which are known to decrease calcium currents as well as entry of calcium into the myocardium [12]. Furthermore different drugs such as β-adrenergic blocking agents and antiarrhythmic agents, which depress cardiac contractile force, were found to decrease Ca^{2+}/Mg^{2+} ATPase activity in heart sarcolemma [6, 7]. On the other hand, both cyclic AMP-protein kinase dependent phosphorylation and electrical stimulation of heart sarcolemma were shown to increase Ca^{2+}/Mg^{2+} ATPase [24, 25]. In this paper we report that the effects of electrical stimulation and cyclic AMP-protein kinase on sarcolemmal membrane phosphorylation as well as Ca^{2+}-ATPase are additive. Such an observation is hoped to explain the molecular mechanism of increased calcium influx through the sarcolemmal membrane of beating heart under the influence of hormones, which are known to produce positive inotropic action as a consequence of cyclic AMP-protein kinase mediated membrane phosphorylation [9]. It is pointed out that Ca^{2+}-ATPase referred here requires millimolar concentrations of Ca^{2+} for activation and utilizes ATP as a substrate and thus should not be confused with Ca^{2+}-stimulated Mg^{2+} dependent ATPase, which requires micromolar concentrations of Ca^{2+} and utilizes Mg^{2+} ATP as a substrate.

Materials and methods

Heart sarcolemmal membranes were prepared from rat ventricles by the hypotonic shock-LiBr treatment method [5]. As reported previously [5] these membranes contained negligible amounts (2 to 4%) of contamination by other subcellular organelles such as mitochondria, sarcoplasmic reticulum and myofibrils. Furthermore, Na^+-K^+ ATPase (12.84 ± 0.74 μmoles P_i/mg/hr) and adenylate cyclase (480 ± 20.5 pmoles cyclic AMP/min/mg) activities in sarcolemmal preparations as determined by methods described elsewhere [12] were enriched by 8 to 10 fold with respect to the heart homogenate enzyme activities.

Sarcolemmal membranes (50—108 μg proteins) were suspended in 1 ml of 50 mM Tris-HCl buffer, pH 7.5 and 1.25 mM $CaCl_2$ at 37 °C for 5 min. The Ca^{2+}-ATPase reaction was started by the addition of 4 mM Tris-ATP. After a 10 min incubation period, unless indicated in the text, the enzyme reaction was stopped by the addition of 1 ml of 12%

trichloroacetic acid (ice cold), the inorganic phosphate liberated estimated and Ca^{2+}-ATPase activity was calculated [5, 12]. Mg^{2+}-ATPase activity was also determined under experimental conditions similar to those employed for Ca^{2+}-ATPase activity except that 1.25 mM $MgCl_2$ was used instead of $CaCl_2$. The electrical stimulation was carried out during ATPase reaction with a Grass SD9 stimulator and platinum electrodes with a total surface area of 49.3 mm^2 and a mutual distance of 7 mm. Optimal parameters for the AC square wave current (24) of 0.6 volts, 2 cycle/sec, 10 msec impulse duration and 0.01 msec impulse delay were employed in this study. In one set of experiments, phosphorylation activity of both unstimulated and electrically-stimulated membranes was determined by using 1 ml of medium containing 50 mM Tris-HCl, pH 7.5, 5 mM $MgCl_2$ and 50 μM [γ-^{32}P]-ATP (260—600 cpm/pmol) at 26 °C. When indicated 10 μM cyclic AMP and 20 μg of protein kinase (freshly dialyzed) was used and the acid stable, alkali labile and hydroxylamine insensitive incorporation of ^{32}P in the membrane fraction was estimated [25]. The results were analyzed by using the Student's "t" test.

Results

Electrical stimulation of sarcolemmal membranes was found to increase Ca^{2+}-ATPase activity (Table 1). The magnitude of this increase in the enzyme activity was not altered by the presence of 20—100 mM NaCl or KCl in the incubation medium (Table 1). Furthermore, the activation of sarcolemmal Ca^{2+}-ATPase by electrical stimulation was not associated with any appreciable changes in the temperature of pH of the incubation medium. ATP hydrolysis due to electrical stimulation in the absence of membranes was rather negligible. Prestimulation of sarcolemma electrically also resulted in an increased Ca^{2+}-ATPase activity and the enzyme reaction was found to be linear in both unstimulated and stimulated membrane preparations (Fig. 1). Electron microscopic examination [5, 15] of the unstimulated and stimulated membranes revealed no apparent changes in the sarcolemmal ultrastructure upon electrical stimulation (Fig. 2).

Table 1

Influence of electrical stimulation of heart sarcolemma on Ca^{2+}-ATPase activity at different concentrations of monovalent cations

Additions	Ca^{2+}-ATPase activity (μmoles Pi/mg/hr)	
	Unstimulated	Stimulated
Control	19.6 ± 0.41	31.35 ± 0.35
20 mM NaCl	20.36 ± 0.41	31.28 ± 0.44
100 mM NaCl	19.66 ± 0.62	31.84 ± 0.90
20 mM KCl	19.76 ± 0.30	30.10 ± 1.58
100 mM KCl	20.43 ± 0.48	32.37 ± 0.64

The osmolarity of the incubation medium was adjusted with sucrose. Results are means ± S.E. of 6 experiments. After a 5 min of preincubation period, Ca^{2+} ATPase reaction was started by the addition of ATP. Electrical stimulation was started at the time of initiating ATPase reaction with ATP and stopped 10 min later when the reaction was terminated by the addition of trichloroacetic acid.

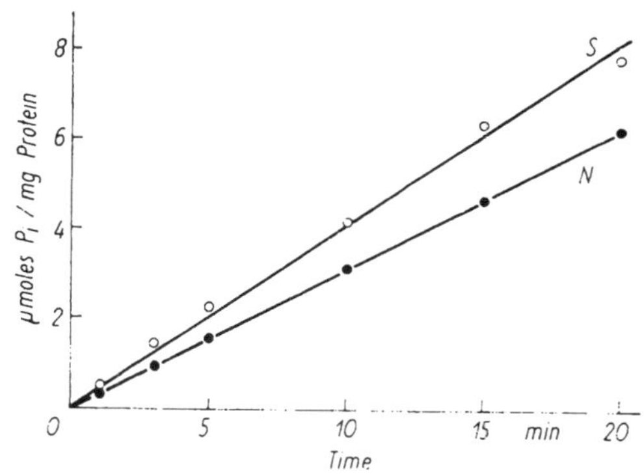

Fig. 1. Influence of 10 min electrical prestimulation on the Ca^{2+}-ATPase activity of rat heart sarcolemma. S: Electrically stimulated membranes. N: Unstimulated membranes. ATPase activity was determined at different times of incubation. The results are average of 6 experiments. Linear regression plot analysis revealed $y = 0.313x - 0.012$ for N and $y = 0.368x + 0.244$ for S.

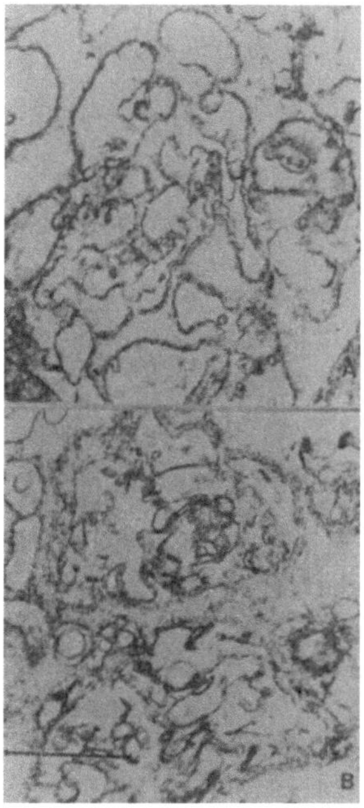

Fig. 2. Electron micrographs of the isolated rat heart sarcolemmal pellets. A. Unstimulated membranes. B. Electrically stimulated membranes. The black bar represents one micron.

In another set of experiments, the effect of cyclic AMP and/or protein kinase on membrane phosphorylation was determined by employing unstimulated and electrically stimulated preparations (Table 2). A considerable amount of ^{32}P was incorporated in the membrane fraction in the absence of protein kinase or cyclic AMP. This may be due to the presence of endogenous protein kinase in the sarcolemmal membranes employed in this study. Although exogenous protein kinase had no influence on membrane phosphorylation, cyclic AMP increased this activity. A marked stimulation of membrane phosphorylation in both unstimulated and electrically stimulated preparations was seen

Table 2

Influence of cyclic AMP dependent phosphorylation on Ca^{2+}-ATPase activity of unstimulated and electrically stimulated rat heart sarcolemma

Additions	Membrane phosphorylation (pmoles P_i incorporated/mg/min)		Ca^{2+}-ATPase activity (μmoles P_i/mg/hr)	
	Unstimulated	Stimulated	Unstimulated	Stimulated
None	—	—	22.0 ± 1.4	26.5 ± 1.5
Mg^{2+} + ATP	155 ± 14.5	200 ± 9.1	23.8 ± 1.3	28.9 ± 1.5
Mg^{2+} + ATP + PK	148 ± 12.5	191 ± 13.3	—	—
Mg^{2+} + ATP + cAMP	197 ± 20.0	267 ± 16.1	23.9 ± 1.4	28.4 ± 1.6
Mg^{2+} + ATP + cAMP + PK	256 ± 29.0	395 ± 27.1	29.0 ± 0.8	36.3 ± 1.2

In one set of experiments acid stable, alkali labile and hydroxylamine insensitive phosphorylation was determined whereas in the other set of experiments Ca^{2+}-ATPase activity was measured under the experimental conditions described above. Each value is a mean of 3 to 4 experiments. Unstimulated or electrically stimulated membranes were employed immediately in these experiments. Membrane phosphorylation activity was determined during the first min of incubation with γ-^{32}P-ATP.

when both cyclic AMP and protein kinase were used. The data in Table 2 also indicate a greater phosphorylation activity in the electrically stimulated membranes in comparison to that in the unstimulated preparations. Time-course studies concerning the effect of cyclic AMP-protein kinase on unstimulated and electrically stimulated sarcolemma revealed that the actions of cyclic AMP-protein kinase and electrical stimulation on membrane phosphorylation were essentially additive (Fig. 3).

The effect of cyclic AMP-protein kinase was also studied on Ca^{2+}-ATPase activities in unstimulated and electrically stimulated sarcolemmal preparations and the results are shown in Table 2. Incubation of membranes with both cyclic AMP and protein kinase was necessary to observe stimulation of Ca^{2+}-ATPase activity. Furthermore, Ca^{2+}-ATPase activity in the electrically stimulated preparations was significantly

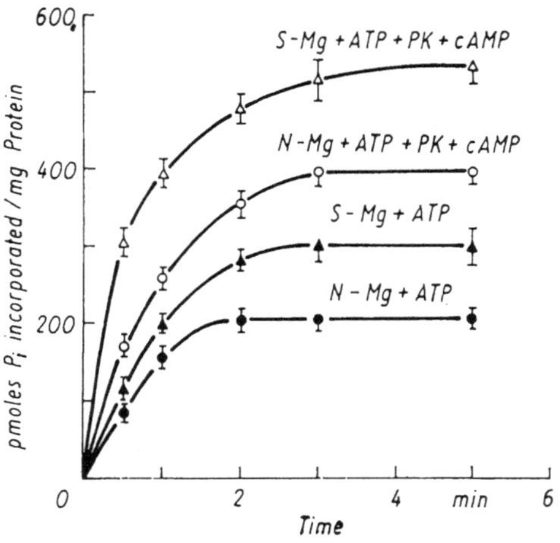

Fig. 3. Time-course of cyclic AMP dependent phosphorylation in unstimulated (N) and electrically stimulated (S) heart sarcolemmal membranes. Phosphorylation activity was measured in these membranes in the absence or presence (Mg + ATP + PK + cAMP). Each value is a mean ± of 4 experiments.

higher than that in the unstimulated membranes under all experimental conditions (Table 2). Mg^{2+}-ATPase activities in unstimulated and stimulated preparations were 15.1 $\pm$ 1.1 and 18.9 $\pm$ 1.1 (μmoles Pi/mg/hr) respectively. Although these activities were not significantly altered upon addition of either cyclic AMP or protein kinase, Mg^{2+} ATPase activities in the presence of both cyclic AMP and protein kinase were 20.8 $\pm$ 1.3 and 25.8 $\pm$ 1.0 (μmoles Pi/mg/hr) for unstimulated and stimulated membranes respectively.

Discussion

We have shown that electrical stimulation of heart sarcolemma increased the Ca^{2+}-ATPase activity. Such an increase cannot be attributed to augmented ATP hydrolysis in the incubation medium due to electrical stimulation since prestimulated sarcolemmal membranes also showed higher Ca^{2+}-ATPase activity in comparison to the control values. Furthermore, electrical stimulation in the absence of sarcolemmal membranes in the incubation medium did not cause any appreciable ATP hydrolysis. It is also unlikely that the observed effect of electrical stimulation was due to membrane aggregation or other apparent alterations because no changes in the sarcolemmal ultrastructure were evident in this study. Since electrical stimulation of synaptosomes has been demonstrated to increase phosphatidylinositol turnover [3] and since phosphatidylinositol hydrolysis by a specific phospholipase C has been shown to increase sarcolemmal Ca^{2+}-ATPase activity [8] it is reasonable to assume that the observed increase in Ca^{2+}-ATPase activity by electrical stimulation may be due to an increase in the sarcolemmal phosphatidylinositol turnover.

The results of this study have revealed that electrically stimulated heart sarcolemma incorporated more ^{32}P in comparison to unstimulated membranes. Furthermore, treatment of membranes with cyclic AMP-dependent protein kinase increased ^{32}P incorporation in both unstimulated and electrically stimulated preparations. In fact, the actions of electrical stimulation and cyclic AMP-protein kinase on membrane phosphorylation were essentially additive in nature. It was interesting to observe that treatment of membranes with cyclic AMP-protein kinase not only increased sarcolemmal Ca^{2+}-ATPase activity in unstimulated preparation, as reported previously [25], but this effect was also additive with that seen due to electrical stimulation. Although pretreatment of sarcolemma with cyclic AMP only increased membrane phosphorylation in both unstimulated and stimulated preparations, Ca^{2+}-ATPase activity in this condition was not increased. Such an effect of cyclic AMP may be due to the presence of endogenous membrane bound protein kinase but this degree of membrane phosphorylation may not be sufficient to cause activation of Ca^{2+}-ATPase and thus exogenous protein kinase may be required for this purpose. It however remains to be determined whether the increased Ca^{2+}-ATPase activity due to cyclic AMP-protein kinase is a result of direct phosphorylation of the enzyme molecule per se or is mediated indirectly through the phosphorylation of some other component in the membrane.

Heart sarcolemma has been shown to possess an ATPase complex which is activated by both Ca^{2+} or Mg^{2+} [1, 15]. Recently, we have been successful in isolating and purifying a Ca^{2+}-dependent ATPase which is not activated by Mg^{2+} whereas the membrane bound enzyme remained after solubilizing Ca^{2+}-dependent ATPase was still activated by either Ca^{2+} or Mg^{2+} [5, 21]. It is the activity of this Ca^{2+}/Mg^{2+} ATPase which seems to be increased by electrical stimulation as well as by cyclic AMP-dependent protein kinase mediated membrane phosphorylation. Such a view is supported by the fact that Mg^{2+} ATPase activity, like Ca^{2+} ATPase activity was increased in the electrically stimulated preparations as well as by cyclic AMP-dependent protein kinase membrane phosphorylation and the effects of these interventions were additive. Furthermore, sarcolemmal Ca^{2+}-ATPase activity was increased by electrical stimulation in the presence of high concentrations of Na^+, which has been shown to exert a marked inhibitory effect on the purified Ca^{2+}-dependent ATPase from heart sarcolemma [21]. It should also be pointed out that like sarcolemmal Ca^{2+}/Mg^{2+} ATPase, the activity of bacterial H^+-ATPase has also been reported to increase upon the application of electric pulses under in vitro conditions [14, 17]. Thus both electric impulses as well as membrane phosphorylation can be seen to regulate the activities of membrane ATPases.

Earlier it was proposed that sarcolemmal Ca^{2+}-ATPase may be involved in opening Ca^{2+} channels in the membrane and thus may permit Ca^{2+}-entry into the myocardial cell along the concentration gradient [8, 9]. Accordingly, ATP should be required for Ca^{2+}-influx upon depolarization of the myocardium. In fact, metabolic dependence of slow phase of the action potential, which is considered to represent calcium current in the cardiac muscle, has been demonstrated [18, 19, 22]. Furthermore, ATP has been shown to increase the duration of action potential, calcium current and myocardial

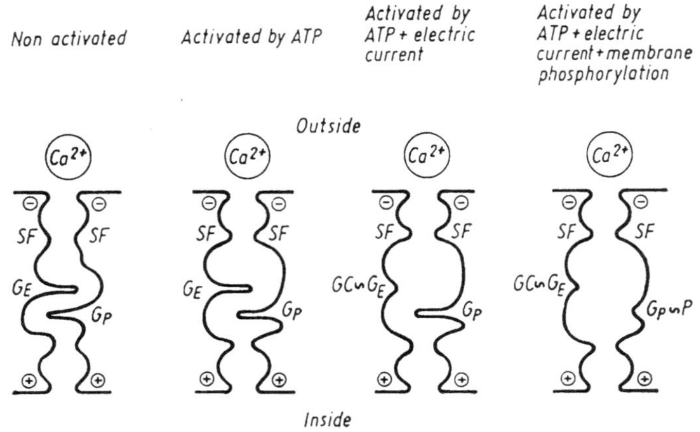

Fig. 4. A hypothetical representation of different stages of calcium channels in heart sarcolemma. This Figure is based on modification of the scheme proposed by REUTER [16]. ⊖ ⊕ — electrical charges at outside and inside of the cell membrane. SF — selective filter. GE — gate operated by electrical current (voltage dependent). GP — gate opened by membrane phosphorylation. GC — gating current. The transition of a non-activated to an activated state of channel may be due to the hydrolysis of ATP in which sarcolemmal Ca^{2+}-ATPase may be intimately involved. Electrical impulse in the form of a gating current may open voltage sensitive gate and this event is associated with Ca^{2+}-influx during the slow phase of the action potential. The fourth state of Ca^{2+}-channel may occur upon depolarization of cell in the presence of hormones which increase intracellular cyclic AMP and where second gate is also opened by membrane phosphorylation due to cyclic AMP-protein kinase. Disappearance of membrane current and dephosphorylation by protein phosphatase will again restore the nonactivated state of the channel.

contractile force [2, 10, 11]. Activation of membrane Ca^{2+}-channels in snail neurons [23] and an increase in Ca^{2+}-influx in isolated intestinal epithelial cells by exogenous ATP has also been reported [13]. From these findings it appears that opening of Ca^{2+}-channels may require energy which is derived from ATP hydrolysis due to activation of sarcolemmal Ca^{2+}-ATPase upon electrical stimulation. Since the Ca^{2+}-ATPase activity of the electrically stimulated preparations was further increased by membrane phosphorylation, it is possible that one site of the Ca^{2+}-ATPase may be regulated by electrical impulses whereas the other is concerned with cyclic AMP-protein kinase mediated phosphorylation. These observations can be viewed to support the concept of REUTER [16] where he has postulated the presence of one voltage sensitive gate and one phosphorylation sensitive gate in Ca^{2+}-channels of the heart sarcolemmal membrane. Thus sarcolemmal Ca^{2+}-ATPase can be considered as a biochemical correlate of the electrophysiological defined Ca^{2+}-channel in the heart membranes and different states of its activation can be represented in a scheme shown in Figure 4. Accordingly, Ca^{2+}-channel may be activated by ATP hydrolysis through the involvement of Ca^{2+}-ATPase, which is considered to be localized in the sarcolemmal membrane transversely. The voltage sensitive gate in the activated state is opened by a gating current upon depolarization of the myocardium and this may permit the entry of Ca^{2+} for the occurrence of cardiac contraction. The membrane phosphorylation, on the other hand, may open the second gate and will thus allow a greater influx of calcium into the myocardial cell upon depolarization and may explain the positive inotropic action of hormones which are known to increase the intracellular concentration of cyclic AMP. The disappearance of the gating current and dephosphorylation by protein phosphatase will again restore the Ca^{2+}-channels to their nonactivated state. Thus sarcolemmal Ca^{2+}-ATPase can be seen to play a key role in the Ca^{2+} gating mechanism for the entry of Ca^{2+} upon depolarization of myocardium as well as upon membrane phosphorylation in the presence of different hormones.

Acknowledgments

This research was supported by a grant from the Medical Research Council. Dr. A. ZIEGELHOFFER was a Visiting Professor supported by the Canadian Heart Foundation and his permanent address is: Institute of Experimental Surgery, Slovak Academy of Sciences, Bratislava, Czechoslovakia

References

[1] ANAND-SRIVASTAVA, M. B., V. PANAGIA and N. S. DHALLA: Adv. Myocardiol. **3** (1982), 359–371

[2] ANTONI, H., G. ENGSTFELD and A. FLECKENSTEIN: Pfluegers Arch. **272** (1960), 91–106

[3] BLEASDALE, J. E. and J. N. HAWTHORNE: J. Neurochem. **24** (1975), 373–379

[4] DHALLA, N. S., M. B. ANAND and J. A. C. HARROW: J. Biochem. **79** (1976), 1345–1350

[5] DHALLA, N. S., M. B. ANAND-SRIVASTAVA, B. S. TUANA and R. L. KHANDELWAL: J. Mol. Cell. Cardiol. **13** (1981), 413–423

[6] DHALLA, N. S., J. A. C. HARROW and M. B. ANAND: Biochem. Pharmacol. **27** (1978), 1281 to 1283

[7] DHALLA, N. S., S. L. LEE, M. B. ANAND and M. S. CHAUBAN: Biochem. Pharmacol. **26** (1977), 2055–2060
[8] DHALLA, N. S., G. N. PIERCE, V. PANAGIA, P. K. SINGAL and R. E. BEAMISH: Basic Res. Cardiol. **77** (1982), 117–139
[9] DHALLA, N. S., A. ZIEGELHOFFER and J. A. C. HARROW: Can. J. Physiol. Pharmacol. **55** (1977), 1211–1234
[10] FLITNEY, F. W., J. F. LAMB and J. SINGH: J. Physiol. (London), **273** (1977), 50–52
[11] GOTO, M., A. YATANI and Y. TSUDA: Rec. Adv. Stud. Card. Struc. Metab. **11** (1978), 37–44
[12] HARROW, J. A., P. K. DAS and N. S. DHALLA: Biochem. Pharmacol. **27** (1978), 2605–2609
[13] KIMMICH, G. A. and J. RANDLES: Am. J. Physiol. **243** (1982), C116–C123
[14] MALONEY, P. C. and S. SCHATTSCHNEIDER: FEBS Letters, **110** (1980), 337–340
[15] PANAGIA, V., J. M. J. LAMERS, P. K. SINGAL and N. S. DHALLA: Int. J. Biochem. **14** (1982), 387–397
[16] REUTER, H. and PORZIG: Advances in Myocardial. **3** (1982), 87–93
[17] ROGNER, M., K. OHNO, T. HAMAMOTO, N. STONE and Y. KAGAWA: Biochem. Biophys. Res. Commun. **91** (1979), 362–367
[18] SCHNEIDER, J. A. and N. SPERELAKIS: J. Surg. Res. **16** (1974), 389–403
[19] SPERELAKIS, N. and J. A. SCHNEIDER: Am. J. Cardiol. **37** (1976), 1079–1085
[20] TAKEO, S., P. DUKE, G. M. M. TAAM, P. K. SINGAL and N. S. DHALLA: Can. J. Physiol. Pharmacol. **57** (1979), 496–503
[21] TUANA, B. S. and N. S. DHALLA: J. Biol. Chem. **257** (1982), 14440–14445
[22] VOGEL, S. and N. SPERELAKIS: Am. J. Physiol. **235** (1978), H46–H51
[23] YATANI, A., Y. TSUDA, N. AKARKE and A. M. BROWN: Nature, **296** (1982), 169–171
[24] ZIEGELHOFFER, A. and N. S. DHALLA: J. Mol. Cell. Cardiol. 10, suppl. 1 (1978), 136
[25] ZIEGELHOFFER, A., M. B. ANAND-SRIVASTAVA, R. L. KHANDELWAL and N. S. DHALLA: Biochem. Biophys. Res. Commun. **89** (1979), 1073–1081

Department of Biochemistry I, Medical Faculty, Erasmus University Rotterdam, The Netherlands

Ca^{2+}-Calmodulin and Cyclic AMP-dependent Phosphorylation of Cardiac Sarcolemma

J. M. J. Lamers

Introduction

In recent years cardiac SL has received much attention, because of its involvement in regulating the availability of Ca^{2+} for the contractile process [11, 28, 39]. In addition it contains receptor sites for hormones that affect cardiac performance. Upon stimulation of the β-adrenergic receptor, SL adenylate cyclase becomes activated resulting in an increase of cellular cyclic AMP concentration [12]. Cyclic AMP in turn activates a protein kinase leading to phosphorylation of SL but also SR and myofibrillar proteins [14, 17, 23, 25, 37, 39, 40, 41, 44]. Phosphorylation of specific proteins in cardiac SL may stimulate the rate of Ca^{2+} extrusion by the Ca^{2+} pump, the voltage-dependent Ca^{2+} channel or even the Na^+/Ca^{2+} antiporter [4, 5, 25, 35, 39, 45].

CaM, the ubiquitous Ca^{2+}-dependent modulator protein, has attracted a great deal of attention in recent years [7]. It is now recognized as the coupling factor of the two second messengers cyclic AMP and Ca^{2+}. Because enzymes regulated by the Ca^{2+}-CaM complex are also substrates for cAMP-PK, e.g. phosphorylase kinase and myosin light chain kinase, cyclic AMP can regulate the action of the Ca^{2+} signal. The recent discovery of Ca^{2+}/CaM-PK in both cardiac SL and SR [19, 25, 26, 29] suggests that cyclic AMP can influence the state of membrane phosphorylation indirectly by changing the cellular Ca^{2+} concentration. The finding of Ca^{2+}/CaM dependent phosphorylation in cardiac SL may well be of importance for elucidating other modes of control of Ca^{2+}-fluxes across SL .

In the present study we have investigated three aspects which are related to the mechanism of β -adrenergic stimulation of the heart. First, the two SL enzymes cAMP-PK and Ca^{2+}/CaM-PK have been studied for their target proteins in both SL and SR. A new example of an interface for interactions of cyclic nucleotide- and Ca^{2+}-mediated events is presented, because both cAMP-PK and Ca^{2+}/CAM-PK can stimulate phosphate incorporation into a 24 kD protein. The reversal of phosphorylation is also induced by using partially purified dog heart protein-Pase. Second, the properties of the SL Ca^{2+}/CaM-PK will be compared with another CaM-dependent system, the Ca^{2+} pumping ATPase, which is also localized in SL. As will be shown the two CaM-dependent systems are inhibited by a potent anti-CaM drug R 24571 in a different manner and the cellular localization of the activating CaM may also be different. Third, the number of Ca^{2+} pump sites has been estimated by following the Ca^{2+}-dependent formation of the ^{32}P enzyme intermediate separated on low pH SDS-PAGE. Herewith the stoichiometric amounts of CaM and several phosphoproteins compared to the phosphoenzyme content could be estimated

Materials and methods

Heat-stable protein kinase inhibitor (PKI) and CaM, purified by the method of DEDMAN et al. [9], were gifts from Dr. H. R. DE JONGE (from our laboratory). cAMP-PK was purchased from Sigma (cat. No. P5511), R24571 was a gift from Dr. H. VAN BELLE (Janssen Pharmaceuticals, Beerse, Belgium), alamethicin was kindly supplied by Dr. J. R. WOODROW from the Public Health Laboratory Service in Salisbury, U. K. protein-Pase was partially purified from dog heart by the method reported by LI and HSAO [30]. The specific activity was about 14 U/ml as assayed by the release of $^{32}P_i$ from ^{32}P-phosphorylase [46], which substrate was kindly supplied by Dr. W. MERLEVEDE (Leuven, Belgium). CaM-deficient brain phosphodiesterase was partially purified following the procedure of DAVIS and DALY [8].

Isolation of purified sarcolemma

SL was isolated from either dog or pig heart by the procedure described by REEVES and SUTKO [34] except that protease inhibitor PMSF was added to all media in 0.5 mM concentration. The preparations were highly enriched in SL ouabain-sensitive Na^+/K^+-ATPase, measured in the presence of 0.4 mg alamethicin/mg protein, amounted to 57 ± 9 (n = 6) and 139 ± 4 (n = 6) μmol/h/mg for pig and dog heart SL respectively. The Ca^{2+} pumping ATPase, which has been unequivocally attributed to SL [5, 25, 39], showed activities of 9 ± 2 (n = 9) and 4.7 ± 0.5 (n = 6) μmol/h/mg, respectively. SR was isolated from dog heart according to the method of HARIGAYA and SCHWARTZ [15] and from the activities of Na^+/K^+-ATPase and Ca^{2+}/Mg^{2+}-ATPase (20.5 ± 2.1 and 24.7 ± 1.7, n = 3, μmol/h/mg, respectively) it can be derived that there was a low SL contamination.

Assay of the protein kinases

Cyclic AMP- and Ca^{2+}/CaM-dependent phosphorylations were carried out by adding 100 μM [γ-^{32}P]-ATP (5—15 Ci/mmol, except the experiment illustrated in Figure 1 was done at 10 μM [γ-^{32}P]-ATP with 10-fold higher specific radioactivity) to 50 μl medium containing 10—20 μg membrane protein, 100 mM KCl, 50 mM Tris maleate (pH 6.8), 5 mM $MgCl_2$, 10 mM theophylline at 25 °C. R24571 was added from a stock solution in DMSO under vigorous mixing shortly (< 5 sec) before addition of membrane vesicles. Termination of reactions, SDS-PAGE, autoradiography and ^{32}P counting were all described in detail previously [23, 25, 27].

Assay of ATPase

Na^+/K^+-ATPase and Ca^{2+}/Mg^{2+} ATPase were determined as in refs. 24 and 25, using the $^{32}P_i$-molybdate extraction in isobutanol previously described by RUITENBEEK [36]. The Na^+/Ca^{2+} antiporter activity was measured in vesicles loaded with 160 mM NaCl, 20 mM MOPS pH 7.5 [24].

Dephosphorylation of prephosphorylated membrane vesicles

SL vesicles were first phosphorylated in 1 ml medium containing 160 mM KCl, 20 mM MOPS pH 7.5, 5 mM $MgCl_2$, 0.1 mM EGTA, 0.107 mM $CaCl_2$, 0.5 mg/ml cAMP-PK, 10 μM cAMP, 0.5 μM CaM and 250 μM [γ-^{32}P]-ATP at 25 °C. After 5 min incubation the membrane vesicles were pelleted at 150000 g (30 min) and twice washed with 15 ml ice-cold 160 mM KCl, 20 mM MOPS pH 7.4. The final pellet was resuspended in 0.42 ml of this buffer and 20 μl of this suspension is added to 30 μl diluted protein-Pase S. Incubations were carried out at 37 °C.

Phosphorylation of the Ca^{2+} pumping enzyme intermediate

Phosphorylations were carried out on ice for 15 sec under the conditions recently described [27]. The phosphoenzyme intermediate was separated on SDS-PAGE by the procedure of Avruch and Fairbanks [1] as described in detail by De Jonge et al. [10]. The amount of ^{32}P-enzyme is defined as the ^{32}P present on a 120 and 200 kD protein at 12 μM Ca^{2+} minus that present in the absence of Ca^{2+} [27].

Estimation of calmodulin content of SL vesicles

An aliquot (100 μl) of SL vesicles was incubated at 95 °C for 10 min and rapidly [18] cooled to 0 °C in an ice bath. This was followed by centrifugation at 15000 g for 15 min at 0–4 °C. Small amounts (30–70 μl) were incubated in 200 μl incubation medium, containing 5 mM $MgCl_2$, 100 mM KCl, 0.2 mM $CaCl_2$, 10 mM Tris (pH 7.5), 3.75 mM β-mercaptoethanol and 10 U/ml activator deficient brain phosphodiesterase [8]. The reaction was stopped after 10 min by placing the tube for 3 min in a boiling water bath. The denatured protein was removed by centrifugation. To the supernatant a 25 μl carrier solution, composed of 30 mM cyclic AMP, adenosine and AMP, was added. Unreacted cyclic AMP was separated from the product AMP on paper chromatography [13]. The extent of phosphodiesterase activation by SL extracts was compared with that found with pure CaM [9].

Results

Cyclic AMP- and Ca^{2+}/CaM-dependent phosphorylation of cardiac membranes

When SL membranes, obtained from dog hearts, were incubated with [γ-^{32}P]-ATP there was a rapid incorporation into specific components (Fig. 1). Cyclic AMP (10 μM) increased 53, 14 and 9 kD phosphorylation, indicating the presence of an endogenous cAMP-PK. A further stimulation was obtained by adding 0.4 mg/mg alamethicin. As previously shown by Jones et al. [18] alamethicin was a potent activator of latent SL enzymic acitivities (e.g. Na^+/K^+-ATPase and adenylate cyclase). The unmasking agent most dramatically increased the intensity of 14 and 26 kD phosphorylation. The right hand panel of Figure 1 shows that an endogenous cAMP-PK is present in cardiac SR and that it was also sensitive to alamethicin. The 9 and 53 kD were visible in both membrane

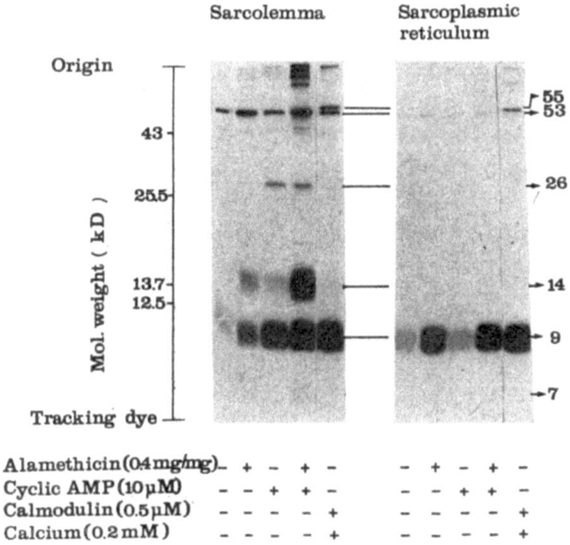

Fig. 1. Endogenous phosphorylation of cardiac SL and SR.

fractions, whereas the 14 and 26 kD seem to be unique for the SL fraction. From other reports [18, 19] it seems likely that the 53 kD phosphoprotein corresponds to the autophosphorylation of the regulatory subunit of this intrinsic cAMP-PK. Phosphorylation patterns depend largely on the conditions used to solubilize the membrane vesicles. The samples shown in Figure 1 all have been boiled for 5 min in SDS. Alternatively, a mild treatment at 37 °C yielded the 9 kD almost entirely in a 24 kD form, which results have been reported earlier [23, 25, 27]. The 9 kD protein easily aggregates into the high molecular weight form of 24 kD by a freeze-thaw cycle of the SDS-denatured membranes.

The foregoing results are all obtained in the presence of 0.1 mM EGTA. If the Ca^{2+}-free concentration is increased in the presence of exogenous CaM, a different type of protein kinase can be demonstrated. Both in cardiac SL and SR there is a Ca^{2+}/CaM-PK which phosphorylated the 9 and 55 kD protein. Previously we demonstrated [27] that alamethicin inactivated the Ca^{2+}/CaM-PK so that its latency could not be investigated. Pig heart SL and SR showed very similar phosphorylation patterns, although the stimulatory effect of cyclic AMP on endogenous protein kinase in pig heart was rather low. It should be noted that the membrane preparations used do contain significant adenylate cyclase activity [27], hence the protein kinase assayed in the absence of extra cyclic AMP probably represented a partially activated enzyme. As shown in Figure 2 the ^{32}P-incorporation into the 9 kD protein of pig heart SL can be estimated by cutting the phosphorylated bands out of the dried gels. The Ca^{2+}-dependent protein kinase reached a half-maximal rate at about 1 μM Ca^{2+} in the presence of 0.5 μM CaM. R 24571 at a concentration of 20 μM did not affect the affinity of the Ca^{2+}/CaM-PK for Ca^{2+} ions, but the maximal rate (Fig. 2). The basal protein kinase activity was not affected by the anti-CaM drug (Fig. 2). This is not surprising since previously PKI has been demonstrated to inhibit this basal activity [27]. Figure 3 gives evidence that R 24571 antagonizes the activation of Ca^{2+}-dependent kinase by CaM in an apparently competitive

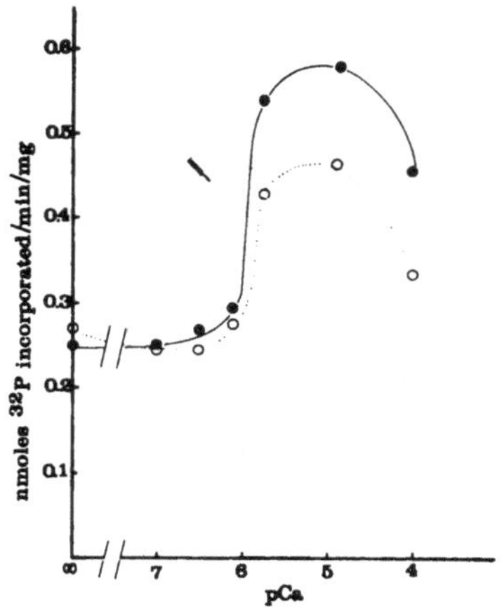

Fig. 2. Effect of R24571 on the Ca^{2+} activation pattern of the Ca^{2+}/CaM-PK present in cardiac SL.

● —— ● Control
○ ····· ○ +20 μM R24571

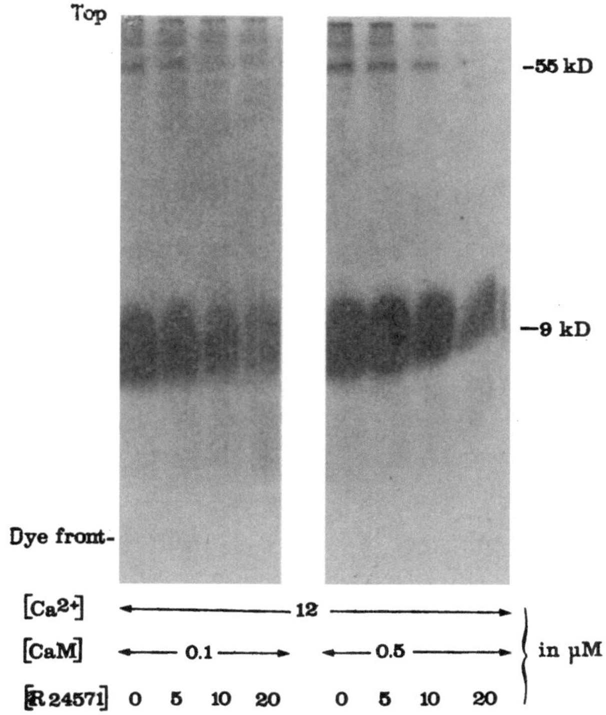

Fig. 3. Effect of R24571 on Ca^{2+}/CaM-PK of cardiac SL: antagonism of the inhibition by CaM.

manner since increasing concentrations of CaM from 0.1 to 0.5 μM completely reversed the inhibition caused by 5 μM R24571. It is important to indicate that the two substrate proteins 55 and 9 kD behaved similarly in all the aspects of the Ca^{2+}/CaM-PK study. This is not the case for the endogenous cAMP-PK, which catalyzed the phosphorylation of only one of these two proteins (9 kD).

Effect of phosphates on phosphorylated SL vesicles

In order to be of physiological significance, the phosphorylation of membrane proteins should be reversible. The results shown in Figure 4 indicate that pig heart SL contain a very low endogenous protein Pase activity in contrast to other species [16, 31]. Using phosphatase S, purified from canine cardiac muscle, we could readily effect the release of ^{32}P from previously phosphorylated SL membranes. The radioactivity profiles obtained when such preparations were fractionated on SDS-PAGE gels (Fig. 4) indicated that non uniform dephosphorylation occurred. Whereas the ^{32}P incorporation into the 9 kD protein is rapidly removed by the protein-Pase, the 14 kD phosphoprotein seems to be

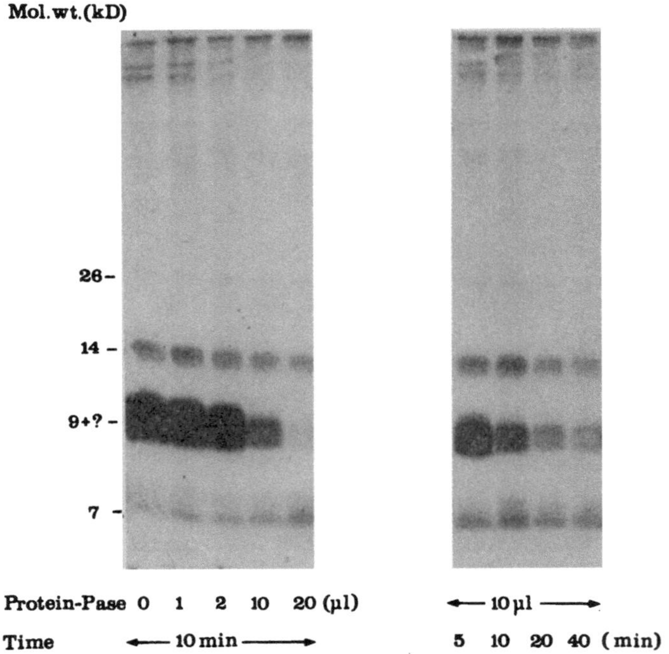

Fig. 4. Dephosphorylation of previously phosphorylated SL by purified protein-Pase S.

resistent to the enzyme. Previously [27] it was shown that the ^{32}P incorporation into 14 kD protein was more resistant to heat-stable protein kinase inhibition, although the phosphorylation was dependent on the presence of cyclic AMP. Another interesting phenomenon, which was evident from the results shown in Figure 4, is the clearcut separation of 2 bands in the 9 kD region. Because these two distinct bands could be demonstrated only a few times, it is possible that a non-reproducible action of a protease could be responsible. On the other hand, this result may be related to the fact that vigorous heat treatment of SR extracts yielded two molecular forms, i.e. 11 and 5.5.kD, which were derived from phospholamban [21].

Cyclic AMP- and Ca^{2+}/CaM-dependent control of SL Ca^{2+} pumping ATPase

As can be seen from Figure 5, the activity of the SL Ca^{2+} pumping ATPase was augmented after phosphorylation of the vesicles by exogenously added cAMP-PK. Although the SL fraction was almost maximally phosphorylated in the presence of cyclic AMP (unpublished results), the addition of soluble cAMP-PK did increase the initial rate of phosphate incorporation. The affinity of the Ca^{2+} pumping ATPase could be shifted from 0.5 to 0.2 μM by cyclic AMP-dependent phosphorylation (Fig. 5). In a previous report it was demonstrated that PKI could prevent the stimulatory effect of cyclic

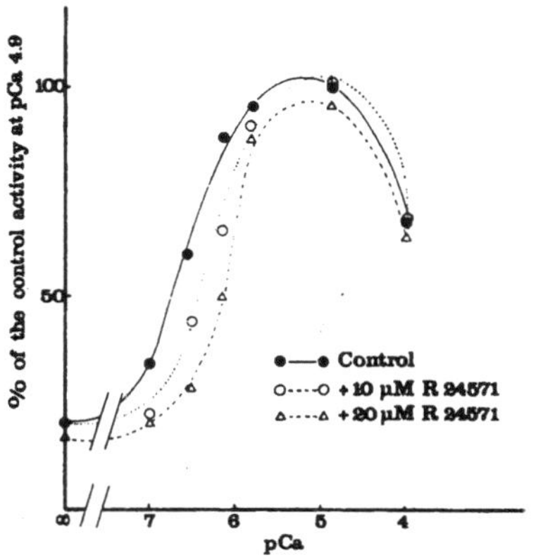

Fig. 5. The effect of cAMP and Ca^{2+}/CaM-PK catalyzed phosphorylation on the SL Ca^{2+} pumping ATPase.

AMP-dependent phosphate incorporation [25]. No effects, neither on V_{max} nor K_a for Ca^{2+}, were observed if vesicles were phosphorylated by the Ca^{2+}/CaM-PK. Thus it is not clear which functional implication the Ca^{2+}/CaM-PK has in cardiac SL. Recently, however, we could demonstrate an inhibitory effect of the anti-CaM drug trifluoperazine on the Ca^{2+} pumping ATPase [25]. This action of trifluoperazine fits into a model analogous to the erythrocyte [33], in which endogenous CaM, tightly bound to the Ca^{2+} pumping ATPase, is essential for most of its enzyme activity. Evidently, CaM is bound to SL more tightly than to erythrocyte membranes, because no effect of exogenous CaM on the Ca^{2+} pumping ATPase (Fig. 5) was observed. Caroni and Carafoli [5] were successful in depleting SL of CaM and could demonstrate that readdition of CaM decreased the K_a for Ca^{2+} from 12 to 0.3 μM of the Ca^{2+} pumping ATPase. The more potent anti-CaM drug R 24571 blocked the Ca^{2+}-dependent activation of the SL Ca^{2+} pumping ATPase (Fig. 6). The V_{max} of the ATPase is only slightly decreased, whereas the K_m (Ca^{2+}) is shifted from 0.4 to 1 μM by the addition of 20 μM R 24571. As a consequence of its hydrophobic character higher concentrations than 25 μM of the drug R 24571 could not be achieved in an aqueous medium. At a Ca^{2+} concentration of 0.7 μM, 20 μM R 24571 produced a 65% inhibition, which could be antagonized by adding exogenously 1 μM CaM (Fig. 7). These data provide evidence that the drug antagonizes the activation of the Ca^{2+} pumping ATPase by CaM in an apparently competitive manner, which was also shown for the Ca^{2+}/CaM-PK. The electrogenic Na^{+}/Ca^{2+} antiporter [5, 24], which is also present in the SL preparation, was less sensitive to R 24571 inhibition compared to the Ca^{2+} pumping ATPase and the Ca^{2+}/CaM-PK (25% inhibition at a concentration of 20 μM R 24571). However, from the results obtained with the Ca^{2+} pumping ATPase

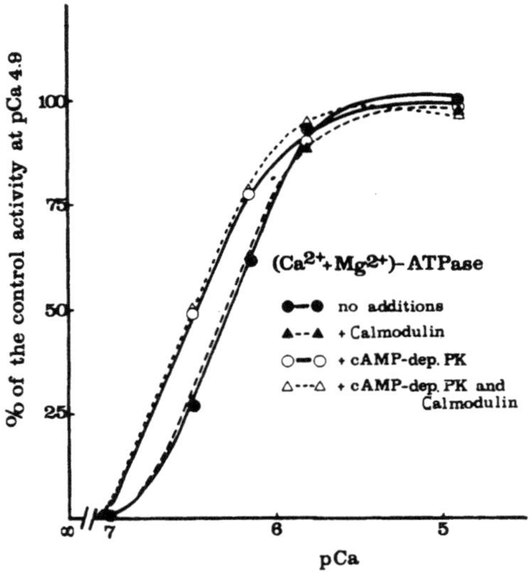

Fig. 6. The effect of R24571 on the Ca^{2+} activation pattern of SL Ca^{2+} pumping ATPase.

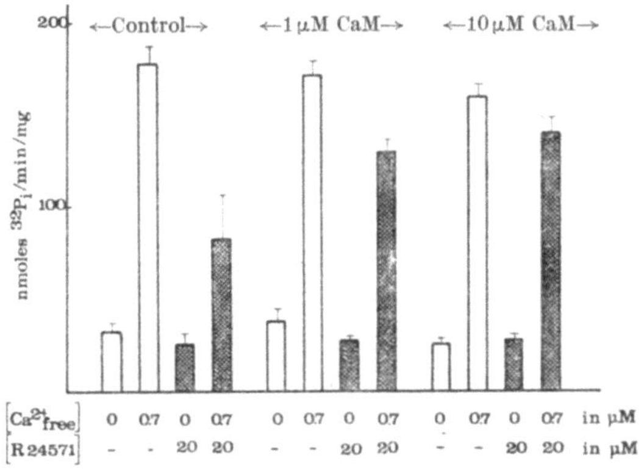

Fig. 7. Effect of R24571 on Ca^{2+} pumping ATPase of cardiac SL: antagonism of the inhibition by CaM.

it is clear that its sensitivity to the anti-CaM drugs critically depended on the Ca^{2+} concentration. The preliminary experiments on the Na^+/Ca^{2+} antiporter have been carried out at 50 μM Ca^{2+}-free concentration (unpublished results).

The amount of phosphoenzyme intermediate of the Ca^{2+} pumping ATPase in relation to the phosphoprotein and CaM content

From the present work it seems likely that both 9 kD and CaM might play a role in regulating the Ca^{2+} pumping ATPase. Moreover, CaM could also exert its action indirectly via 9 kD protein phosphorylation, although no evidence for this proposal has been obtained. Other minor substrate proteins for cyclic AMP- and Ca^{2+}/CaM-PK appeared [14, 26, 53 and 55 kD), which could also be involved in the regulation of the Ca^{2+} pump. Availability of all these proteins in a pure form will permit reconstitution experiments to investigate their possible role in regulating the ATPase. If there is a functional relationship between these proteins and the Ca^{2+} pump it is expected that stoichiometric amounts are present compared to the ATPase monomer. The concentration of the ATPase mono- and dimer can be estimated by recording the Ca^{2+}-dependent ^{32}P incorporation into these protein components, electrophoretically separated on low pH 7.5% SDS-PAGE. The choice of the pH 2.4 is very critical as a higher pH increased the hydrolysis of the acyl-^{32}P intermediate. The results are shown in Table I. The maximal ^{32}P

Table 1

Phosphoprotein and CaM levels in SL vesicles isolated from pig heart

SL preparation No.	9 kD*		14 kD*	120 kD**	
	cAMP-dep.	Ca^{2+}-dep.	cAMP-dep.	Ca^{2+}-dep.	CaM*
	pmoles/mg membrane protein				
1	379	242	111	30	25
2	846	379	92	42	13
3	1346	232	82	147	33
4	1144	332	54	50	33
5	1112	351	96	113	54
6	856	488	68	50	28
mean + S.E.M.	946 ± 138	337 ± 39	83 ± 8	72 ± 19	31 ± 6

* estimated on 15% SDS-PAGE gels (Maizel, J. V., Methods in Virology **5** (1971))
** estimated on 7.5% SDS-PAGE gels (Avruch, J. and G. Fairbanks, Proc. Natl. Acad. Sci. **69** (1972) 1216)
* estimated by addition of heated SL to a CaM-deficient phosphodiesterase

incorporation into the 9 kD protein by cyclic AMP- and Ca^{2+}/CaM-PK was respectively 13 and 5 times higher than the degree of ^{32}P incorporation into the Ca^{2+} pumping enzyme. No clearcut correlations were observed if the relative amounts in separate SL preparations are taken into account. In some membrane preparations the 14 kD phosphoprotein is present near to a 1:1 stoichiometry compared with the phosphoenzyme. The results are in agreement with those obtained by Jones et al. [19]. In their studies the relative concentrations of these protein substrates in SL and SR did not correlate well with the (Ca^{2+} + Mg^{2+})-ATPase activities.

Endogenous CaM content of the membrane has been determined by adding SL extracts to CaM-depleted brain phosphodiesterase. The amount of CaM present could be calculated from extrapolation to activation observed with purified bovine brain CaM. The results obtained with the six membrane preparations are shown in Table I and do suggest a near to 1:2 stoichiometry compared with the phosphoenzyme content.

Discussion

Independently Hui et al. [16], Sulakhe et al. [38] and Krause et al. [22] around 1975 observed that well characterized preparations of cardiac SL contained cAMP-PK activity. Krause et al. [22] estimated the molecular weight of a major substrate protein as 24 kD and this was later confirmed by several other laboratories [17, 18, 23, 35, 41]. The phosphorylation of this protein occurs in response to epinephrine in $^{32}P_i$ perfused rat heart, although the phosphorylation response to epinephrine is not apparently coordinated with the catecholamine-induced inotropic effect [41]. Phosphoproteins of molecular weight lower than 24 kD were also detected [17, 18, 31, 41]. Recently it was shown by us [23, 25] that one of these proteins, the 9 kD, was derived from the 24 kD phosphoprotein. Complete dissociation was reached in 1.7% SDS at 95 °C and partial reassociation occurred after freezing at −20 °C. The latter finding excluded the possibility that the 9 kD protein is a proteolytic product of the 24 kD protein.

CaM has been recognized as a general regulator of Ca^{2+} controlled functions too and some of its effects may be mediated through phosphorylation of proteins. The present communication clearly demonstrates that in cardiac SL from either dog or pig heart a Ca^{2+}-stimulated protein kinase is localized which is completely dependent on exogenous CaM. Earlier it was shown by us [25, 27] that the 9 and 55 kD protein were substrate proteins for this kinase. From the time course of cyclic AMP- and Ca^{2+}/CaM-dependent ^{32}P incorporation it was concluded that two different sites on the 9 kD protein were phosphorylated. Therefore multisite phosphorylation of the 9 kD (or 24 kD) seems to occur and it may not be surprising if any direct correlation between protein phosphorylation and the inotropic effect is not readily apparant by this reason.

MISSELWITZ et al. [32] and JONES et al. [17] have separately purified SL and SR from crude microsomal preparations. The method used for separation, the Ca^{2+}-oxalate precipitation procedure, has been applied on rat and guinea pig heart in our laboratory [23]. The results demonstrated that the 9 and 24 kD phosphoproteins were present in both SL and SR. This has recently been duplicated in independent experiments by JONES et al. [19], although in their report the apparent molecular weights of the proteins involved were 21 and 8 kD. A more rigorous analysis will be required to establish whether the 24 kD protein of cardiac SL and phospholamban are identical. LE PEUCH et al. [29] and KIRCHBERGER et al. [21] recently demonstrated that phospholambam dissociates into monomers of 11 kD molecular weight, a property which is very similar to the 24 kD protein. Thus the 9 kD phosphoprotein described in the present study being localized either in SL or in SR could be identical with the 11 kD phosphoprotein described by others. Evidence presented by LE PEUCH et al. [29] suggested that in cardiac SR a Ca^{2+}/CaM-PK is operative that catalyzes the incorporation of phosphate into phospholamban. This has been confirmed by other reports [19, 20, 27, 29] and is also in agreement with findings in the present communication (compare Fig. 1). Thus it seems not unreasonable to call the SL 24 kD protein a "phospholamban-like" protein [26].

Differences in phosphorylation patterns of cardiac SL and SR were most clear if membranes were treated with the peptide ionophore alamethicin. This agent unmasked endogenous cAMP-PK activity in both types of membranes and provided evidence for the 14 and 26 kD protein to be specifically localized in cardiac SL. Membrane phosphoproteins exclusive to either SR or SL membranes were also previously demonstrated by phosphorylation [17, 19, 23, 27].

The experiments on the Ca^{2+} pumping ATPase mentioned in this and several other reports [5, 16, 25, 38, 45], indicate that cyclic AMP-dependent phosphorylation stimulates the pumping of Ca^{2+} out of the cardiac cell. The abbreviated systole observed upon β-adrenergic stimulation is well explained by this effect on the SL Ca^{2+} pump. On the other hand the group of DEMAILLE [35] provided evidence that phosphate incorporation into the SL 24 kD phosphoprotein, stimulated by cAMP-PK, increased the depolarization-induced Ca^{2+} uptake of the vesicles. According to BARTSCHAT et al. [2] this Ca^{2+} uptake process would serve in vivo for the voltage-dependent Ca^{2+} channel. It is not clear whether the 23 kD phosphoprotein, named calciductin by Demaille's group, is similar to the "phospholamban-like" protein of the present report. Because calciductin was not phosphorylated by Ca^{2+}/CaM-PK [35] it seems to be analogous to the present 26 kD phosphoprotein. From the present results it is not clear which functional implication the Ca^{2+}/CaM-dependent phosphorylation has in SL. Recently CARAFOLI [4] postulated that the Na^+/Ca^{2+} antiporter may be modulated by this type of phosphorylation. At any rate, CaM appears to modulate Ca^{2+} pumping ATPase directly as is shown by its sensitivity to R 24571. The CaM control of the Ca^{2+}-dependent protein kinase and Ca^{2+} pumping ATPase most likely are based on a different mechanism as revealed by the different type of R 24571 inhibition. A tightly bound CaM regulates the ATPase, whereas the Ca^{2+}-dependent protein kinase seems to be dependent on cytosolic CaM.

The most prominently phosphorylated SL protein is the "phospholambam-like" protein of 24 kD molecular weight. This is true for either cyclic AMP- or Ca^{2+}/CaM-dependent phosphorylation of SL and therefore it has been implicated in the functional changes observed. Nevertheless, a role for one or more other phosphorylated proteins with similar Ca^{2+} dependence, for example the 55 kD, and phosphoproteins with similar cyclic AMP dependence (53, 26 and 14 kD) in the regulation of Ca^{2+} transport processes cannot be eliminated.

Ca^{2+} fluxes across cardiac plasma membrane and their modulation by β-adrenergic

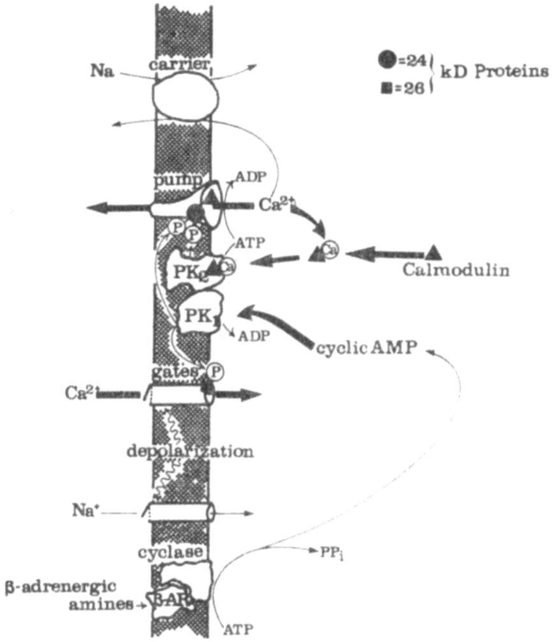

Fig. 8. Schematic diagram depicting Ca^{2+} transport and phosphorylation systems present in cardiac SL.

amines via cyclic AMP- and Ca^{2+}/CaM-dependent processes are schematically depicted in Figure 8. The diagram indicates the Ca^{2+} pump, electrogenic Na^{+}/Ca^{2+} antiporter and the voltage-dependent Ca^{2+} channel that appear to regulate membrane Ca^{2+} fluxes. Cyclic AMP-dependent phosphorylation of the major 24 kD protein increases the Ca^{2+} pump activity, whereas another phosphoprotein of 26 kD molecular weight may activate the voltage-dependent Ca^{2+} channel. CaM may regulate the Ca^{2+} pump directly, as an integral subunit of the enzyme. Depending on the cytosolic Ca^{2+} concentration CaM binds to a protein kinase, which is able to phosphorylate the 24 kD protein. Whether the Ca^{2+} pump or the Na^{+}/Ca^{2+} antiporter are subjected to regulation by this newly discovered kinase remains an interesting topic for future work.

Acknowledgments

I thank Hanny STINIS for her invaluable technical assistence. The secretarial assistence of Cecile HANSON is gratefully acknowledged.

References

[1] AVRUCH, J. and G. FAIRBANKS: Proc. Natl. Acad. Sci. **69** (1972), 1216–1220
[2] BARTSCHAT, D. K., D. L. CYR and G. E. LINDENMAYER: J. Biol. Chem. **255** (1980), 10044 to 10047
[3] VAN BELLE, H.: Cell Calcium **2** (1981), 483–494
[4] CARAFOLI, E.: Proc. Int. Symp. Ca^{2+} modulators, Venice, Italy (1982), in the press
[5] CARONI, P. and E. CARAFOLI: J. Biol. Chem. **256** (1981), 9371–9373
[6] CARONI, P. and E. CARAFOLI: J. Biol. Chem. **256** (1981), 3263–3270
[7] CHEUNG, W. Y.: Science **207** (1980), 19–27
[8] DAVID, C. W. and J. W. DALY: J. Biol. Chem. **253** (1978), 8683–8686
[9] DEDMAN, J. R., J. D. POTTER, R. L. JACKSON, J. D. JOHNSON and A. R. MEANS: J. Biol. Chem. **252** (1977), 8415–8422
[10] DE JONGE, H. R., W. E. J. M. GHIJSEN and C. H. VAN OS: Biochim. Biophys. Acta **647** (1981), 140–149
[11] DHALLA, N. S., A. ZIEGELHOFER and J. A. C. HARROW: Can. J. Physiol. Pharmacol. **55** (1977), 1–22
[12] DRUMMOND, G. I. and D. L. SEVERSON: Circ. Res. **44** (1979), 145–153
[13] DRUMMOND, G. I. and L. DUNCAN: J. Biol. Chem. **245** (1970), 976–983
[14] ENGLAND, P. J.: In: Recently discovered systems of enzyme regulation by vesicle phosphorylation (Ed. P. Cohen), Elsevier North Holland Biomedical Press (1980), 153–173
[15] HARIGAYA, S. and A. SCHWARTZ: Circ. Res. **25** (1969), 781–794
[16] HUI, C. W., H. DRUMMOND and G. I. DRUMMOND: Arch. Biochem. Biophys. **173** (1976), 415–427
[17] JONES, L. R., H. R. BESCH, J. W. FLEMING, M. M. MC CONNAUGHEY and A. M. WATANABE: J. Biol. Chem. **254** (1979), 530–539
[18] JONES, L. R., S. W. MADDOCK and H. R. BESCH: J. Biol. Chem. **255** (1980), 9971–9980
[19] JONES, L. R., S. W. MADDOCK and D. R. HATHAWAY: Biochim. Biophys. Acta **641** (1981), 242–253
[20] KIRCHBERGER, M. A. and T. ANTONETZ: J. Biol. Chem. **257** (1982), 5685–5691
[21] KIRCHBERGER, M. A. and T. ANTONETZ: Biochem. Biophys. Res. Commun. **105** (1982), 152–156

[22] KRAUSE, E.-G., H. WILL, B. SCHIRPKE and A. WOLLENBERGER: Adv. Cyclic Nucl. Res. **5** (1975), 473–490
[23] LAMERS, J. M. J. and J. T. STINIS: Biochim. Biophys. Acta **624** (1980), 443–449
[24] LAMERS, J. M. J. and J. T. STINIS: Biochim. Biophys. Acta **640** (1981), 521–534
[25] LAMERS, J. M. J., J. T. STINIS and H. R. DE JONGE: FEBS lett. **127** (1981), 139–143
[26] LAMERS, J. M. J. and J. T. STINIS: In: Adv. Myocardiology (Eds. V. CHAZOV, V. N. SMIRNOV and N. S. DHALLA) vol. **3** (1982), 289–297
[27] LAMERS, J. M. J. and J. T. STINIS: Proc. 4th Eur. Meeting Int. Soc. Heart Research, Bologna, Italy (1983), in the press
[28] LANGER, G. A.: J. Mol. Cell. Cardiol. **12** (1980), 231–239
[29] LE PEUCH, C. J., J. HAIECH and J. G. DEMAILLE: Biochemistry **18** (1979), 5150–5157
[30] LI, H. C., K.-I. HSIAO and W. W. S. CHAN: Eur. J. Biochem. **84** (1978), 215–225
[31] ST. LOUIS, P. J. and P. V. SULAKHE: Arch. Biochem. Biophys. **198** (1979), 227–240
[32] MISSELWITZ, A.-I., H. WILL, W. SCHULZE, L. WILL-SHAHAB and A. WOLLENBERGER: Biochim. Biophys. Acta **553** (1979), 197–212
[33] MUALLEM, S. and S. J. D. KARLISH: Biochim. Biophys. Acta **597** (1980), 631–636
[34] REEVES, J. P., and J. L. SUKTO: Science **208** (1980), 1461–1464
[35] RINALDI, M. L., C. J. LE PEUCH and J. G. DEMAILLE: FEBS lett. **129** (1981), 277–281
[36] RUITENBEEK, W.: J. Neurol. Sci. **41** (1979), 71–80
[37] STULL, J. T.: Adv. Cyclic Nucl. Res. **13** (1980), 39–93
[38] SULAKHE, P. V., N. L. K. LEUNG and P. J. St. LOUIS: Can. J. Biochem. **54** (1976), 438–445
[39] SULAKHE, P. V. and P. J. St. LOUIS: Progr. Biophys. Molec. Biol. **35** (1980), 135–195
[40] TADA, M. and A. M. KATZ: Annu. Rev. Physiol. **44** (1982), 401–423
[41] WALSH, D. A., M. S. CLIPPINGER, S. SIRKRAMAKRISHNAN and T. E. MC CULLOUGH: Biochemistry **18** (1979), 871–877
[42] WALSH, M. P., C. J. LE PEUCH, B. VALLET, J. C. CAVADORE and J. G. DEMAILLE: J. Mol. Cell. Cardiol. **12** (1980), 1091–1101
[43] WILL, H., T. S. LEVCHENKO, D. O. LEVITSKY, V. N. SMIRNOV and A. WOLLENBERGER: Biochim. Biophys. Acta **543** (1978), 175–193
[44] WOLLENBERGER, A. and H. WILL: Life Sciences **22** (1978), 1159–1178
[45] WOLLENBERGER, A., H. WILL and E.-G. KRAUSE: in: Rec. Adv. Cardiac Struct. Metabol. (Eds. A. Fleckenstein and N. S. Dhalla), University Park Press, Baltimore, vol. **5** (1975), 81–93
[46] YANG, S.-D., J. R. VAN DEN HEEDE, J. GORIS and W. MERLEVEDE: J. Biol. Chem. **255** (1980), 11759–11767

Central Institute of Heart and Circulation Research, Academy of Sciences of the GDR, 1115 Berlin-Buch, GDR, and All-Union Research Center of Cardiology, Academy of Medical Sciences of the USSR, Moscow, USSR

Subunit Analysis and Cross-Linking of Phospholamban in Cardiac Sarcoplasmic Reticulum and Sarcolemma

H. WILL, T. LEVCHENKO and C. KEMSIES

Introduction

A substrate for cyclic AMP-dependent protein kinase in cardiac SR was first described by TADA et al. [12]. The protein was named phospholamban and its M_r was estimated as 22,000. A close functional association of phospholamban and Ca^{2+}-ATPase in cardiac SR was demonstrated by the same authors [4, 11]. Subsequent work by LE PEUCH et al. [6] revealed that phospholamban is a substrate also for a membrane-bound Ca^{2+}- and calmodulin-dependent protein kinase and that the molecule easily dissociates into two halves of M_r 11,000 when SDS and Triton X-100 were present simultaneously. A disintegration into subunits of somewhat smaller size (M_r 9,000) was reported to occur during heat treatment of the SDS-solubilized phosphoprotein (5). A phosphoprotein similar or identical to phospholamban was found also in fragments of cardiac SL [5].

The present work provides a detailed examination of various molecular forms of phospholamban. The analysis is extended to protein species that appear on cross-linking of phospholamban with the bifunctional reagent DTBPI.

Materials and methods

[γ-^{32}P] ATP of specific activity 5—10 C_i/mmole and N-succinimidyl 3-(4-hydroxy, 5-[^{125}I]iodophenyl) propionate (Bolton-Hunter-Reagent) of specific activity 2,000 C_i/mmole were purchased from the Radiochemical Center Amersham, England. Cyclic AMP, ATP and reagents for polyacrylamide gel electrophoresis were from Serva, Heidelberg, BRD. Dimethyl 3,3'-dithiobispropionimidate hydrochloride was synthesized according to [8].

Fragmented SR [3] and fragmented SL [13] were prepared from dog heart ventricle. Catalytic subunit of cyclic AMP-dependent protein kinase was isolated from bovine heart [7] and calmodulin was purified from pig brain [1]. Membranes were phosphorylated as described previously [14] in the absence or in the presence of either 0.5 μM calmodulin together with 0.1 mM $CaCl_2$ or 0.5 μM catalytic subunit or both. Before electrophoresis phosphorylated membranes were solubilized in 5% SDS, 1% β-mercaptoethanol, 0.1 mM EDTA, 50 mM H_3PO_4 adjusted to pH 6.8 with Tris. Iodination of phosphorylated and non-phosphorylated membranes was carried out in 0.5% SDS, 50 mM $NaHCO_3$, 0.05 mM EDTA, pH 6.8, as recommended by SHING and RUOHO [9].

When membranes were phosphorylated for cross-linking experiments, phosphorylated reactions were stopped with a 20-fold volume of ice-cold 0.12 M KCl, 50 mM Hepes, pH 8.0. Membranes were sedimented in a Beckman L 8 centrifuge at 100,000 × g for

40 min. They were subsequently washed with 50 mM Hepes, pH 8.0, and suspended in the same buffer at a protein concentration of 1 mg/ml. DTBPI was added to a final concentration of 10 mM and the cross-linking reaction was allowed to proceed for 1 h at 4 °C. Thereafter unreacted DTBPI was inactivated by adding one tenth the volume of 1 M Tris-HCl, pH 8.0. Polyacrylamide gel electrophoresis was performed in the SDS-urea-system of SWANK and MUNKRES [10] with 12% acrylamide and an acrylamide/N,N'-methylbisacrylamide ratio of 30:1. Following electrophoresis gels were sliced and counted by liquid scintillation spectrometry. Alternatively, gels were stained with Coomassie brilliant blue, destained, dried and autoradiographed with ORWO HS 90 film for 1 to 6 days. Autoradiograms were scanned with a Shimadzu CS 910 dual wavelength scanner.

Results

Heat dissociation of phospholamban

Figure 1 demonstrates the separation of SR phosphoproteins in polyacrylamide gels containing SDS and urea. One major phosphopolypeptide of M_r 6,000 is apparent from autoradiographic pictures when SR membranes were phosphorylated for short time inter-

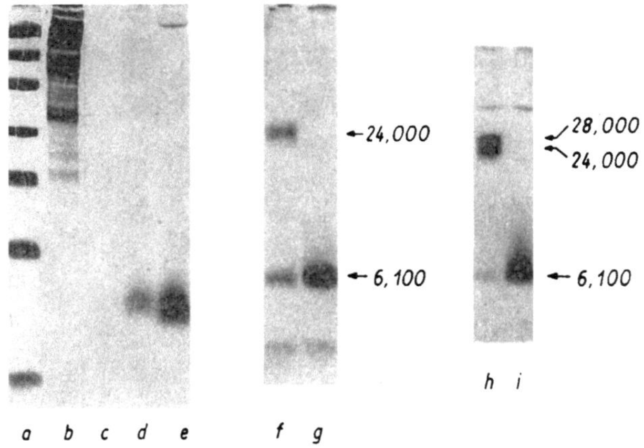

Fig. 1. Electrophoresis of phosphorylated SR in. SDS-urea-polyacryl-amide gels: Coomassie blue staining (b) and autoradiography (c—i). SR membranes were phosphorylated for 90 sec in the presence or absence of 0.1 mM $CaCl_2$, 0.5 μM calmodulin and 0.5 μM catalytic subunit. They were heated in the solubilization solution for 1 min either at 37 °C (lanes f and h) or at 100° (all other lanes). About 50 μg membrane protein was applied per lane.

a) Marker proteins: Phosphorylase b (94,000), serum albumin (67,000) ovalbumin (43,000), carbonic anhydrase (30,000), soybean trypsin inhibitor (20,100), lactalbumin (14,400), glucagon (3,480). Cytochrome c (12,500) and aprotinin (6,500) were used as additional markers (not shown). b) and c) Membranes phosphorylated in the absence of calmodulin and catalytic subunit. d) Membranes phosphorylated in the presence of Ca^{2+} and calmodulin. e) Membranes phosphorylated in the presence of catalytic subunit. f—i) Membranes phosphorylated in the presence of Ca^{2+}, calmodulin, and catalytic subunit.

vals and when they were heated in SDS-solution at 100 °C before electrophoresis. Phosphorylation of the polypeptide is catalyzed both by an endogenous Ca^{2+}- and calmodulin-dependent protein kinase and by added catalytic subunit. A second intense streak of radioactivity appears, when membranes were solubilized at 37 °C rather than at 100 °C (Fig. 1f). While in most experiments the corresponding protein exhibits a M_r of about 24,000, values of about 20,000 and 28,000 have also repeatedly been noted. In few experiments two phosphorylated protein species of M_r 20,000 and 24,000 (Fig. 4) or 24,000 and 28,000 (Fig. 1h) are present together with the 6,000 M_r phosphopolypeptide in the same gel.

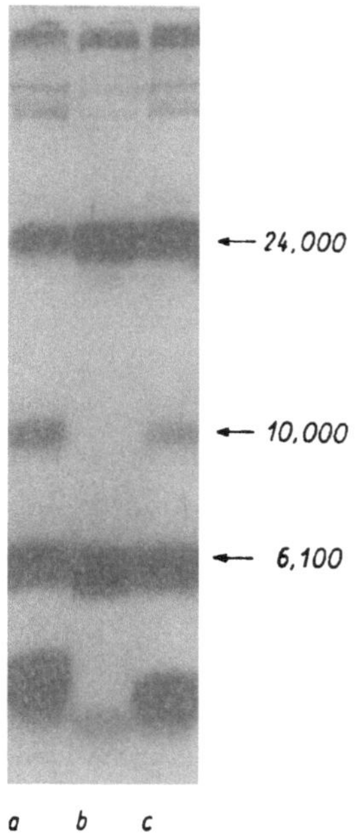

Fig. 2. Phosphoproteins in cardiac SL and SR. SL and SR membranes were phosphorylated for 90 sec in the presence of 0.5 μM catalytic subunit. Solubilization of phosphorylated membranes was performed at room temperature.
a) phosphorylated SL (80 μg), b) phosphorylated SR (20 μg), c) mixture of phosphorylated SL (50 μg) and phosphorylated SR (12 μg).

Phosphoproteins of M_r 6,000 and 24,000 are contained also in fragments of cardiac SL (Fig. 2). The sarcolemmal proteins are phosphorylated by added catalytic subunit and by endogenous Ca^{2+}- and calmodulin-dependent protein kinase. A distinct sarcolemma-bound substrate of cyclic AMP-dependent protein kinase exhibits a M_r of about 10,000. The latter protein is apparently not present in cardiac SR.

The SR phosphoproteins of M_r 20,000, 24,000, and 28,000, which will be referred to as phospholamban oligomers, and the SL phosphoprotein of M_r 24,000 share one property in common: They disappear at higher solubilization temperature. There occurs a rather abrupt change in the relative proportions of ^{32}P-radioactivity bound to the 20–28,000 M_r proteins and to the 6,000 M_r polypeptide within a narrow range of temperature. When membranes were phosphorylated for 90 sec in the presence of Ca^{2+}, calmodulin, and catalytic subunit, the transition temperature ranges between 60° and 70 °C (Table 1). Below this temperature interval a higher amount of ^{32}P-phosphate is associated with the 20–28,000 M_r proteins, while at more elevated temperature radioactivity is found exclusively at a position of the gel corresponding to the 6,000 M_r

Table 1

Effect of temperature on the dissociation of cardiac membrane phosphoprotein (M_r 24000) in SDS-solution

Isolated SR and isolated SL were phosphorylated for 90 sec in the presence of 0.5 μM catalytic subunit, 0.5 μM calmodulin, and 0.1 mM $CaCl_2$. Before electrophoresis solubilized membrane proteins were heated 1 min at the various temperature indicated. The amounts of phosphate incorporated into individual protein species were calculated from radioactivity values of respective gel slices.

Solubilization temperature	Sarcoplasmic reticulum nmoles P_i/mg membrane protein			Sarcolemma nmoles P_i/mg membrane protein			
	6,000-protein	24,000-protein	6,000-protein / 24,000-protein	6,000-protein	10,000-protein	24,000-protein	6,000-protein / 24,000-protein
37°	0.33	1.12	0.29	0.09	0.05	0.13	0.69
50°	0.43	1.02	0.42	0.09	0.05	0.12	0.83
60°	0.62	0.86	0.62	0.14	0.02	0.13	1.08
70°	1.12	0.29	3.86	0.25	0.04	0	∞
80°	1.40	0	∞	0.25	0.04	0	∞
90°	1.40	0	∞	0.24	0.04	0	∞
100°	1.40	0	∞	0.23	0.04	0	∞

polypeptide. The amount of ^{32}P-labeled 10,000 M_r phosphoprotein of SL changes only slightly with heat treatment.

The heat dissociation of phospholamban oligomers is readily reversed by a freezing step. When phosphorylated membranes are solubilized at 100 °C, then frozen, thawed and kept at room temperature before and during electrophoresis, phospholamban oligomers and the 6,000 M_r phosphopolypeptide are present again in comparable amounts (experiments not shown). The conclusion appears justified that one is dealing with a dissociation phenomenon rather than with proteolytic degradation (see also [5]).

Radioiodination of phospholamban

Since the 6,000 M_r phosphopolypeptide is not stained with Coomassie blue an attempt was made to label this as well as other polypeptides of cardiac SR with N-succinimidyl 3-(4-hydroxy, 5-[^{125}I]iodophenyl)-propionate (Fig. 3). A comparison of Figure 1b with Figures 3b and 3e demonstrates that several low molecular weight polypeptides, which are not revealed by the protein stain, are indeed visualized after their derivatization with Bolton-Hunter-Reagent. Unfortunately the phosphopolypeptide of M_r 6,000, which may contain few reactive amino groups only, is labeled to a very low extent. It can hardly be distinguished from neighbouring polypeptides incorporating much more ^{125}I-radioactivity. To further differentiate the phosphopolypeptide from other polypeptides use was made of the relative stability of phospholamban oligomers in SDS-solution. The experimental procedure was as follows: SR membranes were phosphorylated, solubilized at room temperature and subjected to a first gel electrophoresis. After electrophoresis a segment containing phospholamban was cut out from the gel. Proteins included in the segment were extracted and labeled with Bolton-Hunter-Reagent. They were then heated at 100 °C and loaded onto a second gel. The distribution of protein-associated ^{125}I-iodine label in the second gel is shown in Figure 3f and in Figure 4. As can be seen from the autoradiogram and the densitometric scan most of the ^{125}I-radioactivity is

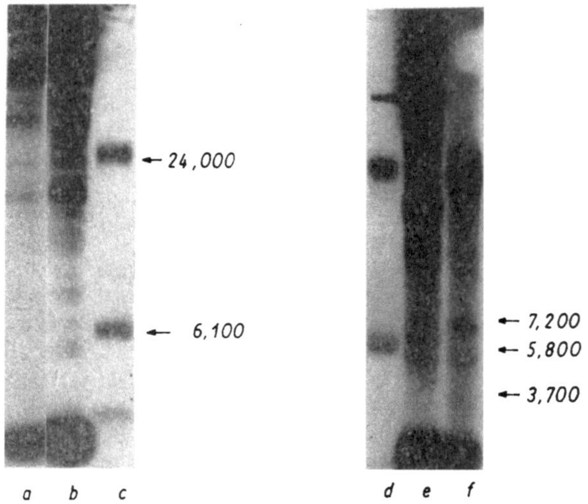

Fig. 3. Labeling of SR proteins with N-succinimidyl 3-(4-hydroxy, 5-[^{125}I]iodophenyl)-propionate.
Iodination of total membrane protein (lanes a, b, and e): Following a 5 min phosphorylation in the presence of 6 mM ATP, 0.1 mM $CaCl_2$, 0.5 μM calmodulin, and 0.5 μM catalytic subunit, SR membranes were solubilized in 0.5% SDS, 50 mM $NaHCO_3$, 0.05 mM EDTA, pH 6.8. A 40 μl aliquot of the solubilization mixture, containing 2 to 6 μg of membrane protein was reacted with Bolton-Hunter-Reagent and either 1 μg (lanes a and b) or 2 μg protein (lane e) were separated by electrophoresis. The exposition time of lane a was 1 day, while lanes b and c were exposed 4 and 6 days, respectively. Iodination of extracted membrane proteins (lane f): SR membranes were phosphorylated as above. They were solubilized at room temperature and subjected to a first gel electrophoresis. Thereafter proteins of M_r 18,000 to 30,000 were extracted with 0.5% SDS, 50 mM $NaHCO_3$, 0.05 mM EDTA, pH 6.8. They were labeled with Bolton-Hunter-Reagent, heated at 100 °C, and subjected to a second electrophoresis. Labeling of phospholamban with ^{32}P-phosphate was carried out in the presence of Ca^{2+} and calmodulin (lane c) or in the presence of catalytic subunit (lane d). Before electrophoresis phosphorylated membranes were solubilized at 37 °C.

bound to proteins of M_r between 18,000 and 30,000. These proteins had been extracted together with phospholamban oligomers from the gel segment selected after the first electrophoretic run. Radioactivity is found in addition, at positions of the gel corresponding to proteins of higher and lower M_r. The lower M_r-proteins are supposed to be derived from phospholamban. The iodinated polypeptide of M_r 5,800 is identical with the phospholamban subunit, that is phosphorylated by Ca^{2+}- and calmodulin-dependent and by cyclic AMP-dependent protein kinases. This polypeptide can likewise be identified from the distribution of ^{32}P-phosphate after reelectrophoresis of ^{32}P-labeled phospholamban oligomers (experiments not shown). The polypeptide moves during reelectrophoresis of extracted phospholamban slightly faster than it moves during electrophoresis of a total membrane mixture. By contrast, proteins of M_r 3,700 and 7,200 cannot be labeled with ^{32}P-phosphate. The possibility then exists that these two proteins represent non-phosphorylatable subunits of phospholamban.

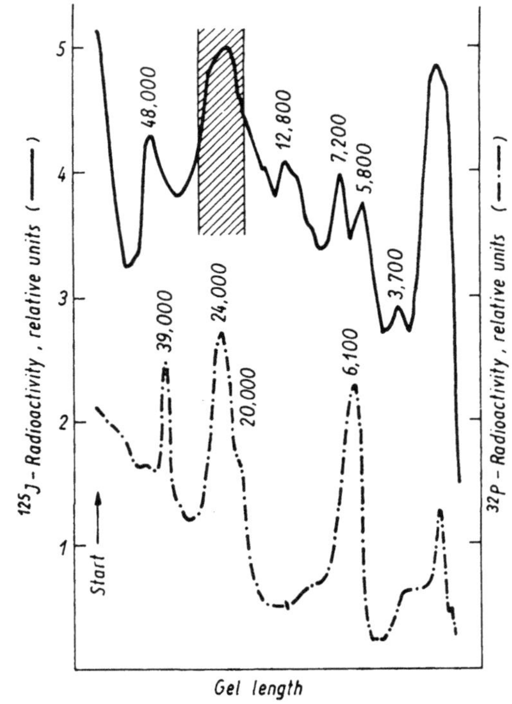

Fig. 4. Densitometric scans of autoradiograms d (·—·—·—) and f (————) from Fig. 3.
The shadowed area corresponds to the segment cut out from the first electrophoretic gel. The ^{32}P-labeled protein of M_r 39,000 is the catalytic subunit of cyclic AMP-dependent protein kinase. For further explanations see legend to Fig. 3.

It should be emphasized that prior phosphorylation of SR membranes (with ATP) is a prerequisite to observe the pattern of iodinated proteins shown in Figures 2f and 3. With non-phosphorylated membranes proteins of M_r 18,000 to 30,000 move to identical positions in repeated electrophoresis. No additional protein species of lower M_r could be detected in respective autoradiograms. It is assumed that SDS easily dissociates non-phosphorylated phospholamban even at room temperature. There are no oligomeric structures of M_r 20—28,000 present in the first gel. There are instead the dissociated subunits of smaller size.

Cross-linking of phospholamban subunits

When phosphorylated SR membranes were incubated with DTBPI, a distinct phosphoprotein of M_r 9,800 appears in addition to the 6,000 M_r phosphopolypeptide (Fig. 5). The newly formed structure is built from the 6,000 M_r phospholamban subunit and a second subunit. DTBPI links both components covalently. The cross-linked complex is broken up again by reduction of the disulfite bond with in the cross-linker molecule (Fig. 5d).

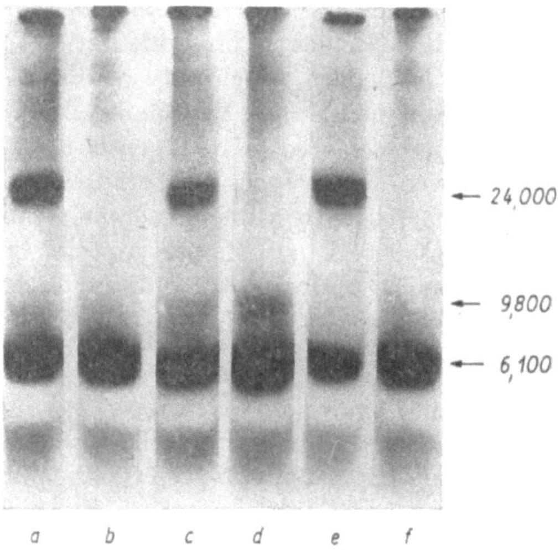

Fig. 5. Cross-linking of phospholamban subunits in SR.
SR membranes were phosphorylated as in Fig. 1d. Phosphorylated membranes were washed and incubated in the absence (lanes a and b) and presence (lanes c—d) of 10 mM DTBPI. Before electrophoresis membranes were solubilized at 37 °C (a, c, e) or 100 °C (b, d, f) in 5% SDS, 0.1 mM EDTA, 50 mM H_3PO_4, pH 6.8, containing (e, f) or not containing 1% β-mercaptoethanol (a—d).

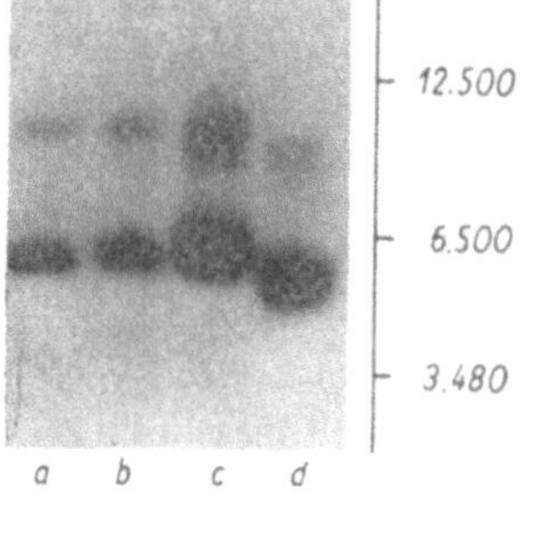

Fig. 6. Cross-linking of phosphoproteins in cardiac SL and SR. Membranes were phosphorylated for 90 sec in the presence of 0.5 μM catalytic subunit. They were washed and incubated in the absence (lane a) and presence (lanes b, c, d) of 10 mM DTBPI. Before electrophoresis membranes were heated 1 min at 100 °C in 5% SDS, 0.1 mM EGTA, 50 mM H_3PO_4, pH 6.8.

a) and b) phosphorylated SL (130 μg), c) mixture of phosphorylated SL (130 μg) and phosphorylated SR (65 μg), d) phosphorylated SR (65 μg).

Figure 6 demonstrates that the phosphoprotein species formed upon exposure of phosphorylated SR to DTBPI exhibits a M_r similar to the 10,000 M_r phosphoprotein of cardiac SL.

Discussion

When biological membranes are solubilized with increasing amounts of detergent conditions are finally reached under which completely delipidated detergent-protein complexes appear along with detergent-lipid mixed micelles. Complete removal of lipid in no way, however, guarantees that single copies of protein exist in solution. Very often residual protein-protein interactions persist, which may or may not have relevance to the proteins native environment in membranes. Phospholamban is one example of a membrane protein that is not easily dissociated by detergents. If solubilization of dog heart membranes with SDS is carried out at room temperature, phospholamban exhibits M_r-values between 20,000 and 28,000. Only at higher temperatures the protein aggregates dissociate and give rise to a 6,000 M_r phosphopolypeptide. It is this polypeptide that is phosphorylated both by cyclic AMP-dependent and by Ca^{2+}/calmodulin-dependent protein kinases.

The behavior of phospholamban in SDS-solution raises two questions:

1. Are the protein species of M_r 20—28,000 homooligomers consisting only of polypeptides of M_r 6,000 or are they heterooligomers built from the 6,000 M_r polypeptide and other hitherto non-identified polypeptides. The latter polypeptides, if they exist, are apparently not prone to phosphorylation.
2. Do phospholamban oligomers really exist in native membranes or should they be regarded solubilization artefacts?

There are no ready answers to both questions. With regard to subunit structure, the present experiments suggest, that phospholamban oligomers might be composed of different types of subunits. This interpretation is based mainly on the experiments with DTBPI: The phosphorylatable subunit of M_r 6,000 is cross-linked to a second subunit of apparently smaller size. There are no protein complexes of M_r higher than 10,000 formed during cross-linking. The formation of such complexes would be expected, if phospholamban oligomers were composed of identical subunits. Furthermore, in experiments, in which phospholamban oligomers were first labeled with ^{125}I-iodine and then dissociated, protein species of M_r 3,700 and 7,200 have been detected in addition to the 6,000 M_r polypeptide. The possible presence of a subunit exhibiting a M_r of about 4,000 may be anticipated also from the M_r values of the three oligomeric forms of phospholamban (20,000, 24,000, and 28,000).

The evidence in favor of a heteropolymeric structure of phospholamban is, however only circumstantial. The M_r of an oligomer as estimated by SDS-polyacrylamide gel electrophoresis must not necessarily equal the sum of molecular weights of the constituting subunits [2]. In the iodination experiments artefacts arising from proteolytic degradation cannot be excluded. Final conclusions about the possible presence of different types of subunits in phospholamban oligomers must await then isolation of phospholamban and subunit analysis of the isolated protein.

Cross-linking experiments are also relevant to the arrangement of proteins in native membranes. It has been demonstrated here that DTBPI links the 6,000 M_r phosphopolypeptide to a second polypeptide. Both polypeptides should be regarded as direct neighbors in membranes of SR. In pursuing this line with a variety of cross-linkers it should be possible to find out all proximate neighbors of the 6,000 M_r phosphopolypeptide. This will allow a more precise answer to the question whether or not phospholamban oligomers exist in native membranes.

A 6,000 M_r phosphopolypeptide and a 24,000 phosphoprotein have also been found in cardiac SL. The two protein species exihibit properties similar to those of phospholamban oligomer and phospholamban subunit in SR. Phosphorylation of both protein species is catalyzed by added cyclic AMP-dependent and by endogenous Ca^{2+}/calmodulin-dependent protein kinases. Heat dissociation of the 24,000 M_r phosphoprotein results in formation of the 6,000 M_r phosphopolypeptide. The amount of ^{32}P-phosphate incorporated into both proteins in SL membranes is, however, much less than the amount of ^{32}P-phosphate incorporated into phospholamban in SR (Table 1). These differences might be intrinsic. They might reflect different levels of prephosphorylation of protein kinase substrates in membranes of SR and SL, respectively. In view of the high purity of the sarcolemmal preparation [13] it is unlikely that the 24,000 M_r and the 6,000 M_r phosphoproteins revealed in these membranes belong to contaminating fragments of SR.

SL membranes contain in addition to the 6,000 M_r and the 24,000 M_r phosphoproteins several other protein kinase substrates that are not present in fragments of SR. The most prominent among them is a protein of M_r 10,000. The protein is phosphorylated by added catalytic subunit. Catalysis by the membrane-bound Ca^{2+}/calmodulin-dependent protein kinase is only little effective. The SDS-solubilized phosphoprotein is not degraded to a significant extent during heat treatment (Table 1). The latter two properties suggest that the 10,000 phosphoprotein is not related to the 6,000 M_r and the 24,000 M_r phosphoproteins. Attention is called, however, to the observation that in SR a phosphoprotein of M_r 9,800 is formed from the 6,000 M_r phosphoprotein by cross-linking. Further experiments are needed to examine possible relationships between the sarcolemmal phosphoprotein of M_r 10,000 and the phosphoprotein appearing upon cross-linking in SR.

Acknowledgment

We thank Dr. P. Westermann from the Central Institute of Molecular Biology, Academy of Sciences of the GDR, for the gift of DTBPI and helpful suggestions.

References

[1] Burgess, W. H., D. K. Jemiolo and R. H. Kretsinger: Biochim. Biophys. Acta **623** (1980) 257–270
[2] Chrambach, A. and D. Rodbard: Science **172** (1971) 440–451
[3] Harigaya, S., and A. Schwartz: Circul. Res. **25** (1969) 781–794
[4] Kirchberger, M. A., M. Tada and A. M. Katz: J. Biol. Chem. **249** (1974) 6166–6173
[5] Lamers, J. M. J. and J. F. Stinis: Biochim. Biophys. Acta **624** (1980) 443–459
[6] LePeuch, C. J., J. Haiech and J. G. Demaille: Biochemistry **18** (1979) 5150–5157
[7] Peters, K. A., J. G. Demaille and E. H. Fischer: Biochemistry **16** (1977) 5691–5697

[8] RUOHO, A., P. A. BARTLETT, A. DUTTON and S. J. SINGER: Biochem. Biophys. Res. Commun. **63** (1975) 417–423
[9] SHING, Y. W. and A. RUOHO: Anal. Biochem. **110** (1981) 171–175
[10] SWANK, R. T. and K. D. MUNKRES: Anal. Biochem. **39** (1971) 462–477
[11] TADA, M., M. A. KIRCHBERGER, D. I. REPKE and A. M. KATZ: J. Biol. Chem. **249** (1974) 6174–6180
[12] TADA, M., M. A. KIRCHBERGER and A. M. KATZ: J. Biol. Chem. **250** (1975) 2640–2647
[13] VETTER, R., H. HAASE and H. WILL: FEBS letters **148** (1982) 326–330
[14] WILL, H., T. S. LEVCHENKO, D. O. LEVITSKY, W. N. SMIRNOV and A. WOLLENBERGER: Biochim. Biophys. Acta **543** (1978) 175–193

IV. Metabolic aspects of myocardial ischaemia

Experimental Cardiology Section, Department of Physiology, Faculty of Medicine, University of Manitoba, Winnipeg, Canada R3E 0W3

Myocardial Membrane Changes Due to Ischaemia-Reperfusion Injury in Dogs Treated With or Without Acebutolol

V. Panagia, J. A. C. Harrow, G. Singh, A. Guerin and N. S. Dhalla

Numerous experimental studies have revealed contractile, metabolic and ultrastructural alterations due to myocardial ischaemia and have reported further cardiac derangements if the reperfusion is instituted after a certain period of coronary occlusion depending upon the animal species [1, 4, 21, 27, 29, 33–35]. Since sarcolemma, sarcoplasmic reticulum and mitochondria, due to their abilities to regulate intracellular calcium, are considered to play an important role in heart function [6, 7, 11], it is conceivable that the ischaemic-reperfusion injury may be associated with disturbances in the functions of these membrane systems. It is therefore the purpose of this study to investigate changes in different membrane systems during myocardial ischaemia as well as after reperfusion of the ischaemic myocardium. In view of the fact that β-adrenergic blocking agents including acebutolol have been shown to reduce ischaemic-reperfusion damage [5, 21, 36], the effects of acebutolol on membrane changes due to myocardial ischaemia and reperfusion were also examined.

Materials and methods

Twenty four mongrel dogs weighing 17 to 24 kg were anesthetized with sodium pentothal (25 mg/kg) intravenously and given artificial respiration throughout the experiment. The anesthesia was maintained by 0.5% halothane, lateral thoractomy was performed to expose the heart, and the left anterior descending artery was dissected for placing silk ligature [5]. Animals were injected saline (untreated) or 5 mg/kg acebutolol (acebutolol-treated) intravenously 5 min before coronary occlusion. Myocardial ischaemia in these groups was induced by occluding the artery for 90 min whereas reperfusion was carried out for 60 min by relieving the coronary ligature after 90 min of coronary occlusion. The control animals in the untreated and acebutolol-treated groups were kept under similar experimental conditions for 90 to 150 min except that the coronary artery was not occluded. The control or ischaemic area of the left ventricle was removed for the isolation and purification of sarcolemmal, mitochondrial and sarcoplasmic reticular membranes according to the procedures described earlier [32]. The methods for the determination of adenylate cyclase, ATPases, calcium accumulation and oxidative phosphorylation activities were the same as reported previously [32]. Use of marker enzymes and inhibitors of some enzyme activities [32] revealed that these membrane fractions were cross contaminated by 2–5% but the degree of contamination in any given fraction was similar in different experimental groups. The results were statistically analyzed by using the Student's "t" test.

Results

The data concerning sarcolemmal changes due to 90 min ischaemia as well as 60 min reperfusion following 90 min ischaemia in untreated and acebutolol treated animals are given in Table 1. Myocardial ischaemia in the untreated animals decreased Na^+—K^+ ATPase activity without changing adenylate cyclase, Mg^{2+} ATPase and Ca^{2+}-dependent ATPase (Ca^{2+}-ATPase) activities. A further depression in Na^+—K^+ ATPase and significant decreases in adenylate cyclase, Mg^{2+} ATPase and Ca^{2+}-ATPase activities were seen in reperfused ischaemic hearts. Acebutolol treatment of the animals was observed

Table 1

Sarcolemmal enzyme activities in ischaemic-reperfused hearts of dogs with or without acebutolol (5 mg/kg) treatment

Preparation	Adenylate cyclase activity (pmol cyclic AMP/mg/min)	ATPase activity (μmol P_i/mg/hr)		
		Mg^{2+} ATPase	Na^+-K^+ ATPase	Ca^{2+}-ATPase
A. **Untreated:**				
Control	270 ± 13	16.2 ± 1.3	9.8 ± 0.7	15.2 ± 1.2
Ischaemic	282 ± 15	15.2 ± 1.5	6.1 ± 0.6*	14.8 ± 1.1
Reperfused	143 ± 17*	12.1 ± 0.6*	3.6 ± 0.9*	11.2 ± 0.7*
B. **Acebutolol Treated:**				
Control	264 ± 15	15.4 ± 0.9	10.5 ± 0.9	15.0 ± 0.8
Ischaemic	255 ± 14	16.1 ± 1.2	8.6 ± 0.5	15.3 ± 0.9
Reperfused	201 ± 11*	14.0 ± 0.8	5.9 ± 0.7*	13.0 ± 1.2

Each value is a mean ± S.E. of 4 experiments. Myocardial ischaemia was induced by occluding the coronary artery for 90 min whereas reperfusion of the ischaemic hearts was carried out for 60 min by removing the occlusion.
* Significantly different from the respective control values ($P < 0.05$)

to fully prevent depression in Na^+—K^+ ATPase activity due to ischaemia as well as in Mg^{2+} ATPase and Ca^{2+}-ATPase activities due to reperfusion. The reperfusion-induced depression in adenylate cyclase and Na^+—K^+ ATPase activities were partially prevented by acebutolol treatment.

Table 2 shows the effect of myocardial ischaemia and reperfusion on calcium binding (studied in the absence of a permeant ion), calcium uptake (studied in the presence of 5 mM oxalate), Mg^{2+} ATPase and Ca^{2+}-stimulated Mg^{2+} dependent ATPase (Ca^{2+}-stimulated ATPase) activities of the sarcoplasmic reticular fraction. Sarcoplasmic reticular calcium binding, calcium uptake and Ca^{2+}-stimulated ATPase activities, unlike Mg^{2+} ATPase activity, were significantly decreased by ischaemia in untreated group and were further depressed upon reperfusion. Treatment of animals with acebutolol completely prevented ischaemic-induced changes and partially prevented reperfusion-induced changes in the calcium transport system of the sarcoplasmic reticulum.

Table 2

Sarcoplasmic reticular calcium transport activities in ischaemic-reperfused hearts of dogs with or without acebutolol (5 mg/kg) treatment

Preparation	Calcium accumulation (nmol/mg/5 min)		ATPase activity (μmol P_i/mg/5 min)	
	Binding	Uptake	Mg^{2+}-ATPase	Ca^{2+}-stimulated ATPase
A. **Untreated**				
Control	66 ± 4.5	1800 ± 205	5.0 ± 0.5	2.4 ± 0.2
Ischaemic	42 ± 3.1*	1209 ± 151*	4.7 ± 0.6	1.5 ± 0.1*
Reperfused	18 ± 2.5*	574 ± 78*	4.8 ± 0.4	0.6 ± 0.1*
B. **Acebutolol Treated**				
Control	56 ± 4.1	1680 ± 170	5.9 ± 0.3	2.1 ± 0.3
Ischaemic	44 ± 3.4	1450 ± 50	5.4 ± 0.2	1.7 ± 0.2
Reperfused	36 ± 2.7*	1076 ± 140*	5.1 ± 0.4	1.3 ± 0.2*

Each value is a mean ± S.E. of 4 experiments. Myocardial ischaemia was induced by occluding the coronary artery for 80 min whereas reperfusion of the ischaemic hearts was carried out for 60 min by removing the occlusion.
* Significantly different from the respective control value ($P < 0.05$)

Table 3

Mitochondrial calcium transport and ATPase activities in ischaemic-reperfused hearts of dogs with or without acebutolol (5 mg/kg) treatment

Preparation	Calcium accumulation (nmol/mg/5 min)		ATPase activity (μmol P_i/mg/5 min)
	Binding		Uptake
A. **Untreated**			
Control	31 ± 2.7	220 ± 17	11.2 ± 0.9
Ischaemic	20 ± 1.6*	213 ± 21	10.9 ± 0.7
Reperfused	47 ± 3.4*	328 ± 26*	10.7 ± 1.1
B. **Acebutolol treated**			
Control	29 ± 3.1	207 ± 15	10.7 ± 0.8
Ischaemic	25 ± 2.5	199 ± 13	10.3 ± 1.4
Reperfused	34 ± 2.7	216 ± 18	9.8 ± 1.0

Each value is a mean ± S.E. of 4 experiments. Myocardial ischaemia was induced by occluding the coronary artery for 90 min whereas reperfusion of the ischaemic heart was carried out for 60 min by removing the occlusion.
* Significantly different from the respective control value ($P < 0.05$)

The results in Tabel 3 indicate that myocardial ischaemia decreased mitochondrial calcium binding (studied in the absence of a permanent ion) without any changes in calcium uptake (studied in the presence of 5 mM P_i and 5 mM succinate) or ATPase activities. On the other hand, mitochondrial calcium binding and calcium uptake activities, unlikely ATPase activity, were significantly increased in reperfusion hearts. These ischaemic and reperfusion-induced changes in mitochondrial calcium transport were completely prevented by acebutolol treatment (Table 3). Mitochondrial ADP: 0 ratio, respiratory control index (RCI) and oxygen consumption (QO_3) were decreased by ischaemia and were further depressed by reperfusion (Table 4). These alterations in mitochondrial oxidative phosphorylation activities due to ischaemia and reperfusion were fully prevented by acebutolol treatment (Table 4).

Table 4

Mitochondrial oxidative phosphorylation activity in ischaemic-reperfused hearts of dogs with or without acebutolol (5 mg/kg) treatment

Preparation	ADP:0 ratio	RCI	Oxygen consumption in state 3 (natom/mg/min)
A. **Untreated**			
Control	2.9 ± 0.2	6.5 ± 0.3	200 ± 9.8
Ischaemic	2.5 ± 0.1*	4.1 ± 0.2*	142 ± 4.2*
Reperfused	1.4 ± 0.3*	2.5 ± 0.3*	102 ± 3.6*
B. **Acebutolol treated**			
Control	3.1 ± 0.2	7.1 ± 0.4	208 ± 11.4
Ischaemic	2.9 ± 0.2	6.9 ± 0.3	192 ± 10.5
Reperfused	2.7 ± 0.2	6.8 ± 0.2	196 ± 10.8

Each value is a mean ± S.E. of 4 experiments. Myocardial ischaemia was induced by occluding the coronary artery for 90 min whereas reperfusion of the ischaemic hearts was carried out for 60 min by removing the occlusion.
* Significantly different from the respective control values ($P < 0.05$)

Discussion

In this study we have demonstrated that myocardial ischaemia in dogs for a period of 90 min decreased sarcolemmal Na^+-K^+ ATPase activity, sarcoplasmic reticular calcium transport activities and mitochondrial calcium binding and oxidative phosphorylation activities. These changes in sarcolemmal Na^+-K^+ ATPase, sarcoplasmic reticular calcium transport and mitochondrial oxidative phosphorylation activities were further attenuated whereas the ability of mitochondria to bind and accumulate calcium was markedly increased upon reperfusing the 90 min ischaemic myocardium for a period of 60 min. Since the myocardial cell damage due to 90 min of ischaemia in dog heart induced by occlusion of the left anterior descending coronary artery has been shown to increase further upon 60 min of reperfusion [27], it is possible that the observed membrane changes may represent biochemical indices for irreversible injury in the ischaemic myocardium. It is also likely that the observed membrane alterations may be involved in the molecular mechanisms for further deterioration of heart function as well as for the genesis of arrhythmias upon reperfusion under the experimental conditions of ischaemia similar to those employed in this study [5, 27]. The observed membrane changes may be due to activation of phospholipase, proteases and lysosomal enzymes during the ischaemic-reperfusion injury [6, 7]. While the ischaemic changes can be conceived to be the consequence of both substrate-lack or oxygen-lack [2, 17, 19], the reperfusion-induced changes may result from the occurrence of intracellular calcium overload [8, 18] as similar alterations have been observed under these experimental conditions.

It was interesting to note that 90 min of ischaemia decreased sarcolemmal Na^+-K^+ ATPase activity without any alterations in adenylate cyclase, Mg^{2+} ATPase and Ca^{2+}-ATPase activities. Depressed sarcolemmal Na^+-K^+-ATPase activity in ischaemic heart disease has also been observed by other investigators [3, 10, 15]. Such a change in the sarcolemmal pump may explain the commonly observed increase in the intracellular Na^+ and loss in the intracellular K^+ from the ischaemic myocardium. Furthermore, it may also account for the occurrence of intracellular calcium overload indirectly due to Na^+-Ca^{2+} exchange mechanism in the cell membrane [7]. Depression in sarcoplasmic reticular calcium binding as well as calcium pump activities and mitochondrial calcium binding in 90 min ischaemic myocardium can also be conceived to participate in the occurrence of intracellular calcium overload. Such observations will help in explaining the inability of the myocardium to relax fully as well as the elevated diastolic tension during prolonged myocardial ischaemia.

Reports in the literature concerning the effect of ischaemic-reperfusion injury on the cardiac sarcoplasmic reticular calcium transport are conflicting [9, 13, 16, 22, 25, 31]. In this study our results indicate a marked defect in the ability of sarcoplasmic reticulum to handle calcium since calcium binding, calcium uptake and Ca^{2+}-stimulated ATPase activities were depressed in both ischaemic and reperfused hearts. Such a defect cannot be accounted for by the presence of some inert protein in the experimental preparations since Mg^{2+} ATPase activity was not altered and the marker enzyme studies revealed an equal degree (2—5%) of cross contamination in the control and experimenta- membranes. This effect on the sarcoplasmic reticulum was different from that on mitochondria because only mitochondrial calcium binding was decreased in the ischaemic hearts whereas both mitochondrial calcium binding and uptake activities were increased in the reperfused myocardium. The observed increase in mitochondrial calcium binding and uptake activities upon reperfusion may be an adaptive mechanism for relieving the cell from the intracellular calcium overload under ischaemic-reperfusion conditions and in fact may account for the impaired ability of the mitochondria to generate energy through a depression in the oxidative phosphorylation activities under ischaemic-reperfusion conditions [14, 23, 30, 34].

The results presented in this study have revealed that pretreatment of animals with a cardioselective β-adrenergic blocking agent, acebutolol, prevented the changes in various membrane functions due to myocardial ischaemia. Furthermore, this agent was capable of fully preventing all the reperfusion-induced membrane changes except those in sarcolemmal adenylate cyclase and Na^+-K^+ ATPase as well as sarcoplasmic reticular calcium pump activities, which were prevented partially. Although endogenous catecholamines are known to be released during myocardial ischaemia-reperfusion injury [20, 26], it cannot be stated with certainty whether the beneficial effects of acebutolol are primarily due to its β-adrenergic blocking activity. Since formation of free radicals during myocardial ischaemia-reperfusion [12] as well activation of membrane disrupting enzymes have been proposed to play a central in the genesis of myocardial cell damage [7], it is possible that the beneficial effects of acebutolol and other β-adrenergic agents for myocardial ischaemic-reperfusion injury may also be due to their actions on such sites.

Summary

Myocardial ischaemia induced by occluding the left anterior coronary artery for 90 min in dogs depressed sarcolemmal Na^+-K^+ ATPase, sarcoplasmic reticulum calcium binding, calcium uptake and Ca^{2+}-stimulated ATPase as well as mitochondrial calcium binding and oxidative phosphorylation activities. Reperfusion of the ischaemic hearts for 60 min further attenuated the changes in sarcolemmal Na^+-K^+ ATPase, sarcoplasmic reticular calcium transport and mitochondrial oxidative phosphorylation activities. Sarcolemmal adenylate cyclase, Mg^{2+}-ATPase and Ca^{2+}-ATPase activities were also decreased but mitochondrial calcium binding and calcium uptake activities were increased upon reperfusing the ischaemic myocardium. All these membrane alterations due to ischaemic-reperfusion injury were fully prevented by treatment of animals with acebutolol except that only partial prevention was observed with respect to changes in sarcolemmal Na^+-K^+ ATPase and adenylate cyclase as well as sarcoplasmic reticular calcium transport activities. These results suggest that changes in sarcolemmal Na^+-K^+ ATPase and sarcoplasmic reticular calcium pump mechanism mayplay an important role in the irreversible ischaemic-reperfusion injury and β-adrenergic agents such as acebutolol may be helpful in ischaemic heart disease due to their ability to protect membrane changes.

Acknowledgments

This research was supported by a grant from the Manitoba Heart Foundation. Dr. G. SINGH was a Visiting Professor from the Department of Pharmacology, Lady Hardinge Medical College, New Delhi, India.

References

[1] ASHRAF, M., F. WHITE and C. M. BLOOR: Am. J. Pathol. **90** (1978), 423–434

[2] BALASUBRAMANIAN, V., D. B. MCNAMARA, J. N. SINGH and N. S. DHALLA: Can. J. Physiol. Pharmacol. **51** (1973), 504–510

[3] BELLER, G. A., J. CONROY and T. W. SMITH: J. Clin. Invest. **57** (1976), 341–350

[4] BIXLER, T. J., J. T. FLAHERTY, T. J. GARDNER, B. H. BULKLEY, H. V. SCHAFF and V. L. GOTT: Circulation 58, Suppl. 1 (1978), 184–193

[5] CHERNECKI, W., P. K. DAS, N. S. DHALLA and G. P. SHARMA: Br. J. Pharmac. **64** (1978), 265–272

[6] DHALLA, N. S., P. K. DAS and G. P. SHARMA: J. Mol. Cell. Cardiol. **10** (1978), 363–385

[7] DHALLA, N. S., G. N. PIERCE, V. PANAGIA, P. K. SINGAL and R. E. BEAMISH: Basic Res. Cardiol. **77** (1982), 117–139

[8] DHALLA, N. S., J. N. SINGH, D. B. MCNAMARA, A. BERNATSKY, A. SINGH and J. A. C. HARROW: In Myocardial Injury, ed. by J. J. Spitzer, Plenum Publishing Corporation, in press (1983).
[9] FEHER, J. J., F. N. BRIGGS and M. L. HESS: J. Mol. Cell. Cardiol. **12** (1980), 427–432
[10] GODIN, D. V., J. M. TUCHEK and M. MOORE: Can. J. Biochem. **58** (1980), 777–786
[11] HESS, M. L.: Circ. Shock **6** (1979), 119–136
[12] HESS, M. L., N. H. MANSON and E. IKABE: Can. J. Physiol. Pharmacol. **60** (1982), 1382–1389
[13] HESS, M. L., M. F. WARNER, A. D. ROBBINS, S. CRUTE and L. J. GREENFIELD: Cardiovasc. Res. **25** (1981), 390–397
[14] KANE, J. J., M. L. MURPHY, J. K. BISSETT, N. DE SOYZA, J. E. DOHERTY and K. D. STRAUB: Am. J. Cardiol. **36** (1975), 218–224
[15] KOBAYASHI, Y., Y. SASAI, N. NAKAMURA and T. KATAGIRI: Jap. Circ. J. **45** (1981), 1256–1263
[16] LEE, K. S., H. LADINSKY and J. H. STUCKEY: Circ. Res. **21** (1967), 439–444
[17] LEE, S. L., V. BALASUBRAMANIAN and N. S. DHALLA: Can. J. Physiol. Pharmacol. **54** (1976), 49–58
[18] LEE, S. L. and N. S. DHALLA: Am. J. Physiol. **231** (1976), 1159–1165
[19] MUIR, J. R., N. S. DHALLA, J. M. ORTEZA and R. E. OLSON: Circ. Res. **26** (1970), 429–438
[20] NADEAU, R. A., and J. DE CHAMPLAIN: Am. Heart J. **98** (1979), 548–554
[21] NAYLER, W. G., R. FERRARI and A. WILLIAMS: Am. J. Cardiol. **46** (1980), 242–248
[22] NAYLER, W. G., J. STONE, V. CARSON and D. CHIPPERFIELD: J. Mol. Cell. Cardiol. **2** (1971), 125–143
[23] PENG, C. F., J. J. KANE, K. D. STRAUB and M. L. MURPHY: J. Cardiovasc. Pharmacol. **2** (1980), 45–54
[24] REIMER, K. A., R. B. JENNINGS and M. L. HILL: Circ. Res. **49** (1981), 901–911
[25] SCHWARTZ, A., J. M. WOOD, J. C. ALLEN, E. P. BORNET, M. L. ENTMAN, M. A. GOLDSTEIN, L. A. SORDAHL and M. SUZUKI: Am. J. Cardiol. **32** (1973), 46–61
[26] SHAHAB, L., A. WOLLENBERGER, M. HAASE and V. SCHILLER: Acta Biol. Med. Germ. **22** (1969), 135–143
[27] SHARMA, G. P., K. G. VARLEY, S. W. KIM, J. BARWINSKI, M. COHEN and N. S. DHALLA: Am. J. Cardiol. **36** (1975), 234–243
[28] SHEN, A. C. and R. B. JENNINGS: Am. J. Pathol. **67** (1972), 417–440
[29] SHEN, A. C. and R. B. JENNINGS: Am. J. Pathol. **67** (1972), 441–452
[30] SORDAHL, L. A., and M. L. STEWART: Circ. Res. **47** (1980), 814–820
[31] TOBA, K., T. KATAGIRI and Y. TAKEYAMA: Jap. Circ. J. **42** (1978), 447–453
[32] TOMLINSON, C. W., S. L. LEE and N. S. DHALLA: Circ. Res. **39** (1976), 82–92
[33] VASDEV, S. C., G. P. BIRO, R. NARBAITZ and K. J. KAKO: Can. J. Biochem. **58** (1980), 1112 to 1119
[34] WEISHAAR, R., K. ASHIKAWA and R. J. BING.: Am. J. Cardiol. **43** (1979), 1137–1143
[35] WEISHAAR, R., G. V. TSCHURTSCHENTHALER, K. ASHIKAWA and R. J. BING: Cardiology **64** (1979), 350–364
[36] ZIEGELHOFFER, A., P. K. DAS, G. P. SHARMA, P. K. SINGAL and N. S. DHALLA: Can. J. Physiol. Pharmacol. **57** (1979), 979–986

Department of Physiology, Medical Faculty of the Technical University, Aachen, FRG

Free Energy of ATP-Hydrolysis as a Limiting Factor of Actin-Myosin Interaction and Ion Pumping in Early Failure of the Heart

H. KAMMERMEIER

The origin of early hypoxic heart failure is still enigmatic. This is already indicated by various hypotheses which were put forward to explain this phenomenon. The main question raises from the fact, that failure occurs if ATP-levels are only slightly or moderately diminished, i.e. by about 20% as compared to the well oxigenated state [1, 11, 15, 19]. On the other hand, under certain conditions, ATP-reduction by 50 to 70% is tolerated without signs of failure [7, 8, 11, 15]. Thus most authors postulated a hypothetical small ATP compartment which provides the energy supply for the contractile proteins [9, 11, 24]. Others postulated that electro-mechanical coupling is failing at various steps [17, 18, 22]. Earlier concepts pointed at the rather good relationship of phosphocreatine breakdown and hypoxic failure, however, causal relationship is contradicted by the fact that phosphocreatine is not the direct substrate of the contractile system.

Our approach was based on the fact that ATP yields very different amounts of energy as defined by the formula of Gibb's free energy or more correctly by a differential term of free energy change or affinity, respectively [5, 6].

$$\Delta G(dG/d\xi) = \Delta G^0_{obs} + R \cdot T \cdot \ln \frac{[ATP]}{[ADP] \cdot [P_i]} \tag{1}$$

$$\Delta G^0_{obs} = 30.5 \text{ kJ} \cdot \text{mol}^{-1}$$

As can be seen from the formula, hydrolysis of ATP reduces the numerator and increases the denominator due to higher concentrations of the split products ADP and inorganic phosphate; even a small extent of the ATP splitting causes marked changes of this ratio, i.e. of the mass action ratio. This is all the more effective as the ratio deviates from unity. In fact the ratio amounts to about 10.000 if true cytostolic concentrations are considered. Thus free energy of ATP-hydrolysis amounts to about 50 to 60 kJ/mol or 12—14 kcal/mol as calculated for example in equation (2).

$$\begin{aligned} dG/d\xi &= 30.500 + 2.577 \cdot \ln \frac{8 \cdot 10^{-3}}{4 \cdot 10^{-9} \cdot 2 \cdot 10^{-1}} \\ &= 54.200 \text{ J} \cdot \text{mol}^{-1} \end{aligned} \tag{2}$$

Most recent estimations of free energy of ATP-hydrolysis agree with these values [5, 23, 26, 50]. This is also in keeping with the fact that isolated mitochondria are capable of synthesizing ATP up to an energy level of 67 kJ/mol [25].

Our approach attempted to find answers for three questions:

- what are the energy levels required for the most important energy consuming processes,
- what are the energy levels of APT-hydrolysis, particularly during the early hypoxic heart failure and,
- is there any mismatch between both?

There are two major groups of energy requiring processes in the myocardium which are directly involved in cardiac function; these are ion pumping mechanisms and the contractile system, i.e. the actomyosin ATPase.

The energy requirement of ion pumping can be calculated according to the formula given in Table 1. It contains the well known osmotic and electric term. We calculated the energy requirement of the three main ion pumping processes of the myocardium, that is, sodium-potassium-ATPase, sarcolemmal Ca^{2+}-ATPase, and sarcoplasmic Ca^{2+}-ATPase. The Table shows that a membrane potential of 90 mV and a concentration ratio of 40 to 1 for potassium results in a small energy requirement for potassium transport of 0.8 kJ/mol. This corresponds to the fact the membrane potential is close to the potassium equilibrium potential. A ratio of 1 to 10 for sodium results in about 14.6 kJ/mol. Including the generally accepted coupling ratio of 3 to 1 a Figure of 46.3 kJ or 11.1 kcal results, which one mol of ATP should provide for maintaining ion pumping. For sarcolemmal Ca^{2+} transport via Ca^{2+}-ATPase the calculation yields about 41 kJ/mol assuming a coupling ratio of 1:1. A higher coupling ratio does not seem to be possible. In contrast, in sarcoplasmic reticulum a coupling ratio of 2:1 is well documented [10]. This ratio seems also possible because of the missing membrane potential. The energy requirement with this coupling ratio results in about 44 kJ/mol or 10.5 kcal/mol

Table 1

Free energy of transmembrane gradients of ions

$$\Delta G = R \cdot T \ \ln \frac{C_i}{C_e} + Z \cdot F \cdot \Delta\Psi$$

R = Gas const.; T = abs. temp.; $C_{i,e}$ = Ion-conc. intra/extracell.; Z = charge; F = Faraday const.; $\Delta\Psi$ = Membrane potential.

	$\Delta\Psi$ mV	C_i/C_e	ΔG kJ/mol	$\Sigma\Delta G$ kJ(kcal)/mol	ATP
Sarcolemma					
K^+	90	40:1	0.8		
Na^+	90	1:10	14.6		
($3K^+/3Na^+$/ATP)				46.3	(11.1)
Sarcolemma					
Ca^{2+}	90	$1:10^4$	41	41.2	(9.8)
(1 Ca^{2+}/ATP)					
Sarcoplas. Ret.					
(2 Ca^{2+}/ATP)	?	$0.5:10^4$	22	43.9	(10.5)

respectively, if an intrasarcoplasmic concentration of 0.5 mM is assumed as estimated by ENDO [cf. 6].

The estimation of energy requirements of the actomyosin ATPase is more difficult, since the various intermediate steps of energy transduction are still hypothetical, particularly with respect to their thermodynamics. There are earlier estimates indicating an energy level of 45 kJ or 10.5 kcal per mol, respectively. But only more recent investigations of DAWSON, GADIAN and WILKIE [5], under utilization of phosphorus nuclear magnetic resonance measurements, yielded direct values on the energy requirement of the frog muscle contractile system.

According to these results the force of contraction of an isolated frog muscle (at 0 °C) very strongly depends on the available free energy. The force of contraction decreases with reduction of free energy and approaches zero in the range of 43 kJ/mol. This corresponds to about 45 kJ/mol at 37 °C. Thus when all processes are considered, the actomyosin ATPase and the transport processes together require energy at a level of 42 to 46 kJ/mol ATP.

The second question raised initially concerned the available free energy of ATP-hydrolysis. The calculation seems simple, however, real cytosolic concentrations are needed. These can be calculated fairly well for ATP and inorganic phosphate, from tissue content using well known data on myocyte compartmentation [27]. However, the cytosolic ADP concentration is lower by about one order of magnitude than tissue content as a consequence of protein binding of ADP and thus cannot be easily calculated from compartmentation data. This problem can not be overcome by NMR-methods either, since free cytosolic ADP-concentrations are below the detection limits. Therefore, all groups interested in cytostolic ADP-concentrations use the creatine kinase equilibrium equation.

$$K_{CK} = \frac{[ATP] \cdot [Cr]}{[ADP] \cdot [PCr] \cdot [H^+]} \quad (3)$$

$$ADP = \frac{[ATP] \cdot [Cr]}{[PCr] \cdot [H^+] \cdot K_{CK}} \quad (4)$$

This approach has the advantage that phosphocreatine and creatine, which are easily estimated without major problems of binding and compartmentation are used for calculation. The disadvantage of introducing H^+-concentration is of minor importance provided that the intracellular H^+-ion concentration remains approximately constant as in our experiments, that is under hypoxic perfusion (4).

The value of equilibrium constant of the creatine kinase was sometimes a matter of discussion since values of $1.5 \cdot 10^8$ to $2 \cdot 10^9$ were used in the literature. However, as described elsewhere [27] all data indicate for physiological conditions (pH and $[Mg^{2+}]$) a value close to 10^9.

The basis of this approach is the existence of equilibrium conditions for the creatine kinase. But, there is general agreement that in cardiac muscle and under most conditions in skeletal muscle as well, deviation from equilibrium can be neglected [3, 5, 6, 12, 20, 21, 23].

The existence of equilibrium conditions for the creatine kinase reaction includes some other interesting aspects. Figure 1 shows a graph of the equation of Gibb's free energy

$$dG/d\xi = -\Delta G^0_{obs} + R \cdot T \cdot \ln \frac{[ATP]}{[ADP] \cdot [P_i]} \qquad dG/d\xi = -\Delta G^0_{obs} + R \cdot T \cdot \ln \frac{[PC]}{[Cr] \cdot [P_i]}$$

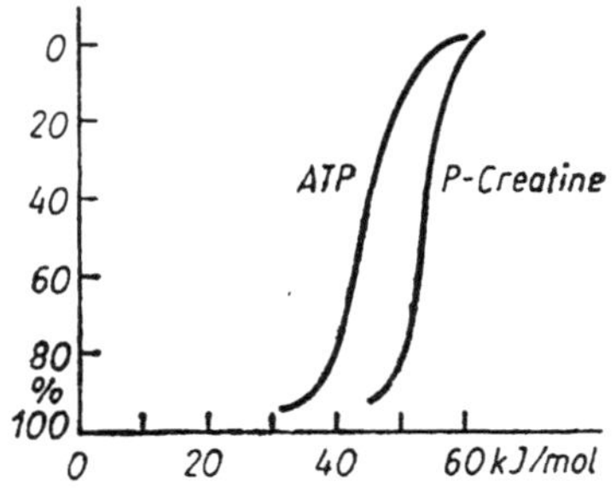

Fig. 1. Relationship between free energy (change) of ATP and phosphocreatine hydrolysis and extent of hydrolysis in a closed system. For calculation physiological, cytosolic concentrations and ΔG^0_{obs} of 30.5 and 43 kJ · mol^{-1} resp. were used.

(change), i.e. the relationship between free energy of ATP hydrolysis and phosphocreatine, respectively and the corresponding extent of hydrolysis. The graphs were calculated using normal cytosolic concentrations of the metabolites involved, but no secondary reactions were included. The curves are very similar to buffer dissociation curves. This, however, could be expected from the respective equations, where ΔG corresponds to pH and ΔG^0_{obs} to pK. One can argue that the ATP-system actually buffers the energy level in the range of 9—11 kcal or 40 to 50 kJ respectively and phosphocreatine in the range of 50 to 60 respectively. The more interesting aspect is that most of the energy of the ATP-system can only be used in the range mentioned. In the physiological range or the range above the needs of the main energy consuming processes, in other words above 46 kJ/mol, the ATP-system can provide only less than half of its total energy content. Thus, if only about 30% of ATP are split, the energy level runs the risk to be lower than required.

In contrast, the free energy of phosphocreatine can be used almost completely in the physiological range. The most interesting aspect results from the fact that equilibrium of the creatine kinase reaction includes that both the ATP-system and the phosphocreatine system are at the same energy level. Thus the different course of phosphocreatine and ATP breakdown in anoxia can be easily explained: If ATP supply ceases and ATP consumption continues, the ATP-system is kept or buffered respectively at a high energy level at the cost of the phosphocreatine system. A distinct ATP-reduction cannot be expected before phosphocreatine is split almost completely. But in this stage the energy level already falls in the range required. Thus from these considerations the metabolic pattern during early hypoxic failure, that is, small reduction of ATP levels and almost complete consumption of phosphocreatine, are throughout compatible with an insufficient energy level.

Our experiments concerning this question were made in isolated perfused rat hearts the mechanical performances of which were recorded in two ways: first by measurement of left intraventricular pressure, and second by estimating force changes developed at the apex with a semi-isometric setup.

The hearts were paced electrically at a rate of 240 or 270/min, respectively. In addition after every twentieth beat a potentiated beat was induced by paired stimulation.

Anoxia was achieved by switching from oxygen/CO_2 gased Krebs-Ringer-medium to a nitrogen/CO_2-gased medium.

The mechanical effects of anoxia in our preparations are shown in Figure 2 (left part). During the first minute of anoxia the systolic pressure decreases by about 50% and thereafter this decrease continues up to the fifth min. Similar changes in performance appear in force of regular beats potentiated by paired stimulation (Fig. 2, lower left). The latter seems of interest, since postextrasystolic potentiation is explained by increased Ca^{2+}-loading of the SR [2]. These findings indicate that major

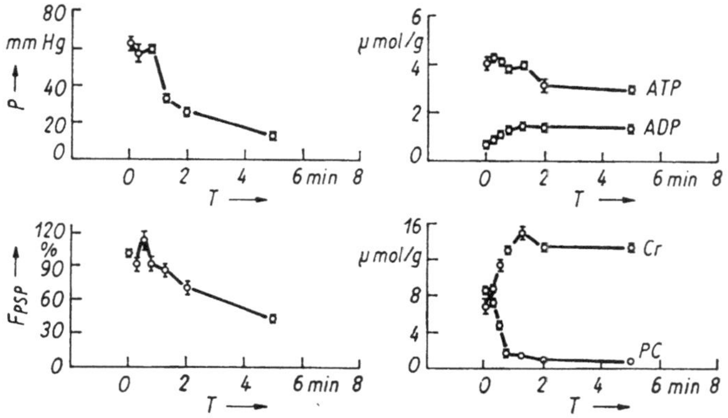

Fig. 2. Mechanical performance and metabolite content of isolated rat hearts during 5 min anoxic perfusion. ($\bar{x}$: ± SEM; N: 5 to 7)

changes of Ca^{2+}-loading of SR do not occur during early anoxia. To obtain additional information on excitation contraction coupling the effect of bolus application of increased extracellular Ca^{2+} was tested. Administration of a 6 mM Ca^{2+}-bolus increases peak systolic pressure, but the extent of increase is almost the same during five min of anoxic perfusion. This observation also indicates that major changes in excitation-contraction coupling do not occur in this phase of anoxic perfusion.

The metabolite content of the hearts was assayed after freeze stop fixation of the hearts and perchloric acid extraction by high performance liquid chromatography [14]. Figure 2 (right part) demonstrates the well known metabolic pattern caused by myocardial anoxia, i.e. moderate reduction of ATP content and corresponding increase in ADP. Phosphocreatine breakdown takes place much more rapidly and is almost completed within the first min of anoxia. This is accompanied by a corresponding increase in tissue creatine content. The course of changes in inorganic phosphate concentration (not shown) is very similar to that of creatine.

The course of free energy of ATP-hydrolysis calculated as aforementioned gives no further information with respect to the initial question. It decreases rather rapidly to values between 45 and 50 kJ/mol during the first minute of anoxia and then continues to decrease slowly in all experimental groups.

The results shown here concern only one experimental group of our study, namely that with unmodified Krebs-Ringer-perfusion. For several reasons the same experimental protocol was carried out with lidocaine containing medium, which was used to facilitate electrical pacing in anoxia and in addition with a medium containing lidocaine and

6 mM Ca^{2+}. The course of mechanical and metabolic changes was very similar in all three groups.

The crucial point as to the question of the role of free energy change of ATP-hydrolysis in early hypoxic failure concerns the relationship of free energy and contractile performance. The there graphs of the three experimental groups (Fig. 3) demonstrate that in the range of 50 to 60 kJ/mol contractile performance is almost unchanged. This range corresponds to normoxic conditions and to 15 to 30 sec of anoxia. In the range of

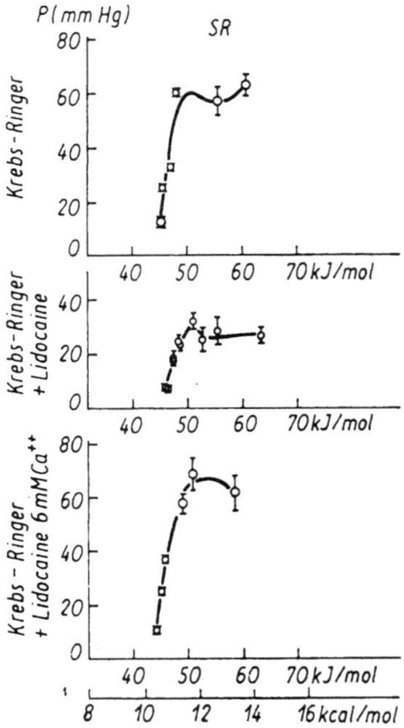

Fig. 3. Free energy (change) of ATP hydrolysis during early hypoxic failure of isolated perfused rat hearts under different experimental conditions. Failure occurs at a level of about 45 kJ · mol^{-1}, i.e. at the level necessary for actomyosin interaction and ion pumping.
($\bar{x}$: ± SEM; N: 5 to 7)

50 to 45 kJ/mol a steep reduction of contractile performance occurs, which can be extrapolated to about 45 kJ/mol for complete cessation of contractile function in all three experimental groups.

As mentioned above the needs for ion pumping is in the range of 42 to 46 kJ/mol and that of the contractile system at 45 kJ/mol. According to these graphs this is the same range, which is reached during early hypoxic failure. Thus, during early hypoxic failure free energy of ATP hydrolysis apparently is reduced to a level, which indicates a real mismatch of the energy levels of supply and demand.

References

[1] ALBERTY, R. A.: In: Horizons of bioenergetics (Ed. A. San Pietro), Howard Gest. N.Y. (1972)
[2] ANTONI, H., R. JACOB and R. KAUFMANN: Pflügers Archiv **306** (1969), 33–57
[3] BEIS, I. E. and E. C. NEWHOLME: Biochem. J. **152** (1975), 23–32
[4] COBBE, S. M. and P. A. POOLE-WILSON: J. Molec. Cellul. Cardiol. **12** (1980), 761–770
[5] DAWSON, M. J., D. G. GADIAN and D. R. WILKIE: Nature **274** (1978), 861–866

[6] Dawson, M. J., D. G. Gadian and D. R. Wilkie: J. Physiol. **299** (1980), 465—484
[7] Feinstein, M. B.: Circul. Res. **10** (1962), 333—346
[8] Giesen, J., R. Müller and H. Kammermeier: Basic Res. Cardiol. **75** (1980), 780—801
[9] Gudbjarnason, S., P. Mathes and K. G. Ravens: J. Molec. Cellul. Cardiol. **1** (1970), 325—339
[10] Hasselbach, W.: Topics in Current Chemistry **78** (1979), 3—56
[11] Hearse, D. J.: Amer. J. Cardiol. **44** (1979), 1115—1121
[12] Hassinen, I. E. and K. Hiltunen: Biochim. Biophys. Acta **408** (1975), 319—330
[13] Isselhard, W.: Pflügers Archiv **271** (1960), 437—460
[14] Jüngling, E. and H. Kammermeier: Analyt. Biochem. **102** (1980), 358—361
[15] Kammermeier, H.: Verhandl. Deutsch. Gesell. Kreislauff. **30** (1964), 206—211
[16] Kammermeier, H. and J. Doering: Pflügers Archiv **274** (1961), 14
[17] Katz, A. M., F. Messineo, J. Miceli and P. A. Nash-Adler: Life Science **28** (1981), 1103 to 1107
[18] Kübler, W. and A. M. Katz: Amer. J. Cardiol. **40** (1977), 467—471
[19] Kübler, W. and P. G. Spieckermann: J. Molec. Cellul. Cardiol **1** (1970), 351—377
[20] McGilvery, R. W. and Th. W. Murray: J. Biol. Chem. **249** (1974), 5845—5850
[21] Mommaerts, W. F. H. M.: Physiol. Reviews **49** (1969), 427—508
[22] Nayler, W. G., P. A. Poole-Wilson and A. Williams: J. Molec. Cellul. Cardiol. **11** (1979), 683—706
[23] Nishiki, K., M. Erecinska and D. F. Wilson: Amer. J. Physiol. **234** (1978), 73—81
[24] Pool, P. E., J. W. Covell, C. A. Chidsey and E. Braunwald: Circul. Res. **19** (1966), 221 to 229
[25] Slater, E. C., J. Rosiny and A. Mol: Biochim. Biophys. Acta **292** (1973), 534—553
[26] Wilson, D. F., K. Nishiki and M. Erecinska: Trends in Biochem. Sci. **6** (1981), 16—19
[27] Kammermeier, H., P. Schmidt and E. Jüngling: J. Molec. Cellul. Cardiol. **14** (1982), (267—278)

Central Institute of Heart and Circulation Research, Academy of Sciences of GDR, Berlin-Buch, GDR, and Department of Biochemistry, University of Bristol Medical School, Bristol, U. K.

Isoproterenol-Induced Protein Phosphorylation in the Isolated, Ischaemic Rat Heart*

E.-G. KRAUSE, P. J. ENGLAND and S. BARTEL

Introduction

During cardiac ischaemia caused by coronary artery ligation *in situ* there is an increase in intracellular cyclic 3′, 5′ adenosine monophosphate (cyclic AMP), which is probably induced by release of catecholamines from sympathetic nerve terminals in the heart (see [16]). In the normally perfused heart catecholamines cause increased Ca^{2+} fluxes leading to increased contractility [12]. This is associated, and may indeed be brought about by increased phosphorylation of membrane and contractile proteins [4, 5, 29, 35]. The contractile proteins troponin I (TN-I) and C-protein are both phosphorylated *in vitro* and *in vivo* by cyclic AMP-dependent protein kinase, while myosin P-light chain is phosphorylated by a specific Ca^{2+}-calmodulin-dependent protein kinase (see [6]). Phospholamban, an 11000 mol weight protein of the sarcoplasmic reticulum, is phosphorylated by a cyclic AMP-dependent as well as Ca^{2+}-calmodulin-dependent protein kinase *in vitro* [13, 22] and possibly *in vivo* [14, 21].

In heart ischaemia and anoxia is characterized by a rapid reduction in contractile response [30], although the intracellular concentrations of ATP and H^+ ions are initially unchanged from the aerobic state [10] and the level of cyclic AMP is elevated [36]. It has been suggested that a reduction in the Ca^{2+}-influx across the sarcolemma may occur during ischaemia and anoxia, which may be correlated with a decrease in the phosphorylation of membrane proteins [28]. A decreased phosphorylation of TN-I was observed in infarcted canine heart muscle [1], whereas according to CUMMINS et al. [2] a 50 per cent increase in the phosphorylation of P-light chain was observed only after 30 min of ischaemia.

The purpose of this study was to investigate wether the reduced contractile response following the onset of ischaemia was reflected in alterations in protein phosphorylation. Furthermore the catecholamine responsivness of the acute ischaemic tissue was studied, as a reduction or loss of cyclic AMP accumulation induced by isoproterenol during acute ischaemia have been recently described [15, 27].

Methods and materials

Hearts from Wistar rats (220—260 g) were perfused by the Langendorff technique using modified Krebs-Henseleit bicarbonate-buffered medium containing 11 mM glucose and gassed with O_2:CO_2 (19:1) [4] at a flow rate (maintained by roller pump) of 12 ml/min. Following a 5 min preperfusion the hearts were perfused with a medium containing

* This research was supported by a grant from the Wellcome Trust of Great Britain

0.5 MBq $^{32}P_i$ per ml for 15 min in a recycling system. The hearts were then switched back to non-radioactive medium for measurement of contractile response for 1 min. Ischaemia was induced by reducing the flow to 0.5 ml/min. For anoxic perfusion the flow rate was kept at 12 ml/min, but the medium was gassed with N_2:CO_2 (19:1). D,L-isoproterenol (70 pmole in 0.15 M NaCl) was injected as a 5 µl bolus into the aortic cannula after various periods of ischaemia as indicated in Figure 1, and the hearts freeze-clamped 20 seconds later. Hearts not injected with isoproterenol were also freeze-clamped at the end of the perfusion. Changes in contractile force were monitored with a force displacement transducer (Ormed Engineering, Welwyn Garden City, Herts, U.K.) attached to the apex of the heart.

Analysis of protein phosphorylation

Samples of frozen hearts were prepared for polyacrylamide gel electrophoresis in the presence of sodium dedecyl sulphate essentially as described by [11]. Electrophoresis was carried out by the method of [18] using either a combination of a 5 and 12.5% gel or a 5—15% gradient gel of polyacrylamide. Following staining with Coomassie Brilliant Blue the gels were dried, and ^{32}P in protein bands determined by densitometric scanning after autoradiography of the gels. The specific radioactivity of ^{32}P-γ-ATP in the frozen hearts was measured as described by [7], and used to correct the densitometric values for each heart.

Metabolites and other assays

Metabolites were assayed spectophotometrically by the following methods: ATP and creatine phosphate according to [20], lactate according to [9]. Cyclic was purified by column chromatography and assayed by protein-binding displacement as described by [15]. The proportion of phosphorylase in the **a** form was assayed according to [4]. Protein was determined by the Biuret method. All data are expressed as mean ± S.E.M (no. of observations).

Results and discussion

Contractile and metabolic responses to ischaemia

The contractile performance of the heart, measured as contractile force, defined as the difference between the developed tension at systole and diastole, rate of relaxation and frequence of beating, all showed a rapid deterioration from the onset of ischaemia, similar to that described by MANNING et al. [23]. As shown in Figure 1 contractile force and rate of relaxation fell to less than 50 per cent of control after 15 s, and thereafter decreased to 25 and less than 10 per cent, respectively, after 4 min. A very similar decrease in these parameters was also observed when hearts were perfused with anoxic medium (data not shown), where the flow rate was maintained at 12 ml/min. The response of these parameters to isoproterenol varied depending on period of ischaemia.

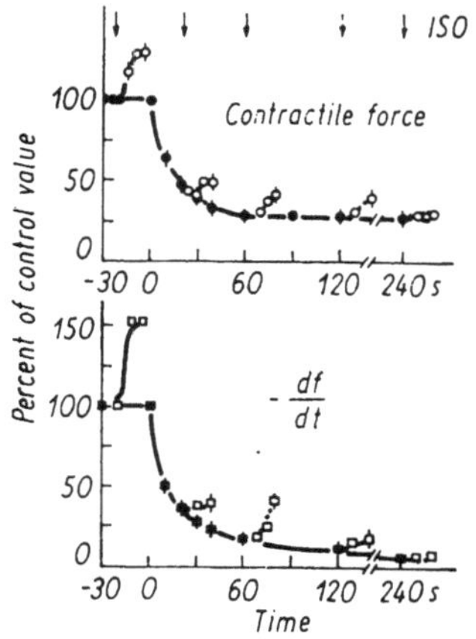

Fig. 1. The effect of ischaemia on the contractile force and relaxation rate of perfused heart, and the response to isoproterenol.
(• , ■) untreated hearts; (○ , □) changes following a bolus injection of isoproterenol.

When isoproterenol was given in the control period, there was an increase in contractile force and rate of relaxation of approximately 30 and 50 per cent, respectively. These response progressively decreased by ischaemia, and were almost completely lost after 4 min. Similar changes were also observed in the frequency of contraction (data not shown).

The intracellular concentration of ATP remained constant throughout the period of ischaemia, at a value of 21.2 ± 0.5 μmol/g protein (n = 95), and was unchanged on injection of isoproterenol (see Fig. 2). The creatine phosphate concentration was 25.6 $\pm$ 2.4 μmol/g protein (n = 10) in control perfusion, but fell rapidly to 9.29 ± 3.1 μmol/g (n = 6) during the first 90 s of ischaemia. There was no further decrease during the subsequent 3.5 min (see Fig. 2). When isoproterenol was injected either to control hearts

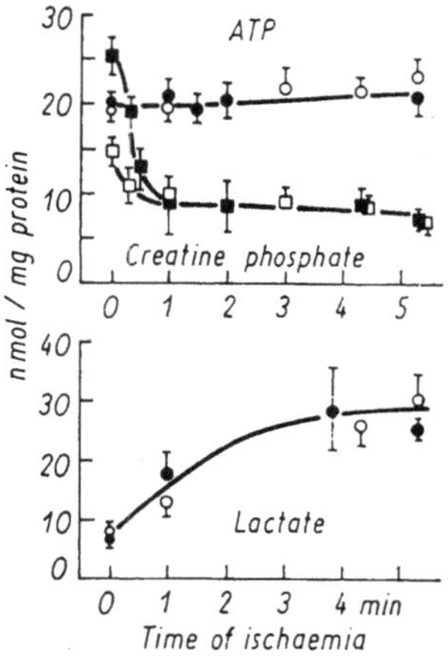

Fig. 2. The effect of ischaemia on the levels of ATP, creatine phosphate, and lactate, and the response to isoproterenol.
For symbols see legend of Fig. 1.

or during the first 40 s of ischaemia the creatine phosphate concentration fell during the 20 s of exposure to catecholamine to 14.8 and 11.4 μmol/g, respectively. At longer periods of ischaemia there was no change in creatine phosphate on exposure to isoproterenol. The total lactate content of control hearts was 8.14 ± 1.4 μmol/g protein (n = 11), which rose to 26.1 ± 3.7 μmol/g (n = 5) during the first 4 min of ischaemia. There was no significant effect of isoproterenol on lactate levels. In preliminary experiments start-

Phosphorylation of proteins during ischaemia

ing a reperfusion of the hearts with a flow rate of 10 ml/min after a period of 5 min of ischaemia, the levels of lactate were normalized (6.39 ± 2.3 μmol/g; $n = 7$) within a period of 80 s.

Three proteins labeled with ^{32}P were selected for measurements in this study: TN-I, myosin P-light chain, and a protein of apparent mol. wt. 11000 (11 K protein). The 11 K protein may be the monomer of phospholamban [21] or a protein of sarcolemmal origin [19, 32, 33] which can be phosphorylated *in situ*. This 11 K protein co-migrated with a ^{32}P-labeled protein present in a cardiac preparation enriched in microsomal or sarcolemmal vesicles (J. Huggins and P. J. England, unpublished data), indicating at least a partial membrane origin. The identities of TN-I and myosin P-light chain were established by co-migration with pure samples of these proteins. The phosphorylation of phosphorylase was calculated from the proportion of the enzyme in the **a** form. Figures 3 and 4 show the effect of ischaemia on the phosphorylation of 11 K protein, TN-I, and phosphorylase. In control perfusions there was a low level of phosphorylation of TN-I, phosphorylase, and the 11 K protein (this was often undectable). Myosin P-light chain showed a substantial phosphorylation of 0.5–0.6 mol of phosphate/mol. Isoproterenol in control perfusion increased the phosphorylation of TN-I, phosphorylase and the 11 K

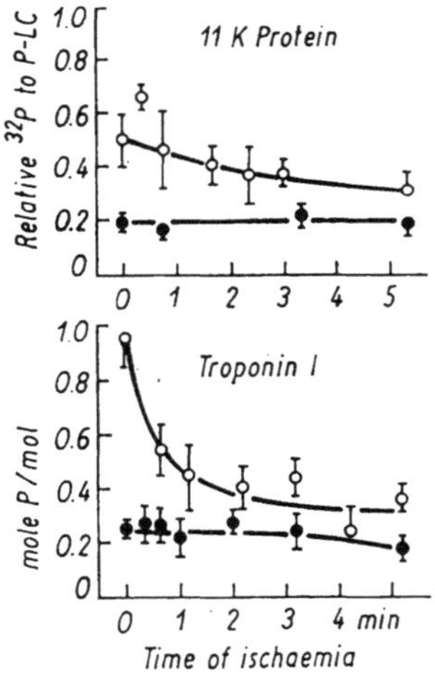

Fig. 3. Phosphorylation of troponin I and a 11 K protein in perfused control and ischaemic rat hearts, and the effect of isoproterenol.
Hearts injected with a bolus of isoproterenol and freeze clamped 20 sec later.
For symbols see legend of Fig. 1.

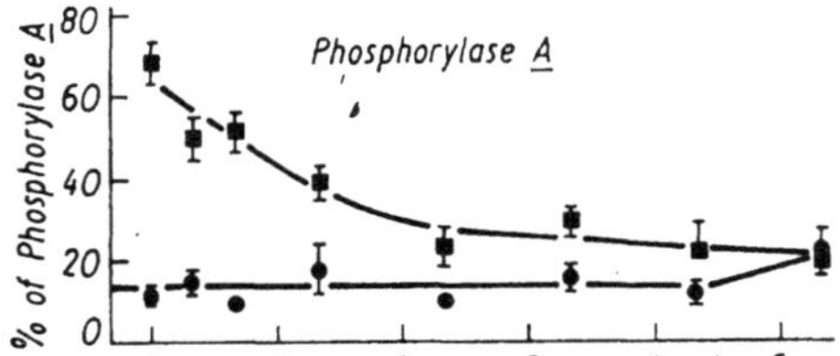

Fig. 4. The effect of ischaemia on the amount of phosphorylase **a** and the effect of isoproterenol.
(●) untreated hearts; (■) hearts injected with a bolus of isoproterenol and freeze clamped 20 sec later (from Krause and England [14]).

protein, but not the myosin P-light chain phosphorylation state. The results on TN-I and P-light chain phosphorylation after administration of catecholamine are in quantitative agreement with previous studies [4, 11, 29].

Ischaemia by itself caused no changes in the phosphorylation of any of the proteins studied. Thus the phosphorylation state of the examined proteins are probably not causally related to the rapid deterioration in contractile performance of the heart following ischaemia. However there was a gradual decrease in the isoproterenol-induced phosphorylation of TN-I, phosphorylase and the 11 K protein with increasing period of ischaemia. There was no significant change in phosphorylation of myosin P-light chain in any of these experiments (data not shown). The decrease in the phosphorylation of TN-I, phosphorylase and 11 K protein is paralleled with the decrease or loss of the responsivness of the acute ischaemic heart to accumulate cyclic AMP induced by isoproterenol [15]. Figure 5 shows the observed correlation between TN-I phosphorylation and the content of cyclic AMP in control and ischaemic hearts with and without exposure to

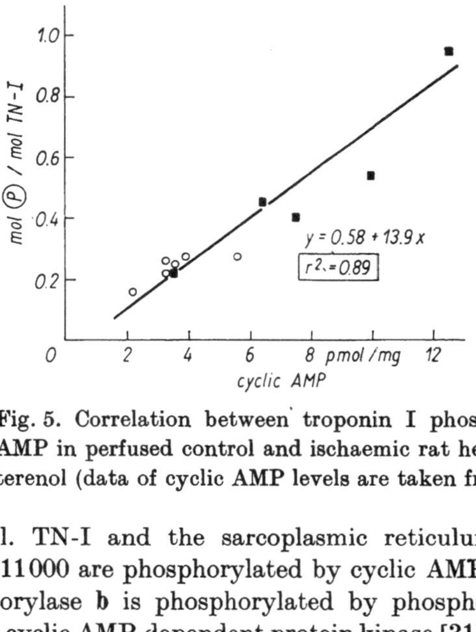

Fig. 5. Correlation between troponin I phosphorylation and the levels of cyclic AMP in perfused control and ischaemic rat hearts after a bolus injection of isoproterenol (data of cyclic AMP levels are taken from [14]).

isoproterenol. TN-I and the sarcoplasmic reticulum and/or sarcolemma protein(s) of mol · wt. 11000 are phosphorylated by cyclic AMP-dependent protein kinase [6, 19, 32]. Phosphorylase **b** is phosphorylated by phosphorylase kinase, whose activity is increased by cyclic AMP-dependent protein kinase [31]. A reduction or loss in the responsivness to isoproterenol at the level of cyclic AMP would therefore be expected to cause a decrease in the phosphorylation of these three proteins, and was observed in the present study. A decrease in cyclic AMP concentration and TN-I phosphorylation with ischaemia has also been reported in dog heart by Antipenko et al. [1].

Myosin P-light chain, since it is phosphorylated by a Ca^{2+}-calmodulin-dependent protein kinase [26], would not be expected to be responsive to changes in cyclic AMP. It has been previously shown [11] that the levels of cardiac P-light chain phosphorylation remain constant during a number of inotropic interventions, including those which raise intracellular Ca^{2+}. Therefore the changes in phosphorylation of this protein as shown by Cummins et al. [2] in heart tissue following a period of 30 min of ischaemia, probably only reflect subsequent alterations of the contractile protein in the heart without physiological relevance.

The isoproterenol-induced rise in cyclic AMP is generally accepted to be the result of an activation of the membrane-bound β-adrenergic receptor/adenylate cyclase system. It is therefore probable that in the ischaemic heart the rapid loss of increased cyclic AMP concentration accompanied by a failure of the subsequent reactions at the level of protein phosphorylation is the result of an inhibition of the receptor/cyclase system, rather than an activation of phosphodiesterase. Studies on isolated membrane preparations have indicated no changes in the β-adrenergic receptor number and their affinity for catecholamines after short periods of ischaemia [24]. The effect of ischaemia on the cyclic AMP synthesis as well as protein phosphorylation is also not explainable by a decrease in the concentration of ATP, as the total tissue concentration was unchanged throughout the studied ischaemic period. The increased inhibition of cyclic AMP accumulation during the fourth and fifth minute of ischeamia was, however, correlated with an increase in lactate concentration. As lactate has been reported to inhibit isolated adenylate cyclase [17], a similar mechanism could be occuring in the intact ischaemic tissue. This suggestion is supported by results demonstration that in anoxic conditions or after a reperfusion of ischaemic hearts the isoproterenol-inducable increase in cyclic AMP was maintained or rapidly restored, respectively (unpublished data).

An alternative explanation for the effect of ischaemia could involve the antiadrenergic action of adenosine [3, 27], which was not measured in this study. Furthermore the effects of ischaemia could involve alterations in adenylate cyclase activity, via changes in the lipid composition of the cell membrane. Adenylate cyclase has been shown [8] to be inhibited by endoperoxides produced during prostaglandin biosynthesis, which may be increased during ischaemia by a stimulated release of arachidonic acid from sarcolemmal phospholipids [25]. A rapid decrease in the activity of adenylate cyclase was recently demonstrated using membrane fractions isolated from ischaemic rat hearts [34].

There is strong evidence that cyclic AMP is connected with serious pathological effects of catecholamine stimulation in the ischaemic heart [16]. The loss or attenuation of isoproterenol-induced cyclic AMP accumulation may thus prevent additional sympathetic stimulation and further deterioration of cardiac function. The significance of phosphorylation and/or dephosphorylation of proteins in this process remains to be clarified. The rapid reduction in contractile response of the acute ischaemic heart, however, seems not to involve an detectable alteration in the phosphorylation of studied proteins: troponin I, myosin P-light chain, and the 11 K protein.

References

[1] ANTIPENKO, A. E., O. G. CHONCHAROV, B. F. OROVIN and V. R. PEPINOVA: Voprosy Med. Khimii **27** (1981), 492–495

[2] CUMMINS, P., R. CROME, D. M. YELLON and D. J. HEARSE: J. Molec. Cellul. Cardiol. **13** (1981), 18

[3] DOBSON, J.: Circul. Res. **43** (1978), 785–792

[4] ENGLAND, P. J.: Biochem, J. **160** (1976), 295–304

[5] ENGLAND, P. J.: In: Recently discovered systems of enzyme regulation by reversible phosphorylation (ed: P. J. Cohen), Elsevier/North-Holland Biomedical Press (1980), 153–170

[6] ENGLAND, P. J., D. MILLS, PASK, H. T. and S. A. JEACOCKE: this volume

[7] ENGLAND, P. J., and D. A. WALSH: Anal. Biochem. **75** (1975), 429–435

[8] GORMAN, R. R., M. HAMBERG and B. SAMUELSSON: J. Biol. Chem. **250** (1975), 6460–6463

[9] Hohorst, H. J., F. H. Kreutz and T. Bücher: Biochem. Z. **332** (1959), 18–29
[10] Jacobus, W. E., I. H. Pores, S. K. Lucas, L. M. Weisfeldt and J. T. Flaherty: J. Molec. Cellul. Cardiol. **14** (1982), Suppl. 3, 13–20
[11] Jeacocke, S. A. and P. J. England: Biochem. J. **188** (1980), 763–768
[12] Katz, A. M.: The Physiology of the Heart, Raven Press, New York (1977)
[13] Katz, A. M.: Cold Spring Harbor Conf. Cell. Prolif. **8** (1981), 849–858
[14] Krause, E.-G. and P. J. England: J. Molec. Cellul. Cardiol. **14** (1982), 611–613
[15] Krause, E.-G. and A. Wollenberger: Adv. Cyclic Nucleotide Res. **12** (1980), 49–61
[16] Krainias, E. G. and R. J. Solaro: Nature **298** (1982), 182–184
[17] Krishna, N., J. Gorsti and G. Krishna: Pharmacologist **15** (1973), 158–162
[18] Laemmli, U. K.: Nature **277** (1970), 680–685
[19] Lamers, J. M. J.: this Volume
[20] Lamprecht, W., P. Stein, F. Heinz and H. Weisser: In: Methoden der enzymatischen Analyse (ed.: H. U. Bergmeyer) Akad. Verlag Berlin (1970), 1734–1737
[21] Le Peuch, C. J., J.-C. Gaillex and J. G. Demaille: FEBS letters **114** (1980), 165–168
[22] Le Peuch, C. J., J. Haiech and J. G. Demaille: Biochemistry **18** (1979), 5150–5157
[23] Manning, A. S., D. J. Hearse, S. C. Dennis, G. R. Bullock and D. J. Coltart: Europ. J. Cardiol. **11** (1980), 1–21
[24] Mukherjee, C., T. M. Wong, L. M. Buja, R. J. Lefkowitz and J. T. Willerson: J. Clin. Invest. **64** (1979), 1423–1428
[25] Owens, K., D. L. Pang and W. B. Weglicki: Biochem. Biophys. Res. Commun. **89** (1979), 368–373
[26] Pires, E. N. V., S. V. Perry and M. A. W. Thomas: FEBS letters **41** (1974), 292–296
[27] Schrader, J., G. Baumann and E. Gerlach: In: Catecholamine and the Heart (ed.: W. Delius, E. Gerlach, H. Grobecker, and W. Kübler), Springer Verlag, Berlin Heidelberg New York (1981), 142–151
[28] Sperelakis, N. and J. A. Schneider: Amer. J. Cardiol. **37** (1976), 1079–1085
[29] Stull, J. T., C. F. Sanford, D. R. Manning, D. K. Blumenthal and C. W. High: Cold Spring Harbor Conf. Cell Prolif. **8** (1981), 823–840
[30] Theroux, P., D. Franklin, J. Ross and W. S. Kemper: Circul. Res. **35** (1974), 896–908
[31] Walsh, D. A., J. P. Perkins, C. O. Brostrom, E. S. Ho and E. G. Krebs: J. Biol. Chem. **246** (1971), 1968–1976
[32] Will, H., T. Levchenko and C. Kemsies: this Volume
[33] Will, H., T. S. Levchenko, D. O. Levitzky, V. N. Smirnov and A. Wollenberger: Biochim. Biophys. Acta **543** (1978), 175–193
[34] Will-Shahab, L. and I. Küttner: this Volume
[35] Wollenberger, A. and H. Will: Life Sciences **22** (1978), 1159–1178
[36] Wollenberger, A., E.-G. Krause and G. Heier: Biochem. Biophys. Res. Commun. **36** (1969), 664–670

Department of Cardiology, Parma University, Parma, Italy

The Functional and Metabolic Consequence of Myocardial Ischaemia and Reperfusion. Effects of Verapamil

R. Ferrari and O. Visioli

Introduction

In this article some of the metabolic and functional changes seen during myocardial ischaemia and reperfusion will be discussed. The experiments have been carried out using isolated Langendorff perfused rabbit's hearts in which the rate of coronary flow can be precisely regulated and held constant. Three different degrees of ischaemia lasting for 30, 60 and 90 minutes have been investigated, after which the effects of post-ischaemic reperfusion have been followed. Relevant to these findings, this review will consider: (1) events during the early stages of ischaemia, (2) events during prolonged period of ischaemia, (3) events on reperfusion in relation to different periods of ischaemia, (4) mitochondria and reperfusion damages, (5) effects of slow Ca^{2+} channel antagonist on the ischaemic and reperfusion damage.

Events during the early stages of ischaemia

During mitochondrial ischaemia the rate of oxygen uptake in the cell decrease considerably. This causes an impairment in the oxidation of mitochondrial NADH or other reduced coenzymes, molecular oxygen being the terminal electron acceptor of the electron transport chain. There is, therefore, a reduction of the passage of electrons to oxygen in the inner mitochondrial membrane, leading to a reduction or abolition of the membrane potential, which according to Mitchell's [15] chemiosmotic hypothesis, is essential for ATP synthesis. The immediate result of this sequence of events is: a reduced or abolished mitochondrial ATP synthesis and an accumulation of metabolic products which cannot be oxidised completely to CO_2 and H_2O and are not washed out of the tissue because of the coronary flow reduction. They include NADH, $FADH_2H^+$, CO_2 acyl CoA and lactate. The increased NADH, H^+, CO_2 and lactate content of the ischaemic cell induces a fall of intracellular pH. Intracellular acidosis has two effects which very rapidly bring about an alteration of the normal contractile behaviour of the myocardial cell: (1) protons decrease the affinity of the contractile apparatus for Ca^{2+} and (2) elevated intracellular H^+ inhibits the sarcolemma channels responsible for the passage of Ca^{2+} ions into the cell during the action potential. Together these actions lead to a decline of active tension generation.

Figure 1 shows that when the coronary flow of the isolated and perfused rabbit hearts was reduced from the unrestricted rate of 25 ml/min to 3 ml/min, developed pressure rapidly fell to close to zero. Contractile activity of the hearts had completely ceased ten minutes after reducing the coronary flow to 1 ml/min or 0 ml/min despite an increase in the pacemaker stimulus to 5 V. 90 minutes after the reduction of coronary flow to 3 ml/min the developed pressure was still 13% of control activity. The fact the myocardial contractility is reduced the early phase of ischaemia, however, does not means that tissue ATP content is reduced immediately after the onset of ischaemia. On the contrary from the results shown in Figure 2 it appears that after 30 minutes of ischaemia ATP

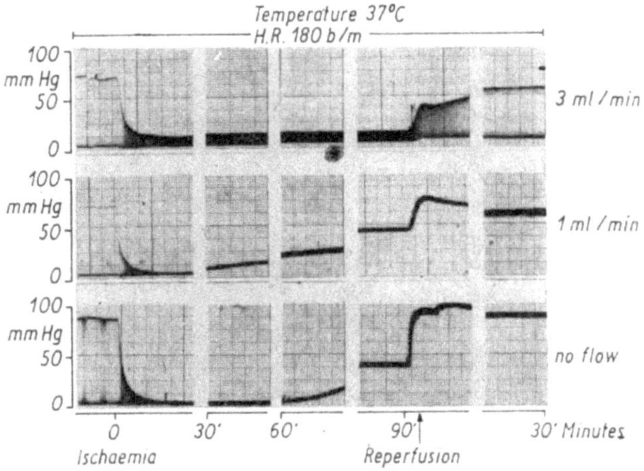

Fig. 1. Mechanical records from four electrically paced (180 b/min) Langendorff-perfused rabbit hearts. Ischaemia was induced by reducing coronary flow from 25 ml/min to 3 ml/min, or 1 ml/min or 0 for 90 minutes after which the hearts have been reperfused for 30 minutes.

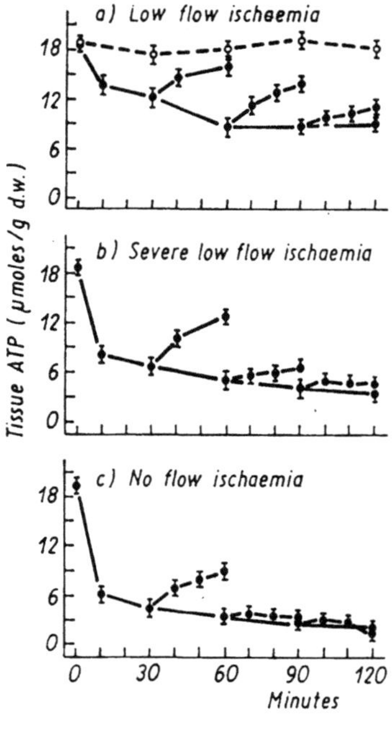

Fig. 2. Effect of different degress of ischaemia and subsequent reperfusion on tissue ATP content. Low flow ischaemia: coronary flow 3 ml/min; severe low flow ischaemia: coronary flow 1 ml/min, no flow ischaemia: coronary flow 0 ml/min. The data are expressed as mean ± S.E.

content was as much as 83%, 69% and 55% of control values, depending on the degree of coronary flow reduction.

There are at least three reasons which can explain these findings: (1) the maintenance of contraction utilises approximately 75% of the total ATP production of the myocardial cell. Therefore the ischaemic-induced cessation of contraction removes an enormous energy drain on the cell, although some ATP is still used by the ischaemic cell to drive a variety of other processes, (2) a reduced amount of ATP during the early phase of ischaemia can be generated by anaerobic glycolysis and by the residual oxidative metabolism and (3) ATP can also be generated from CP in the myocardial cell functions as a reservoir and as transmitter of energy (Moreadith et al. [16]), being converted to ATP at the site of ATP hydrolysis. CP is formed by direct enzymatic transfer of a phosphate group from ATP to creatine when ATP is at a high concentration; for example, at the outer surface of the inner mitochondrial membrane under aerobic condition. Whenever the ATP concentration falls, thus raising the ADP concentration, the phosphate groups of CP are transferred back to ADP, producing ATP. It can be argued, therefore, that myocardial CP levels, rather than ATP content, provide a more reliable index of energy available during the early stage of ischaemia. Figure 3 shows that the decline of CP after 30 minutes of ischaemia was always greater than the decline of ATP.

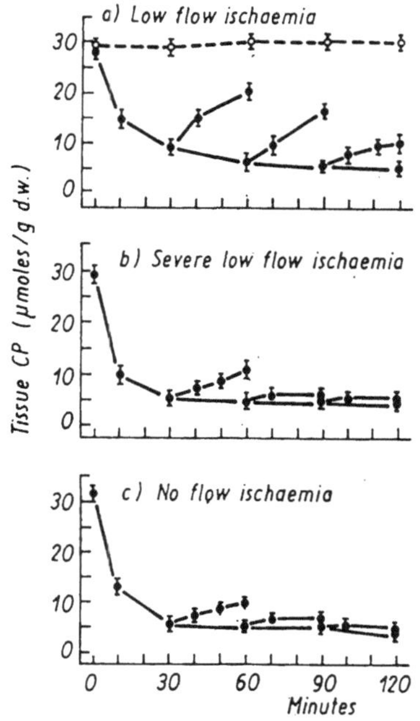

Fig. 3. Effect of different degres of ischaemia and subsequent reperfusion on tissue CP content. Low flow ischaemia: coronary flow 3 ml/min; severe low flow ischaemia coronary flow 1 ml/min; no flow ischaemia: coronary flow 0 ml/min. The data are expressed as mean ± S.E.

It should be emphasized here that, although these series of events are the consequences of a reduced or abolished rate of mitochondria oxidation, this does not mean that the processes of respiration or energy coupling in the mitochondrial respiratory chain are altered. Under early ischaemic condition these processes do not occur (or occur at reduced rate) simply because the cellular uptake of oxygen is abolished or severely reduced. In our experiments after 30 minutes of ischaemia, mitochondrial yield was unchanged. Once isolated after 30 minutes of ischaemia, the mitochondria were still able to

Table 1

Effect of different degrees of ischaemia and subsequent reperfusion on rate of oxygen consumption of isolated mitochondria

Duration of Ischaemia (Min) before Reperfusion	30	60	90	120
	QO_2 (n atoms O_2/mg prot./min)			
Series A: After ischaemic perfusion				
Aerobic	264 ± 21.7 (4)	275 ± 31.0 (4)	242 ± 22.0 (5)	251 ± 19.5 (5)
Moderate low flow ischaemia (3 ml/min)	232 ± 9.9 (6)	212 ± 6.9 (5)	203 ± 23.0 (6)	210 ± 31.2 (3)
Severe low flow ischaemia (1 ml/min)	227 ± 8.7 (5)	189 ± 21.1 (3)	197 ± 19.0 (4)	171 ± 21.0 (3)
No flow ischaemia	231 ± 13.1 (4)	202 ± 19.7 (5)	192 ± 20.1 (6)	159 ± 19.0 (3)
Series B: 30 min after reperfusion				
Moderate low flow ischaemia (3 ml/min)	240 ± 11.0 (4)	227 ± 8.1 (4)	200 ± 15.2 (5)	
Severe low flow ischaemia (1 ml/min)	236 ± 12.1 (4)	176 ± 23.0 (4)	187 ± 17.3 (4)	
No flow ischaemia	249 ± 31.0 (3)	209 ± 13.3 (4)	121 ± 12.0 (6)	

The data are expressed as mean ± S.E. The number of experiments is reported in brackets.

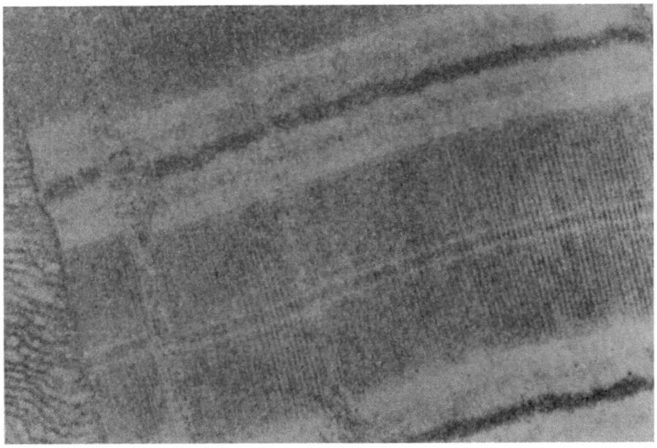

Fig. 4. Longitudinal section of rabbit heart muscle perfusion fixed after 30 minutes of ischaemia. Note the perfect structure of the myofibrils and the relax state of them.

use oxygen for ADP phosphorylation (Table 1, NAYLER et al. [19]). Reperfusion of the hearts made ischaemic for 30 minutes always resulted in some recovery of ATP and CP content (Fig. 2 and 3) suggesting that a significant proportion of the mitochondrial population, at least, have retained the capacity to oxidise substrate and to form ATP. Similarly the non-contractile state of ischaemic myocardial cell does not mean that the cell lost the capacity of generating active force. When examined at the ultramicroscope the myofibrils appears to be normal even after 30 minutes of ischaemia (Fig. 4). Simply it means that the conditions to bring about an active contraction, mainly the presence of a Ca^{2+} concentration of 10^{-5} M and sufficient ATP to support myosine-ATPase in the contractile proteins are not met. Restoration of such conditions after 30 minutes of ischaemia resulted in a recovery.

Events during prolonged period of ischaemia

Extending the ischaemic period to 30, 60 and 90 minutes resulted in a progression of ischaemic damage, as diastolic pressure increased (Fig. 1) and ATP and CP levels further decreased (Fig. 2 and 3). The oxidative phosphorylation capacity of mitochondria isolated from hearts after prolonged period of ischaemia was either unchanged or slightly reduced, depending on the degree of coronary flow reduction (Table 1). The progression of ischaemic damage seems to be delayed by the presence of residual coronary flow. When coronary flow was reduced 78% from control values for 120 minutes, ATP and CP levels together with the mitochondrial QO_2 were better maintained than when coronary flow was completely abolished for the same period of time.

It is possible that during low flow ischaemia (C.F. = 3 ml/min) the hearts reached a new state where the rate of cellular ATP hydrolysis is reduced by the depressed mechanical activity to match in part, at least, the lower ATP production. During low flow ischaemia possibly some aerobic and anaerobic ATP production is still occurring. Under ischaemic condition, however, several metabolic pathways continue to utilise the free energy provided by ATP. They include reactions involved in the maintenance of ion distribution and cell volume (LANGER, [13]), enzyme reactions such as adenylcyclase (DOBSON and MAYER [4]), myokinase (BERNE and RUBIO [1]), fatty acid synthetase (WOOD et al. [26]) and protein kinase (LARNER [14]). In addition, ATP is essential for maintenance of normal cell structure, biosynthesis of proteins, nucleic acids, comples carbohydrates and lipids and also for mitochondrial oxidative phosphorylation, as the entry of glucose into the glycolytic pathway and the activation of fatty acid require ATP.

In the flow ischaemia group, the residual ATP production (Fig. 2) may be just sufficient to maintain the structural integrity of the mitochondria which, when isolated after 90 or 120 minutes, had retained the capacity of oxidative phosphorylation (Table 1). The same amount of ATP however may not be sufficient to prevent the increase in resting tension an abnormality which depends by both, ATP and cytosolic calcium (Fig. 1). It is interesting to note here that after 90 minutes of severe ischaemia (total ischaemia, or 1 ml/min ischaemia) mitochondrial calcium was slightly increased, when tissue calcium was unchanged (Fig. 5). This was not the case for the 3 ml/min group. The finding that the ischaemic mitochondria had accumulated some calcium suggests that: (a) the ischaemic mitochondria are capable of maintaining a membrane potential, which is the driving force of mitochondrial calcium transport (NICHOLLS et al. [20]); (b) the cytosolic calcium concentration is somewhat elevated, the extra-mitochondrial calcium concentration being the major factor determining calcium accumulation, (CARAFOLI et al. and SCARPA et al. [22]). This also suggests that the ischaemic episode induces an alteration of the intracellular calcium homeostasis.

Because of the existence of Ca^{2+} gradients across the cell and subcellular membranes,

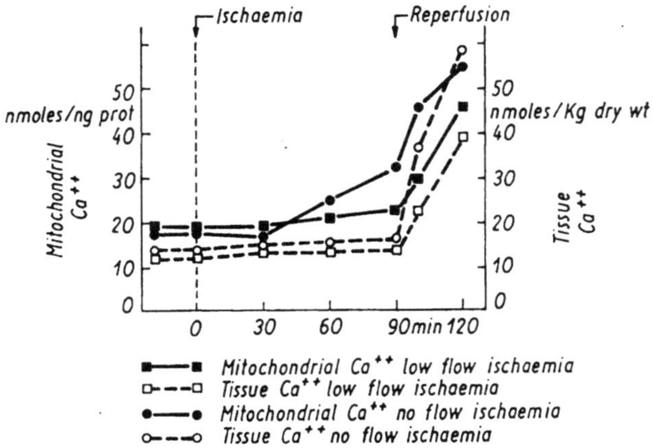

Fig. 5. Effect of 90 minutes of low flow ischaemia (coronary flow 3 ml/min) and no flow ischaemia and reperfusion on tissue and mitochondrial calcium content. Calcium content was measured by the atomic absorption spectrophotometry. Mitochondria were isolated in absence of EDTA and in the presence of 5 μM of ruthenium red in an attempt to reduce mitochondrial calcium accumulation during the extraction procedure.

maintainance of the normal calcium homeostasis implies movements of Ca^{2+} against these gradients and therefore it is an energy dependent process (NAYLER et al. [17, 18]). Since the severe impairment of oxygen delivery which occurred during 1 ml/min or 0 ml/min ischaemia, resulted in a rapid depletion of high energy phosphate reserves, it is quite likely that during an ischaemic episode the tissue level of ATP would fall beyond the level required for the maintenance of cytosolic Ca^{2+}. It has been reported (HARRIS [8]) that the Michaelis constants of different animals for the various fractions which influence calcium movement in the myocardium lie in the range of 5—25 μM and the highest is that of Ca^{2+} activate-ATPases of the sarcolemma. This function is, therefore, likely to be most sensitive to a fall in the concentration of ATP. This will results in an increase of the cytosolic-calcium concentration which will be transported into the mitochondria in an attempt to maintain the normal cytosolic calcium concentration (FERRARI et al. [5]).

Events on reperfusion in relation to different periods of ischaemia

Reperfusion after 30 minutes of ischaemia resulted in a recovery of mechanical function (data not shown) and ATP and CP content (Fig. 2 and 3). The recovery of developed pressure and of high energy phosphate groups was inversely proportional to the severity of coronary flow reduction. ATP and CP, however were not completely restored to aerobic control levels (Fig. 2 and 3). Reperfusion after prolonged period of low flow ischaemia (60 or 90 minutes) resulted in a restoration of active pressure generation and of ATP and CP level (Fig. 1, 2 and 3), the recovery being inversely correlated with the duration of the ischaemic episode. Reperfusion after prolonged period of more severe (1 ml/min) or total ischaemia resulted in a tissue and mitochondrial Ca^{2+} overload (Fig. 5). Mitochondria virtually lost their capacity to phosphorylate ADP (Table 1).

There was no recovery of ATP, CP or active pressure generation (Figs. 1, 2 and 3). Diastolic pressure, which rose rapidly during the early stages of reperfusion, remained elevated (Fig. 1).

From these results it would appear that whether or not reperfusion is beneficial or detrimental to the ischaemic myocardium depends upon the duration and severity of the ischaemic period. Increasing the severity and the duration of the ischaemic period reduces the recovery of normal myocardial function on reperfusion. A prompt recovery of mechanical and metabolic function on reperfusion was always present after 30 minutes of severe coronary flow reduction (1 ml/min) or abolition. After this short period of ischaemia, there was some residual ATP content, ATP being considerably depleted only after 60 or 90 minutes of severe ischaemia. The presence of a residual coronary flow rate of 3 ml/min able to maintain some aerobic and anaerobic metabolism enabled some recovery during reperfusion even after prolonged period of ischaemia (60—90 minutes). In particular in these groups, mitochondrial function after reperfusion was either unchanged or improved, but never worsened (Table 1).

The most likely explanation for these results is that the residual ATP content of these ischaemic hearts was sufficient to support the basic cellular function such as control of cell volume, maintenance of ionic homeostasis and preservation of ultrastructure. The readmission of flow at this stage of the ischaemic damage, when cellular membrances are presumably still intact, some cellular supplies of ATP are available, and pathways of electron transport and oxidative phosphorylation are simply blocked and not damaged should result in a rapid re-energization of the electron transport pathway. This, in turn, leads to a restoration of oxidative phosphorylation and ATP production with a resumption of contractile activity.

The restoration of ATP content on reperfusion, however, was incomplete even after a short period of ischaemia (30 minutes). This is probably due to a reduction of adenine nucleotide pool of the ischaemic cell rather than to a defect of the mitochondrial ATP producing capacity. Jennings et al. [11] reported that during the early state of ischaemia adenosine monophosphate (AMP) accumulates, while ATP decreases. AMP is then dephosphorylated to form adenosine which is lost from the cell and further degradated (Berne et al. [1]).

This results in destruction of much of the adenosine nucleotide pool of the ischaemic cell. Destruction occurs because net resynthesis of adenine nucleotides under ischaemic condition is limited being an ATP requiring process.

Reperfusion of the ischaemic myocardium after 90 minutes of total or 1 ml/min ischaemia did not lead to a re-establishment of cell function. On the contrary, it produced massive tissue and mitochondrial calcium accumulation with a further decline in mitochondrial function (Fig. 5 and Table 1). There was no recovery of active tension generation or of high energy phosphate groups (Fig. 1, 2 and 3).

A number of mechanisms have been suggested to explain these findings. In particular, it has been proposed that when faced with the possibility of producing ATP via oxidative phosphorylation or accumulating calcium, cardiac mitochondria will preferentially perform the latter task, causing a further deterioration of ATP synthesis (Hearse [9] and Ferrari et al. [6]). Thus it appears that mitochondrial function plays an important role in the molecular mechanism of reperfusion damage after prolonged period of ischaemia.

Mitochondria and reperfusion damage

With the readmission of coronary flow there is clearly an abundant supply of external calcium to enter the myocardium. In our experiments tissue calcium content was increased after 30 minutes reperfusion following prolonged ischaemia (total or 1 ml/min ischaemia) (Fig. 5). This indicates that there was an alteration of the cell membrane leading to a breakdown of the permeability barrier to ions such as calcium. The mechanism for this breakdown is unclear. It may be related to abnormalities occurring during the period of ischaemia which becomes manifest only during reperfusion. They include: (a) disruption of the sarcolemma as consequences of severe depletion in cytosolic ATP or (b) detergent effect of acyl CoA and free fatty acids accumulated during ischaemia or (c) activation of phospholipases (Chien et al. and Vasdev et al. [24]). Alternatively the increased permeability of the sarcolemma during reperfusion may results directly from the re-introduction of coronary flow. Ganote [7] suggested that on reoxygenation contraction of the myocardial cell pulls apart the sarcolemmal membrane altering its permeability. The sudden readmission of oxygen to the cell after a period of ischaemia may generate free radicals leading to a peroxidation of membrane lipids.

Whichever the mechanism is involved, the influx of calcium leads to an increased calcium concentration at the time when mitochondria are re-energized by the readmission of O_2. Cytosolic ADP concentration is also increased (Jennings et al. [10]). Under these circumstances the ischaemic mitochondria which are still able to function can use the restored membrane potential either to phosphorylate ADP or to accumulate calcium, thus buffering the cytosol. The amount of ATP produced or calcium accumulated will depend on the equilibrium between these two reactions. It has been shown (Williams et al. [25]) that in the presence of 1 mM free magnesium, which is a physiological concentration, the equilibrium between mitochondrial calcium transport and ATP synthesis seems to be shifted towards ATP synthesis. Magnesium acts as a physiological modulator of mitochondrial calcium transport. These results of Williams et al. [25] may be interpreted as suggesting that in the presence of magnesium, the rate of ATP synthesis would be maintained at free calcium concentration far in excess of these found in the normal myocardial cell.

When considering the situation *in vivo* during post ischaemic reperfusion, we have to take into account that: (a) reperfusion induces a large release of magnesium with a consequent decrease of the cytosolic concentration of this ion (Shen et al. [23]), (b) calcium enters the cell abnormally causing a very significant elevation of the cytosolic concentration and (c) the influx of calcium from the extracellular fluid is continuous. Under these circumstances the equilibrium between mitochondrial ATP production and calcium accumulation is very likely to be shifted towards calcium transport. Mitochondria would begin to accumulate calcium at maximal rate in an attempt to buffer the cytosolic calcium. With a continuous influx of calcium from the extracellular fluid this would inevitably lead to a massive accumulation of calcium, causing mitochondrial damage. Under these conditions ATP production would not be able to compete effectively for respiratory energy and the situation would be made worse by the fact that intracellular magnesium levels continuously decrease on reperfusion, so favouring the accumulation of calcium. As a consequence of this series of events, little or no ATP will be produced during postischaemic reperfusion (Fig. 2).

Effects of slow Ca^{2+} channel antagonist on the ischaemic and reperfusion damage

Substances which may inhibit the slow calcium channel may be useful in life to protect ischaemic myocardium by affecting the functioning of cardiac and smooth muscle cells and of the cells of the pacemaker, nodal and conducting tissue (NAYLER et al. [19]).

Figure 6 shows some of the effects exerted by verapamil, a prototype of the so called "calcium antagonist" on tissue ATP content and on the percentage of increase of mitochondrial calcium, both measured at the end of ischaemia. The experiments have been carried out using isolated Langendorff perfused rabbits' hearts. Three different degrees of ischaemia lasting for 30, 60 and 90 minutes have been investigated and the effects of verapamil were studied using the more severe ischaemic condition which is no flow ischaemia.

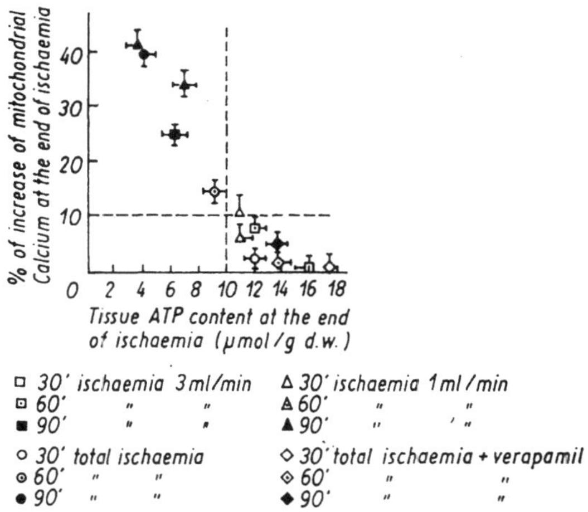

Fig. 6. Relationship between tissue ATP content and % increase of mitochondria calcium content at the end of ischaemia. Results represent the mean ± S.E.

Clearly an inverse relation existed between the ATP content at the end of the ischaemic period and percentage of mitochondrial calcium overload at the end of ischaemia. The greater the depletion in ATP content the greater was the mitochondrial calcium accumulation at the end of ischaemia (Fig. 6). Presence of verapamil was able to maintain the tissue ATP content despite the prolonged period of ischaemia and this resulted in no mitochondrial Ca^{2+} accumulation, which is to say, that verapamil has been able to maintain the myocardial homeostasis for calcium. Thus, it seems that the positive effect of verapamil depends on its ability to spare ATP during ischaemia. If sufficient ATP remains available during ischaemia to maintain membrane ultrastructure and Ca^{2+} into the cell. Under these conditions readmission of oxygen during reperfusion should results in a rapid re-energization of the electron transport pathway, restoration of oxidative phosphorylation and ATP production and translocation into the cytosol with a resumption of contractile activity. Figure 7 shows that this was the case for the verapamil treated hearts, the rise in diastolic pressure during ischaemia being diminished with a greater recovery of developed pressure during reperfusion. From Figure 7 also it appears that in the hearts which received verapamil the rate of fall of developed pressure was greater than in control hearts.

This effect which is related to the ability of verapamil to reduce the slow calcium current leading to a reduction of myocardial contraction is extremely important. The rate of fall in CP and ATP during ischaemia is dependent on physical activity and the rate of ATP hydrolysis existing before or at the onset of ischaemia (KÜBLER et al. [12], REIBEL et al. [21]). Therefore, verapamil, by reducing active force development during the early stages of ischaemia, decreases the rate of consumption of ATP. Thus sufficient ATP remains available during ischaemia to maintain membrane ultrastructure and intracellular Ca^{2+} homeostasis. Under these conditions diastolic pressure will not rise and reperfusion will lead to a recovery of myocardial function (Fig. 7).

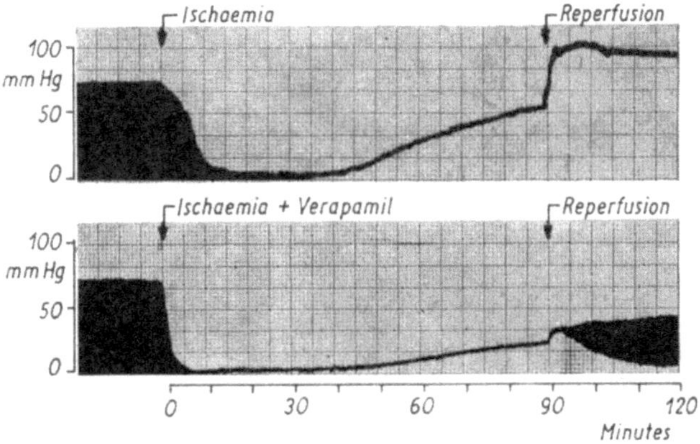

Fig. 7. Mechanical records from two electrically paced (180 b/min) Langendorff perfused rabbit hearts. Control hearts were made ischaemic by reducing coronary flow to 1 ml/min. Verapamil was administered in the perfusate (1 mg/l) at the time of ischaemia. Notice the more rapid decline of developed pressure in the verapamil-receiving hearts.

Acknowledgments

This study was supported by a grant CNR CT 80.00606.04. The Authors would like to thank G. LAUCCI and G. CORUZZI for the technical and secretarial assistance in preparing this publication.

References

[1] BERNE, R. M. and R. RUBIO: Circ. Res. **23** (1974), 109–120
[2] CARAFOLI, E. and A. L. LEHNINGER: Biochem. J. **122** (1971), 681–690
[3] CHIEN, K. R., J. ABRAMS, A. SERRONI, J. T. MARTIN and J. L. FARBE: J. Biol. Chem. **253** (1978), 4809–4817
[4] DOBSON, J. G. Jr. and S. E. MAYER: Circ. Res. **33** (1973), 412–140
[5] FERRARI, R., A. J. WILLIAMS and W. G. NAYLER: J. Mol. Cell. Cardiol. **11** (1979), 13
[6] FERRARI, R., F. DI LISA, R. RADDINO and O. VISIOLI: In: Advances in beta-blocker Therapy II (Ed. A. Zanchetti) (1981), 21–39

[7] GANOTE, C. E. and J. P. KALTENBACH: J. Mol. Cell. Cardiol. **11** (1979), 389–406
[8] HARRIS, P.: Eur. J. Cardiol. **3** (1975), 157–163
[9] HEARSE, D.: J. Mol. Cell. Cardiol. **9** (1977), 607–617
[10] JENNINGS, R. B., H. K. HAWKINS, J. E. LOWE, M. L. HILL, S. KLOTMAN and K. A. REIMER: Amer. J. Pathol. **92** (1978), 187–214
[11] JENNINGS, R. B. and K. A. REIMER: Amer. J. Pathol. **102** (1981), 241–255
[12] KUBLER, W. and P. G. SPIECKERMANN: J. Mol. Cell. Cardiol. **1** (1970), 351–367
[13] LANGER, G. A.: J. Mol. Cell. Cardiol. **12** (1980), 231–239
[14] LARNER, J.: Circ. Res. **38**, suppl. I, (1978), 2–7
[15] MITCHELL, P.: Chemiosmotic coupling in oxidative and photosynthetic phosphorylation. Glynn Research Ltd., Bodmin U.K. (1966)
[16] MOREADITH, R. W. and W. E. JACOBUS: J. Biol. Chem. **257** (1982), 899–905
[17] NAYLER, W. G.: Amer. J. Pathol. **102** (1981), 262–270
[18] NAYLER, W. G., R. FERRARI and A. WILLIAMS: Amer. J. Cardiol. **46** (1980), 241–248
[19] NAYLER, W. G. and P. A. POOLE-WILSON: Basic. Res. Cardiol. **76** (1981), 1–15
[20] NICHOLLS, D. G. and M. CROMPTON: FEBS Lett. III (1980), 261–268
[21] REIBEL, D. K. and M. J. ROVETTO: Amer. J. Physiol. **234** (1978), H620–H624
[22] SCARPA, A. and P. GRAZIOTTI: J. Gen. Physiol. **62** (1973), 756–772
[23] SHEN, A. C. and R. B. JENNINGS: Amer. J. Path. **67** (1909), 441–452
[24] VASDEV, S. C., C. P. BIRO, R. NARBAITZ and K. KAKO: Can. J. Biochem. **58** (1980), 1112–1119
[25] WILLIAMS, A. J., J. S. CRIE and R. FERRARI: Circulation 62 suppl. III (1980), 177
[26] WOOD, J. M., A. E. HUTCHINGS and N. BRACHFELD: J. Mol. Cell. Cardiol. 4 (1972), 97–111

Laboratory of Metabolic Regulation, Experimental Unit, Institute for Clinical and Experimental Medicine, Prague, Czechoslovakia

The Role of Calcium in Myocardial Ischaemia

B. Mosinger

One of the major problems of myocardial ischaemia is currently the role of calcium in ischaemic injury. Recognized originally by Shen and Jennings [15] and Jennings [10], it became important both to theoretical cardiology und practical medicine due to the increasing use of calcium antagonists in clinical cardiology and cardiac surgery [6, 13, 16]. The starting questions can be formulated as follows:

1. Is there a causal relation between myocardial calcium overload during post-ischaemic reperfusion and ischaemic injury?
2. To what extent is ischaemic injury related to extracellular calcium concentration?

To answer these questions the following methods were used. Briefly, isolated rat hearts were perfused with constant non-recirculating flow using modified Krebs-Henseleit solution [11] gassed with 95% O_2 plus 5% CO_2 and adding 5.5 mM glucose. Transient complete ischaemia of global type lasted 5—30 min and the damage was monitored by the rate of lactate dehydrogenase (LDH) release into the effluent during reperfusion [12]. Aortic and perfusion pressures were continuously recorded from the side-arm of an aortic cannullae. The results were expressed as the means $\pm$ standard error, if not indicated otherwise, and statistically highly significant differences marked by asterisks.

External calcium and LDH release

By altering calcium concentration in the perfusate, LDH release into the effluent after 30 min ischaemia accelerated as soon calcium concentration roses to a certain level. Curve peaks shifted to the left and appeared at shorter intervals (Fig. 1). With 5 or 7.5 mM Ca concentration in the medium focal to massive necroses became visible even with the naked eye at the end of experiments. Between the total amount of enzymes released within 30 min of reperfusion and Ca concentration in the medium a non-linear relation was found (Fig. 2). The relation could be linearized by plotting the logarithm of LDH rate against Ca concentration. Extrapolating a straight line to LDH axis, we obtain a value fairly far from zero; in other words, even a medium with a zero Ca concentration seemed to be incapable to prevent ischaemic damage. This prediction was tested experimentally.

In control a medium with 2.5 mM Ca concentration throughout the experiment was used. In a second and third group calcium was omitted from medium either in reperfusion phase only or both in ischaemic and reperfusion phase. As can be seen in Figure 3,

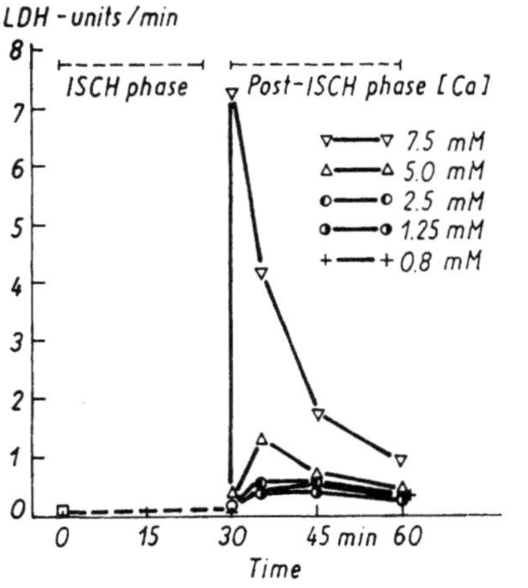

Fig. 1. Effect of various calcium concentrations in perfusion medium on LDH release rate.
The concentration of calcium as indicated in Fig. was present troughout each experiment. There was no effect of calcium on LDH release before ischaemia. A fixed flow around 9 ml/min was maintained by a peristalic pump which was stopped during the ischaemic phase, (n = 8 in each group).

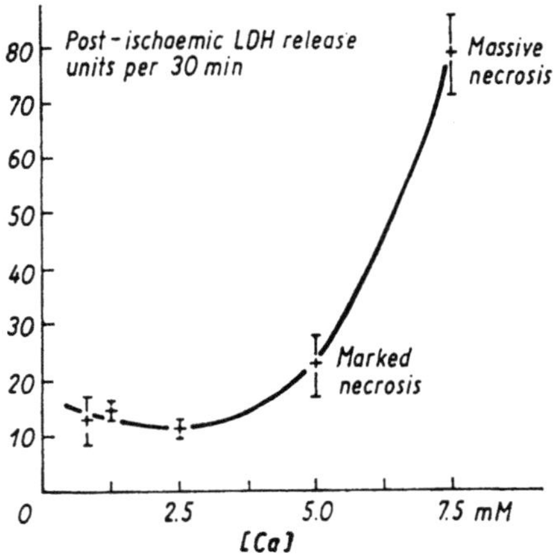

Fig. 2. Total amount of LDH released per 30 min after 30 min ischaemia.
Coronary flow the same as indicated in Fig. 1. Peak LDH released corresponds to the enzyme content of around 35% of myocytes population, (n = 8 in each group).

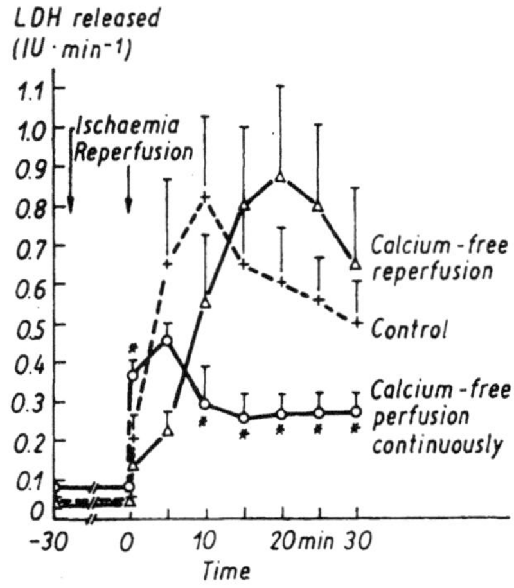

Fig. 3. Rate of LDH release during postischaemic reperfusion using zero calcium concentration in medium.
Control groups was perfused with medium containing 2.5 mM concentration of calcium. The other two groups had zero calcium either only in reperfusion phase or 10 min before, during and after ischaemia, (n = 5–8 in each group).

this was the only group showing a significant decrease but not abolition of ischaemic damage. Note that aside from a delay of curve maximum, the absence of calcium only in the reperfusion phase had no effect on the total LDH release.

Different effect of calcium according the phase of its action was seen also in another 4 group experiments using a perfusion medium with a 2.5 and 7.5 mM Ca concentration. Each of them was present either in a single or both ischaemic and reperfusion phase. As can be seen in Figure 4, the degree of ischaemic damage (LDH leakage, resp.) was dependent on Ca concentration varying before and not within reperfusion.

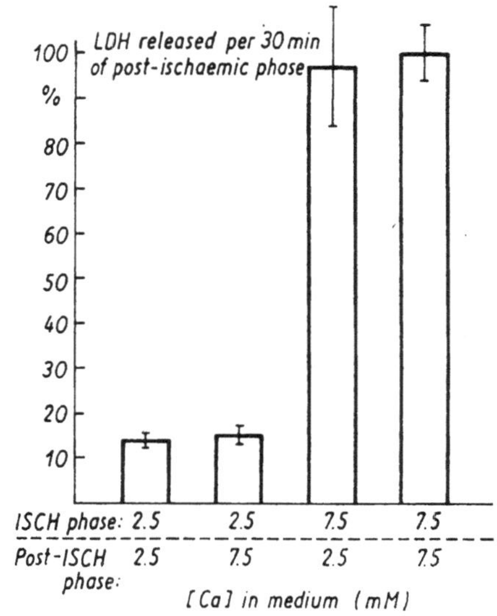

Fig. 4. LDH release after 30 min ischaemia due to permutation of different calcium concentration in medium in different ischaemic phases.
The results are expressed in percent of the highest value of total LDH released during 30 min after ischaemia, (n = 6—12 in each group).

Ischaemia versus calcium paradox

Previous experiments showed that an omission of calcium from reperfusion medium delayed (Fig. 3) and increasing the Ca concentration in perfusion medium precipitated the LDH release maximum (Fig. 1). In the following series of experiments the phenomenon of maximum shift-which might be just accidental-was verified in calcium overload without ischaemia, i.e. in calcium paradox [1, 17] and in ischaemia with constant Ca concentration. As can be seen in Figure 5, a gradual increasing of calcium overload leads not only to increased myocardial damage but also to a shift of maxima to the left. On the other hand, Figure 6 shows that the extension of ischaemic injury due to gradual prolongation of coronary flow arrest delays the time of onset of maxima. Ischaemia exceeding 15 min led to a further prolongation of enzyme release but resulted (in individual case) in appearing of two or more peaks in a way indicating a stochastic rather than a deterministic process (not shown).

Experimental data in Figures 5 and 6 were fitted by curves derived from a mathematical model. As follows from its parameters, growing Ca concentrations result above all in increased permeability of cellular membranes, whereas extension of ischaemia results in increase of damaged cellular population with a concomitant slow-down and heterogenity of the cellular components wash-out rate. The latter effect seems to be attributable to increasing myocardial contracture and/or rigor [7].

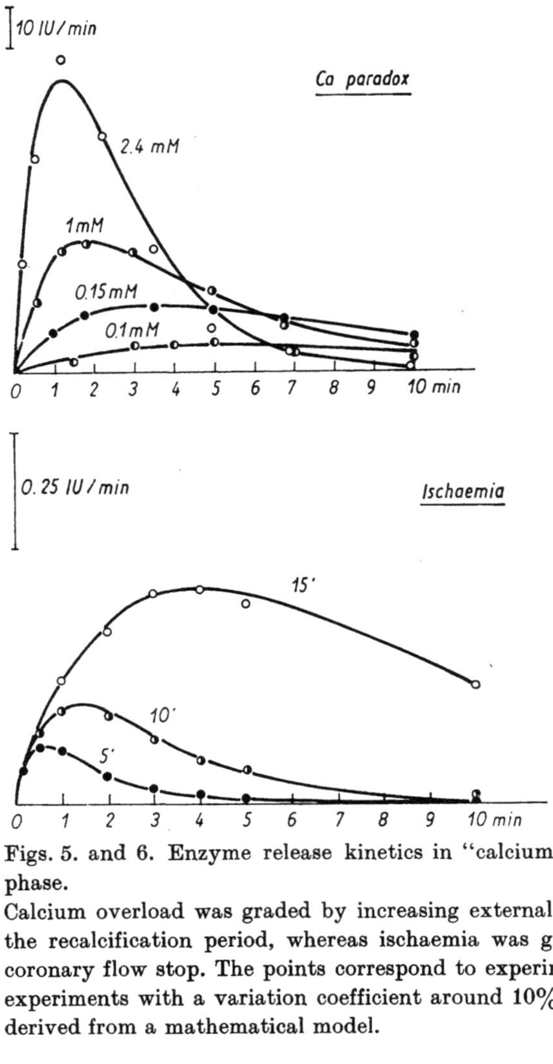

Figs. 5. and 6. Enzyme release kinetics in "calcium paradox" and post-ischaemic phase.
Calcium overload was graded by increasing external calcium concentration during the recalcification period, whereas ischaemia was graded by the length (min) of coronary flow stop. The points correspond to experimental data (means from 4—8 experiments with a variation coefficient around 10%) and solid lines connect data derived from a mathematical model.

Calcium, coronary resistance and ischaemic injury

In most experiments ischaemic injury was associated with an increased coronary resistance. Assuming and exponential relation, the obtained data expressed as a ratio of perfusion pressures before and after ischaemia on the one hand and LDH release on the other showed a very close correlation. Interestingly, the nature of this relation did not change with the use of perfusion medium containing 2.5 mM or 0 mM calcium concentration (Fig. 7).

Immediately after the onset of reperfusion we observed a transient overshoot of coronary resistance lasting several seconds. The inserted part in Figure 8 shows a schematic illustration of a typical course of perfusion pressures: 1 denotes the pre-ischaemic perfusion pressure, 2 denotes the maximum of transient perfusion pressure elevation

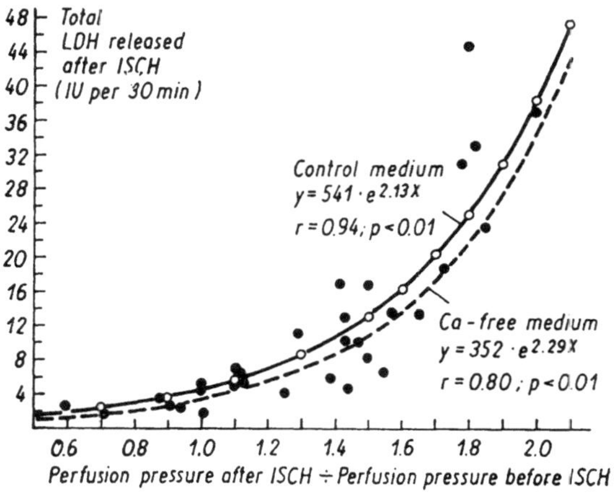

Fig. 7. Post-ischaemic perfusion pressure and LDH release.
The best data fitting was found by assuming an exponential relationship between perfusion pressure and LDH release.

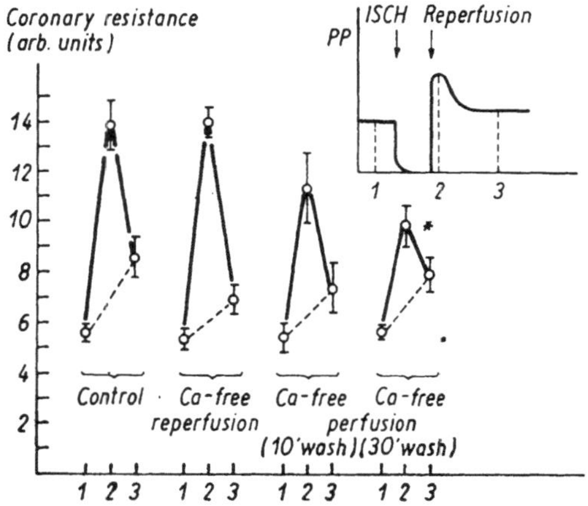

Fig. 8. Biphasic coronary resistance as observed immediatelly after reperfusion.
A typical time course or perfusion pressure before and after the start of reperfusion is shown in the inserted part of the Fig.
Data obtained in individual phases were statistically evaluated and compared to control, (n = 5—12 in each group).

and 3 a more or less balance state of perfusion pressure after reperfusion. The data obtained during these phases and converted to arbitrary units of coronary resistance (the ratio of instantaneous perfusion pressure and coronary flow) were compared in 4 group experiments. The respective experimental designs are described in Figure 8. Note that coronary resistance during reperfusion rose in phase 3 in all groups irrespective of the presence (2.5 mM) or absence of calcium in the perfusion medium.

Groups 3 and 4 where the hearts were perfused with a calcium-free medium also 10 or 30 min before ischaemia, showed a distinct tendency to a decrease of transient resistance in phase 2.

Even though the reason for the biphase change in coronary resistance during reperfusion is not quite clear, its increase as a whole is most probably due to myocardial contracture developing during ischaemia [2]. Since myocardial contracture depends both on ATP depletion and intracellular calcium increase [7, 8, 14], ischaemic contracture seems to develop even under conditions of a zero external calcium concentration.

Obviously the transient resistance in phase 2 reflects best the degree of contracture developed during the ischaemic phase. It can be therefore inferred that contracture decreased only if the heart was exposed to calcium — free medium before reperfusion. This resembles previously shown calcium-free perfusion effect on the LDH release.

Table 1

Flow-dependent LDH release in post-ischaemic phase

The meaning of "transient overflow" is described in the text. Note that the difference in LDH release during the first minute of reperfusion increased more than 20 times due to higher rate of reperfusion.

	Before	ISCH	Low-flow reperfusion time (min)						LDH released per 30 min
	−30	1	5	10	15	20	25	30	
Coronary flow ml/min	9.5 ± 0.08	2.3 ± 0.3	2.7 ± 0.35	2.7 ± 0.36	2.7 ± 0.36	2.7 ± 0.36	2.7 ± 0.36	2.7 ± 0.36	—
LDH released mU/min (n = 5)	27.4 ± 5.6	107 ±21.7	64 ± 21	125 ± 30	144 ± 26	121 ± 26	103 ± 24	94 ± 23	3,303 ± 682
	High-flow reperfusion								
Coronary flow ml/min	9.3 ± 0.06	12.9 ± 0.5	14.5 ± 0.13	14.3 ± 0.06	14.3 ± 0.06	14.3 ± 0.06	14.3 ± 0.06	14.3 ± 0.06	—
LDH released mU/min (n = 7)	30 ± 9.3	360 ± 40	686 ± 84	795 ± 102	739 ± 104	560.1 ± 121	491 ± 84	422 ± 59	18,378 ± 2,449
	Transient overflow reperfusion								
Coronary flow	9.3 ± 0.06	15.5 ± 0.26	9.3 ± 0.13	9.3 ± 0.13	9.3 ± 0.13	9.3 ± 0.13	9.3 ± 0.13	9.3 ± 0.13	—
LDH released mU/min (n = 5)	31 ± 8	24,914 ± 4,729	7,167 ± 661	2,315 ± 125	1,282 ± 68	868 ± 35	590 ± 39	457 ± 28	81,152 − 6,560

Flow-dependent modulation of reperfusion phase

The results summarized in Figures 3 and 4 might suggest that the reperfusion phase is only a passive and rigid expression of a latent injury sustained already during the ischaemic phase. In the other experiments, however, several factors were found that can modulate the course of the reperfusion phase given a constant calcium concentration in the medium.

One of the important factors permitting to alter the degree of damage during reperfusion both in a positive and negative sense is a simple change of reperfusion rate and/or reperfusion pressures. Table 1 summarizes the results showing a distinct difference in LDH release during a continued low-flow and high-flow reperfusion. However, even a short-term coronary flow elevation may have a very pronounced effect as seen in the group "transient overflow reperfusion". In the respective experiments a jump reflow with a maximum 1 ml/s in the first second, rapidly and exponentially decreasing with a half-time about 4 s was used so that average flow rate during first minute increased only from 9.3 to 15.5 ml/min (Table 1). Despite that this mean flow did not virtually differ from the permanently elevated flow in the "high-flow reperfusion" group, it led to a dramatic exacerbation of ischaemic damage. Even though the damage must have developed within a few seconds of the onset of reperfusion, its consequences could be observed throughout the following 30 min.

Several factors may be implicated in this flow-dependent post-ischaemic damage, including the lipoperoxidative mechanism [5], but the most plausible explanation seems to be a volume expansion of myocardial cells due to disturbed volume regulation induced by ischaemia [3, 19]. This explanation is supported by the finding that a decrease of sodium concentration to 20 mM is associated with a significant regression of damage after ischaemia of the same duration and at the same calcium concentration as in controls.

Latent injury seen to develop during the ischaemic phase is apparently subject to a separate mechanism of its own in which ATP depletion and elevation of ionized intracellular calcium with a subsequent contracture might play a dominant role.

References

[1] Alto, L. E. and N. S. Dhalla: Amer. J. Physiol. **237** (1979), H713—H719

[2] Bricknell, O. L. and L. H. Opie: Circul. Res. **43** (1978), 102—115

[3] Buja, L. M. and J. T. Willerson: Amer. J. Pathol. **103** (1981), 79—95

[4] Ganote, Ch. E., S. Y. Liu, S. Safavi and J. P. Kaltenbach: J. Mol. Cell. Cardiol. **13** (1981), 93—106

[5] Guarnieri, C., F. Flamingi and C. M. Caldarera: J. Mol. Cell. Cardiol. **12** (1980), 797—808

[6] Hearse, D. J.: J. Mol. Cell. Cardiol. **9** (1977), 605—616

[7] Hearse, D. J., P. B. Garlick and S. M. Humphrey: Amer. J. Cardiol. **39** (1977), 986—993

[8] Humphrey, S. M., J. B. Gavin and P. B. Herdson: J. Mol. Cell. Cardiol. **12** (1980), 1397—1406

[9] Jennings, R. B.: Acta med. scand. Suppl. **587** (1975), 83—92

[10] Jennings, R. B.: Circul. 53, Suppl. 1 (1976), 26—29

[11] Krebs, H. A. and K. Henseleit: Hoppe-Seyler's Zeitschr. physiol. Chemie **210** (1932), 33—66

[12] Mosinger, B., J. Stejskal, M. Tutterová and H. Vavřínková: Europ. J. Cardiol. **615** (1978), 389—402

[13] NAYLER, W. G., and P. A. POOLE-WILSON: Basic Res. Cardiol. **76** (1981), 1–15
[14] NAYLER, W. G., P. A. POOLE-WILSON and A. WILLIAMS: J. Mol. Cell. Cardiol. **11** (1979), 683–706
[15] SHEN, A. C. and R. B. JENNINGS: Amer. J. Pathol. **67** (1972), 441–452
[16] WEISHAAR, R. E. and R. J. BING: J. Mol. Cell. Cardiol. **12** (1980), 993–1000
[17] ZIMMERMANN, A. N. E. and W. C. HULSMANN: Nature (London) **211** (1966), 646–647

Department of Biomedical Sciences, University of Tampere, Tampere, Finland

The Effect of Cyclic GMP-Elevating Nitrogenous Compounds on Myocardial Glycolysis

T. Metsä-Ketelä, P. Vuorinen and K. Laustiola

Introduction

The effects of cyclic AMP on carbohydrate metabolism are well known [19, 22]. There are at least three main sites of action; phosphorylase kinase, glycogen synthetase and phosphofructokinase (PFK). The first two actions, which lead to increased glycogenolysis and to decreased glycogen synthesis, respectively, are mediated by cAMP-dependent protein kinase mediated phosphorylation. The effect of cAMP on PFK is a direct one. Thus, cyclic AMP has been thought to mediate the stimulatory effect of β-stimulation on myocardial carbohydrate metabolism.

Cyclic GMP frequently seems to have actions opposite to those of cAMP [7]. However, very little is known regarding the metabolic effects of this nucleotide. On the other hand, many vasodilatating and anti-anginal drugs such as sodium nitroprusside (SNP), nitrite and nitroglycerin stimulate guanylate cyclase, Schultz et al. [20, 21], and it has even been proposed that their vascular smooth muscle relaxing effects are mediated by cGMP [8, 14]. The common feature in the activation of guanylate cyclase by these compounds might be the release of nitric oxide [17]. It has also been suggested that S-nitroso-thiols are the active intermediates of nitroglycerin and sodium nitrite [13].

There is some evidence that drugs which increase the level of cGMP may counteract the metabolic effects of hypoxia. Abiko et al. [1] and Ichihara and Abiko [10] have studied the metabolic effect of nitroglycerin after a coronary ligation in dog heart *in situ*. Nitroglycerin antagonized the stimulatory effect of coronary ligation on carbohydrate metabolism. The mechanism of the action remains unknown. β-blockade produced a very similar response, but the authors think that the mechanisms of these actions are different. In their study, cyclic nucleotides were not measured. We have earlier reported that SNP reduces the atrial lactate production with simultaneous increase in cGMP level, [16]. In the present study, we have further investigated the possible role of cGMP in the regulation of myocardial glycolysis.

Material and methods

Ad libitum-fed male Wistar rats (weighing 250—300 g) were sacrified by dislocation of the neck. The hearts were immediately excised, immersed and washed free from blood in tyrode solution containing 1000 IU/l heparin at room temperature (pH 7.4). The atria were separated from the ventricles in heparinized tyrode bubbled continuously with pure oxygen. A polyester suture was tied to the apex of both atria and they were transferred to an organ bath (20 ml, 30 °C) with continuous Tyrode flow (1.3 ml/min) bubbling with pure oxygen. Oxygen saturation was monitored with a CLARK electrode and kept at maximum during the stabilization period of 45 min (about 95% saturation). Hypoxia was induced by interruption of oxygenation of the incubation medium, which led to an oxygen saturation of 50% within 3 to 4 min. The tissues were freeze-clamped.

Determinations

L-lactate was determined enzymatically [9]. Cyclic GMP was measured by radioimmunoassay [5]. Cyclic GMP in neutralized perchloric acid supernatants was separated from disturbing cAMP by DOWEX®-50W-chromatography.

Soluble guanylate cyclase was partially purified from bovine hearts by modifying the purification procedure previously described for hepatic soluble guanylate cyclase by [4]. Guanylate cyclase activity was determined as described by [6]. Protein was assayed according to [15].

Results

Effects of sodium nitroprusside

In high oxygen saturation (HiOxSa) SNP dose dependently reduced the atrial lactate level (Fig. 1). The maximum decrease was obtained at the concentration of 10^{-5} M SNP. The maximum cGMP response was attained at the concentration of 10^{-3} M SNP. In hypoxia (Fig. 2), the control level of lactate was elevated to 14.6 ± 1.4 nmol/mg prot and the maximum reduction caused by SNP was seen at the concentration of 10^{-3} M. The same dose of SNP also produced the maximum effect on cyclic GMP.

In HiOxSa (Fig. 3), the maximum effects of 10^{-4} M SNP on lactate and cGMP were seen 3 min after administration.

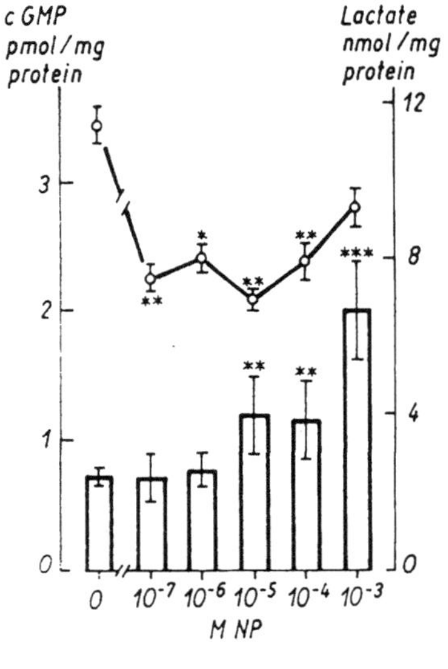

Fig. 1. Concentration response curves of nitroprusside (NP) (incubation time with NP 4 min) in high oxygen concentration (HiOxSa) on the levels of cyclic GMP (bars) and lactate (○ — ○) in isolated rat atria.
Means (± SEM) of 6—12 preparations are given *$p < 0.05$, **$p < 0.01$, ***$p < 0.001$ when compared to the control (○) values

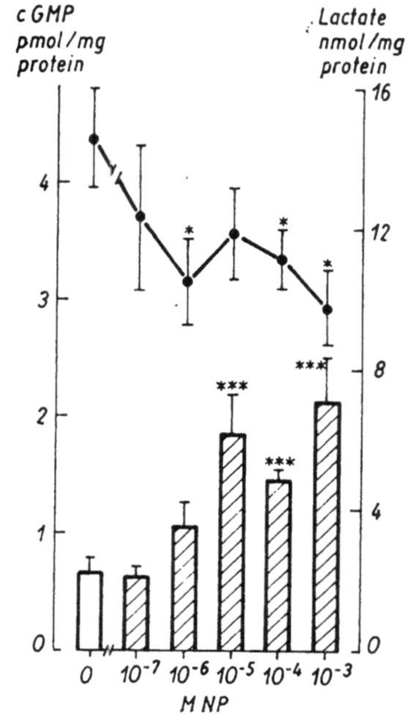

Fig. 2. Effect of nitroprusside (NP) concentration (preincubation time of NP 1 min, hypoxia time 3 min) on the levels of cyclic GMP (control — open bar, NP — hatched bars) and on the lactate production (• — •) in isolated rat atria.
Means (± SEM) of 6—12 preparations are given *p < 0.05, **p < 0.001, ***p < 0.001 when compared to the control (•)

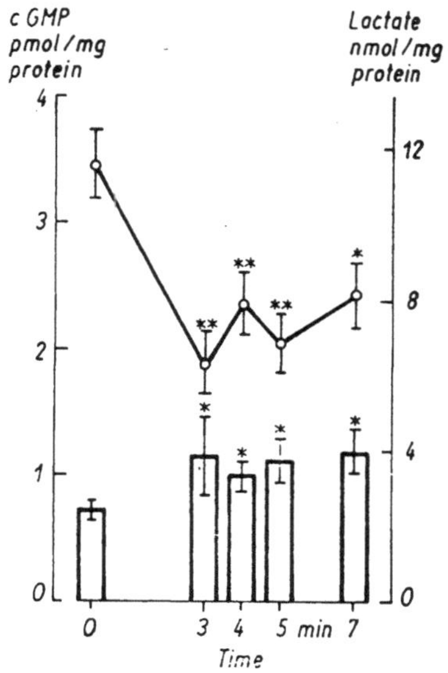

Fig. 3. Time course of the effect of nitroprusside (10^{-4} M) in high oxygen concentration (HiOxSa) on the levels of cyclic GMP (bars) and lactate (○ — ○) in isolated rat atria.
Means (± SEM) of 6—12 preparations are given *p < 0.05, **p < 0.01 when compared to control (○) values

In hypoxia (Fig. 4)., the effects of SNP (10^{-4} M) on the lactate and cGMP levels reached their maximum 3—4 min after the onset of hypoxia.

Effects of 8-bromo-cGMP

In HiOxSa, 8-bromo-cGMP reduced dose dependently the atrial lactate level from 10.6 ± 0.6 nmol/mg prot to 6.0 ± 0.6 nmol/mg prot (Fig. 5). In hypoxia, the maximum effect was obtained at the concentration of 10^{-4} M.

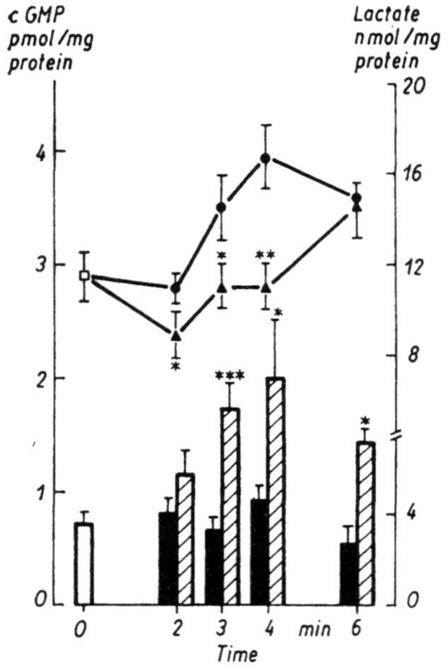

Fig. 4. Time course of the effects of hypoxia and nitroprusside (NP) (10^{-4} M) in hypoxia on the levels of cyclic GMP (shaded bars — hypoxia, hatched bars — NP in hypoxia) and lactate (• — • — hypoxia, ▲ — ▲ — NP in hypoxia) in isolated rat atria.
Means (± SEM) of 6—12 preparations are given *$p < 0.05$, **$p < 0.01$, ***$p < 0.001$ when compared to the control (□) values

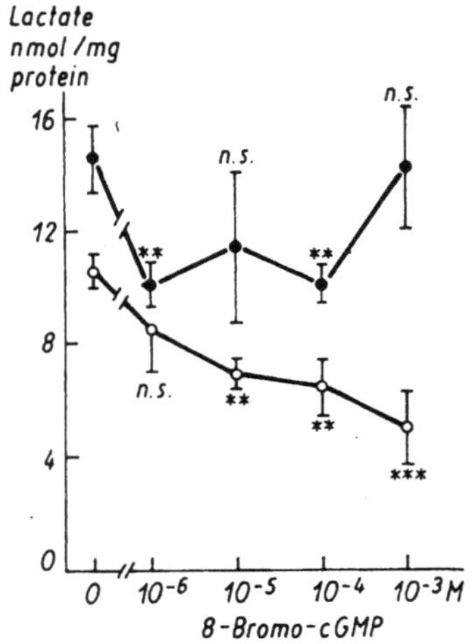

Fig. 5. Concentration response curves of 8-bromo-cGMP in high oxygen concentration (HiOxSa) (○ — ○) and in hypoxia (• — •) on the level of lactate in isolated rat atria.
Means (± SEM) of 6—12 preparations are given *$p < 0.05$, **$p < 0.001$, ***$p < 0.001$ when compared to the control (○ and •) values

Effects of nitroglycerin

Nitroglycerin alone was a weak stimulator of bovine myocardial guanylate cyclase (Table 1), but cysteine could potentiate its stimulation markedly. Similarly, in atria preparation cysteine potentiated the effects of nitroglycerin on atrial lactate and cGMP levels (Table 2).

Table 1

Effects of reducing agents on bovine myocardial guanylate cyclase activation by nitroglycerin

Addition	Guanylate cyclase activity pmol/mg prot/min MN ± SE
Control	3.9 ± 0.7
1 mM nitroglycerin	7.0 ± 0.3
1 mM nitroglycerin + 2.5 mM ascorbate	7.0 ± 0.3
1 mM nitroglycerin + 2.5 mM GSH	9.4 ± 0.3
1 mM nitroglycerin + 2.5 mM cysteine	21.8 ± 0.5

Table 2

Effects of nitroglycerin and cysteine on rat atrial lactate and cGMP levels

Addition	Lactate nmol/mg prot MN ± SE, n = 6 – 12	cGMP fmol/mg prot MN ± SE, n = 6 – 12
Control, HiOxSa	11.1 ± 0.7	827 ± 63
Control, Hypoxia	15.1 ± 1.0	776 ± 54
1 mM nitroglycerin, HiOxSa	10.4 ± 0.7	718 ± 54
1 mM nitroglycerin, Hypoxia	16.0 ± 1.6	870 ± 47
1 mM nitroglycerin + 5 mM cysteine, HiOxSa	9.9 ± 0.8	1049 ± 92*
1 mM nitroglycerin + 5 mM cysteine, Hypoxia	12.1 ± 0.8*	1053 ± 90*

* $p > 0.05$

Discussion

In the present study, we have demonstrated that the myocardial cGMP level has a negative correlation to the lactate levels both in oxygenated and non-oxygenated spontaneously beating rat atria. Thus vasodilatating and anti-anginal drugs such as SNP and nitroglycerin may have direct metabolic effects on the myocardium by elevating the cGMP level.

Murad et al. [17] have suggested a mechanism by which a nitrogenous compound could activate guanylate cyclase. The common intermediate is nitric oxide formed from nitrogenous compound by oxidation, reduction of by spontaneous degradation. SNP has been proposed to release nitric oxide in a spontaneous reaction, while the effect of nitroglycerin is more complicated. Whether nitric oxide interacts directly with guanylate cyclase to produce activation, or whether another intermediate product is involved, is not known [17]. Ignarro et al. [12] have suggested that nitric oxide, nitrates, nitrites and nitroso compounds activate guanylate cyclase through formation of S-nitrosothiol intermediates with sulfhydryl compounds.

According to our results, the activation of myocardial guanylate cyclase with nitroglycerin can be potentiated with cysteine. Cysteine also potentiates the effect of nitroglycerin on the atrial cGMP level. Sodium nitroprusside however, can increase the atrial cGMP level without administration of cysteine. Whether cysteine can potentiate the effect of nitroglycerin on guanylate cyclase and atrial cGMP level through formation of a S-nitrosothiol intermediate or by increasing the release of nitric oxide from nitroglycerin remains unclear.

Sodium nitroprusside, nitroglycerin together with cysteine and 8-bromo-cGMP decreased lactate production in both HiOxSa and hypoxia in spontaneously beating rat atria. The time course and dose dependence of these effects might suggest that cGMP is responsible for the decreased level of tissue lactate. BEITNER et al. [2] have studied the effect of cGMP on glycolytic enzymes. They have shown that cGMP may antagonize the stimulatory effects of cAMP and other allosteric activators on phosphofructokinase (PFK) in enzyme preparations from the rat heart and skeletal muscle. This effect was mot pronounced under conditions in which the enzyme was partially inhibited by ATP or by citrate. Furthermore, in diaphragm muscle, dibutyryl-cGMP also has opposite effects to dibutyryl-cAMP on glucose-1.6-diphosphate level and on the activation of glucose-1.6-diphosphate phosphatase, as well as on PFK, BEITNER et al. [3]. Thus we suggest that cGMP mediates the effect of SNP and nitroglycerin on tissue lactate level seen in this study.

It has recently been demonstrated that hypothermia reduces the tissue level of lactate, inhibits NADH accumulation, and preserves the ATP level during ischaemia [11]. This could be due to low-rate glycolysis, as no glycolytic inhibition develops. The effect of SNP and nitroglycerin through cGMP on tissue lactate level demonstrated in this study could result from low-rate glycolysis similar to that described in hypothermia. In our view, this could be the metabolic effect of all guanylate cyclase stimulating antianginal nitrogenous compounds.

MURAD et al. [17, 18] have proposed that cGMP may function as a feed-back inhibitor of the redox state. The results presented in this study may indicate that cGMP, by inhibition of an overdrive of anaerobic metabolism and lactate accumulation, could readjust the redox state in a more favourable direction for the ischaemic myocyte.

References

[1] ABIKO, Y., K. ICHIHARA and T. IZUMI: Perspectives Cardiovas. Res. **3** (1979), 155–169
[2] BEITNER, R., S. HABERMANN and T. CYCOWITZ: Biochim. Biophys. Acta **482** (1977), 330–340
[3] BEITNER, R. and T. J. COHEN: FEBS Lett **115** (1980), 197–200
[4] BRAUGHLER, J. M., C. K. MITTAL and F. MURAD: Proc. Natl. Acad. Sci. USA **76** (1979), 219–222
[5] BROOKER, C., J. F. HARPER, W. L. TERASAKE and R. D. WOYLEN: Adv. Cyclic Nucleotide Res. **10** (1979), 1–33
[6] GARBERS, D. L. and F. MURAD: Adv. Cyclic Nucleotide Res. **10** (1979), 57–67
[7] GOLDBERG, N. D., M. K. HADDOX and S. E. NICOL: Adv. Cyclic Nucleotide Res. **5** (1975), 307–330
[8] GRUETTER, C. A., D. Y. GRUETTER, J. E. LYON, P. J. KADOWITZ and L. J. IGNARRO: J. Pharmacol. Exp. Ther. **219** (1981), 181–186
[9] HOHORST, H.-J.: In: (Bergmeyer H. U., ed.) Methoden der enzymatischen Analyse II. Weinheim: Verlag Chemie GmbH (1970), 1425–1429

[10] Ichihara, K. and Y. Abiko: Experentia **31** (1975), 477–479
[11] Ichihara, K., J. D. Robishaw and J. R. Neely: Acta Med. Scand. (Suppl) (1981), 13
[12] Ignarro, L. J., J. C. Edwards, D. Y. Gruetter, B. K. Barry and C. A. Gruetter: FEBS Lett **110** (1980), 275–278
[13] Ignarro, L. J. and C. A. Gruetter: Biochim. Biophys. Acta **631** (1980), 221–231
[14] Kukovetz, W. R., S. Holzmann, A. Wurm and G. Pöch: Naunyn-Schmiedeberg's Arch Pharmacol. **310** (1979), 129–138
[15] Lowry, O. H., N. J. Rosebrough, A.-L. Farr and R. J. Randall: J. Biol. Chem. **193** (1951), 265–275
[16] Metsä-Ketelä, T., K. Laustiola, E.-M. Lilius and H. Vapaatalo: Acta Pharmacol. Toxicol. **48** (1981), 311–319
[17] Murad, F., W. P. Arnolds, C. K. Mittal and I. M. Braughler: Adv. Cyclic Nucleotide Res. **11** (1979), 17–204
[18] Murad, F., C. Mittal, W. Arnold and J. M. Braughler: Adv. Pharmacol. and Therapeutics **3** (1979), 123–132
[19] Nimmo, H. G. and P. Cohen: Adv. Cyclic Nucleotide Res. **8** (1977), 145–266
[20] Schultz, K. D., K. Schultz and G. Schultz: Nature **265** (1977), 750–751
[21] Schultz, K. D., E. Böhme, V. A. W. Kreye and G. Schultz: Naunyn-Schmiedeberg's Arch. Pharmacol. **306** (1979), 1–9
[22] Sutherland, E. W., G. A. Robison and R. W. Butcher: Circulation **37** (1968), 279–306

Department of Pharmacology, University Medical School Szeged, Hungary

Possible Pharmacological Measures for the Prevention of Sudden Death in Acute Local Myocardial Ischaemia

L. Szekeres, I. Leprán, I. Krassói, J. Pataricza, É. Udvary, M. Koltai and P. L. Vághy

Sudden death following acute myocardial infarction is mainly the result of ventricular fibrillation which mostly develops from early ventricular arrhythmias appearing within a few minutes after the onset of local myocardial ischaemia [8].

A rational therapeutic approach protecting against these life threatening early post-infarction arrhythmias is based on the following principles:

1. Protection against ischaemia induced electrophysiological changes (antiarrhythmic drugs, calcium-antagonists).
2. Reduction of the ischaemia induced increased symphathetic drive by central or peripheral adrenergic blockade.
3. Reduction of the speed of development as well as the extent of ischaemic changes.

Measures belonging to the first two groups listed above act mainly on the nonischaemic myocardium and the borderline area, unless applied preventively before the onset of myocardial ischaemia. These interventions are more or less known by the clinicians and have occasionally been tested in clinical trials.

Much less is known about the therapeutic interventions which may diminish the size of the ischaemic area. Therefore the present paper is dedicated to this type of drugs.

We have tested the following therapeutic interventions: treatment with a nonsteroid antiinflammatory agent (sulfinpyrazone); or a diet rich in linoleic acid; and these were compared to a β-adrenoceptor blocking drug (pindolol) and a membrane stabilizing antiarrhythmic agent (lidocaine). This latter was included, since clinical trials concerning a short term protective effect of this drug against early postinfarction arrhythmias proved to be promising [5, 6].

To test the therapeutic value of a treatment, the conventional coronary ligation model in anesthetized dogs has been used. This model does not seem to be satisfactory in every respect, since anesthesia eliminates pain, depresses autonomic reflexes and together with the stress of surgical manipulation considerably alters sensitivity to drugs. To eliminate these shortcomings, we have developed a conscious rat infarction model which is described in detail elsewhere [4]. Briefly, in a preliminary surgery a loose ligature of atraumatic silk is stitched under the left coronary artery. The ends of the silk loop were pulled through an intrathoracally placed polyethylene tube and, after closing the chest, it was fixed under the skin. Seven days after surgery, occlusion of the coronary artery was performed by tightening the loose ligature in the conscious animal under ECG control. This gives the possibility to follow the rate of survival, the occurrence and type as well as the time of onset and duration of early postinfarction arrhythmias. As the protective action of sulfinpyrazone, pindolol and lidocaine is a function of an adequate therapeutic blood level, we have found it satisfactory to administer one single dose of these drugs before occlusion. On the other hand, linoleic acid rich (LAR) diet, containing 12% sunflower oil instead of normal fat had to be given for a longer period of time, for a week or more.

All these interventions significantly increased the survival rate, reduced the occurrence and duration of arrhythmias and prolonged the time to the onset of arrhythmias. It is striking that the LAR diet considerably increased survival already after one week feeding (Table 1).

Table 1

Effect of lidocaine, pindolol, sulfinpyrazone and linoleic acid rich (LAR) diet on survival rate and incidence of arrhythmias in the early phase of coronary occlusion in conscious rats

Treatment		Dose mg/kg	n	Survival rate %	Occurence of arrhythmias %				Arrhythmias in survivors		
					None	VF	VT	other	n	onset after occlusion min	duration min
Control			29	31	0	72	76	58	9	3.74	6.55
Lidocaine i.v. 10 min before occl.		2.0	14	64*	29**	21**	50	50	9	10.30***	2.44*
Pindolol i.v. 10 min before occl.		0.015	19	63*	16*	32**	68	58	12	8.61***	3.65
Control			18	33	0	78	94	50	6	4.91	7.25
Sulfinpyrazone p.os		10	10	80*	10	20*	80	60	8	6.27	3.54
1 hour before occl.		50	20	65*	20*	15*	80	40	7	8.65*	2.57*
Control			26	19	0	88	96	42	5	5.13	4.85
LAR	1 week		15	60**	20*	47**	53***	60	9	9.07	4.09
DIET	2 weeks		11	64**	18	36**	64**	45	7	8.90	3.19
	4 weeks		11	64**	27**	36**	64**	45	7	10.3*	3.48
	12 weeks		21	81***	43***	28***	48***	33	17	10.6*	2.19

One could imagine that the severity of heart rhythm disturbances is related to the size of ischaemic area and antiischaemic interventions might exert their antiarryhthmic effects by reducing the size of ischaemic area.

To test these possibilities the ischaemic area was determined by means of Evans blue staining 10 minutes after the occlusion of the left anterior descending coronary artery in dogs [9]. The results indicate that the occurrence and severity of heart rhythm disturbances are indeed related to the size of ischaemic area (Table 2).

The infarcted area has been determined in rats 16 hours after coronary occlusion by nitrotetrazolium blue staining of the sliced heart. The wet weight of the infarcted

Table 2

Occurrence and severity of heart rhythm disturbance and size of the ischaemic (occluded) area in anesthetized dogs

Occurrence and severity of arrhythmia		weight of ischaemic area / total heart weight
no arrhythmia	10	0.185 ± 0.017
Ventricular extra beats	7	0.234 ± 0.022 (+ 26.5%)
Ventricular fibrillation	6	0.318 ± 0.039 (+71.8%)

myocardium, remaining unstained, was expressed as percent of the total wet weight of the ventricles. The results indicate that antiischaemic measures used in this study did not reduce the infarct size as compared to controls (data not shown).

Therefore, we had to assume that some transitory increase of the ischaemic area, not reflected by the infarct size, might be present and perhaps this could favourably be influenced by antiischaemic treatment.

In order to examine this hypothesis, a method suitable to detect and visualize early ischaemic alterations of the myocardium is needed. It has been demonstrated that in conscious rats the early postocclusion arrhythmias appear between the 5th and the 8th minute after coronary occlusion [3]. It is known, however, that the earliest morphological changes are manifested only after 20—30 minutes of ischaemia and histochemical methods, such as glycogen staining, demonstrate metabolic alterations only after 10 to 20 minutes of ischaemia [2].

Therefore, an *ex vivo* perfusion technique for determination of the ischaemic area has been elaborated. Coronary occlusion was performed in three different groups of rats under pentobarbitone (45 mg/kg) anesthesia and the hearts were excised at the 3rd minute when, according to ECG records, arrhythmias did not yet appear, at the 6th minute when the most severe arrhythmias were present, and at the 20th minute after occlusion when the acute phase characterized by arrhythmias was already over. The hearts were perfused retrogradely from the aorta with 5 ml 4% formaldehyde in isotonic NaCl solution.

The blood could be washed out of the normal myocardium whereas the ischaemic area remained dark red, delineated by a sharp borderline in spite of the fact that coronary occlusion has been reopened before perfusion.

Table 3 shows the size of ischaemic area as a function of time elapsed after coronary occlusion. Accordingly, the 3rd and 30th minute values as well as the size of the 16th hour infarcted area were significantly different from the 6th minute ischaemic area, when the most severe arrhythmias appeared. We are of the opinion that the coincidence of early postocclusion arrhythmias and of the transitory increase of the ischaemic area is not an accidental phenomenon.

This assumption is further corroborated by our finding that the antiischaemic interventions protecting against lethal arrhythmias were also able to eliminate the transitory increase of the ischaemic area appearing at the 6th minute after occlusion (Fig. 1).

Table 3

The size of the ischaemic as well as the infarcted area after coronary artery occlusion in rats

	Time	n	Size, %	p
Ischaemic area	3. min	8	21.6 ± 3.11	< 0.01
	6. min	12	34.8 ± 2.30	
	20. min	7	17.8 ± 2.13	< 0.001
Infarcted area	16. h	8	22.7 ± 4.20	< 0.01

Results are given as mean ± S.E.
'p' value indicate statistically significant difference from the 6th min ischaemic area

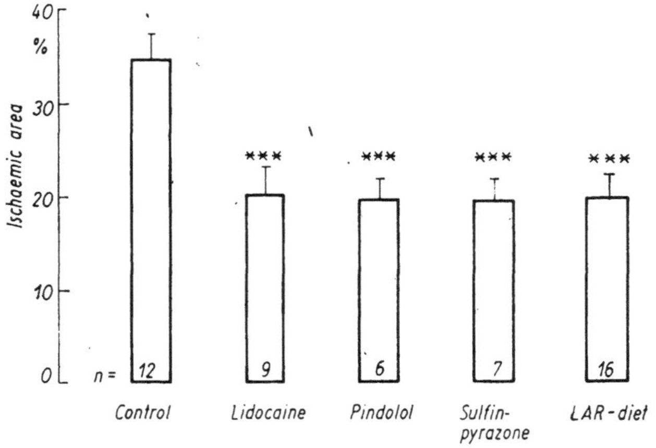

Fig. 1. Effect of lidocaine, pindolol sulfinpyrazone and linoleic acid rich (LAR) — diet on the extent of the ischaemic area in the 6th min after coronary occlusion in anesthetized rats.

These results raise further questions — of which the most important ones are: What is the explanation of this short lasting however so important early increase in the size of the ischaemic area, and how antiischaemic drugs can prevent it?

To explore the possible factors, the antiischaemic action of sulfinpyrazone was analyzed in detail. Repeated occlusions of the left anterior descending coronary artery were performed in anesthetized dogs. The effect of sulfinpyrazone on the ischaemia induced ST segment elevation measured on the epicardial ECG is demonstrated on Figure 2. It is noteworthy that, in spite of the i.v. injection of this drug, the maximal inhibition of the ST segment elevation was demonstrated only 90 minutes after the drug administration.

Sulfinpyrazone did not affect the normal coronary flow but reduced the pacing induced elevation of the ST segment in the epicardial ECG measured in the area perfused dy a critically constricted left descending coronary artery. A maximal protection apbeared only 90 minutes after the i.v. administration of the drug (Fig. 3). It is also shown

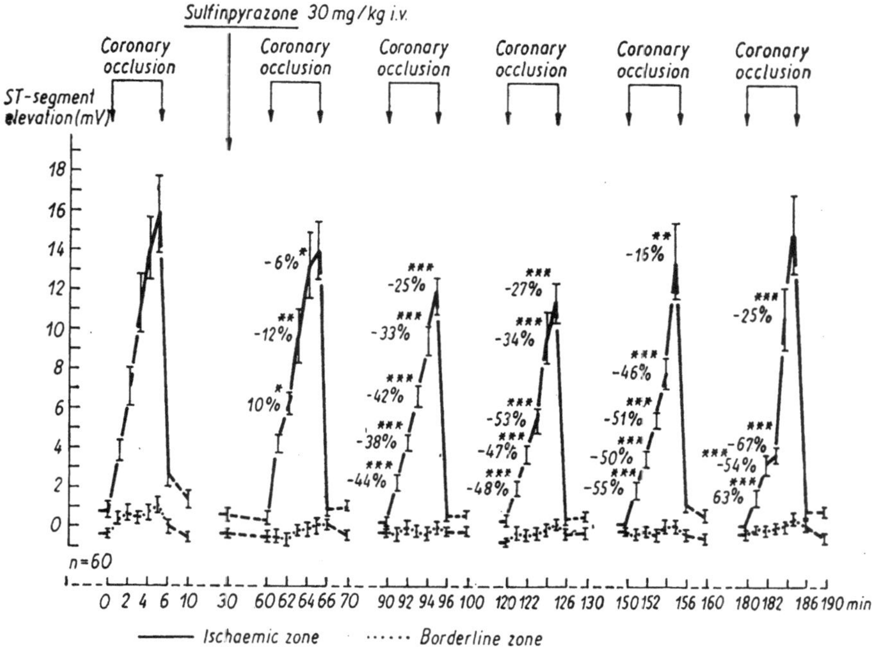

Fig. 2. Effect of sulfinpyrazone on coronary occlusion induced epicardial ST segment elevation in anesthetized, open-chest dogs.

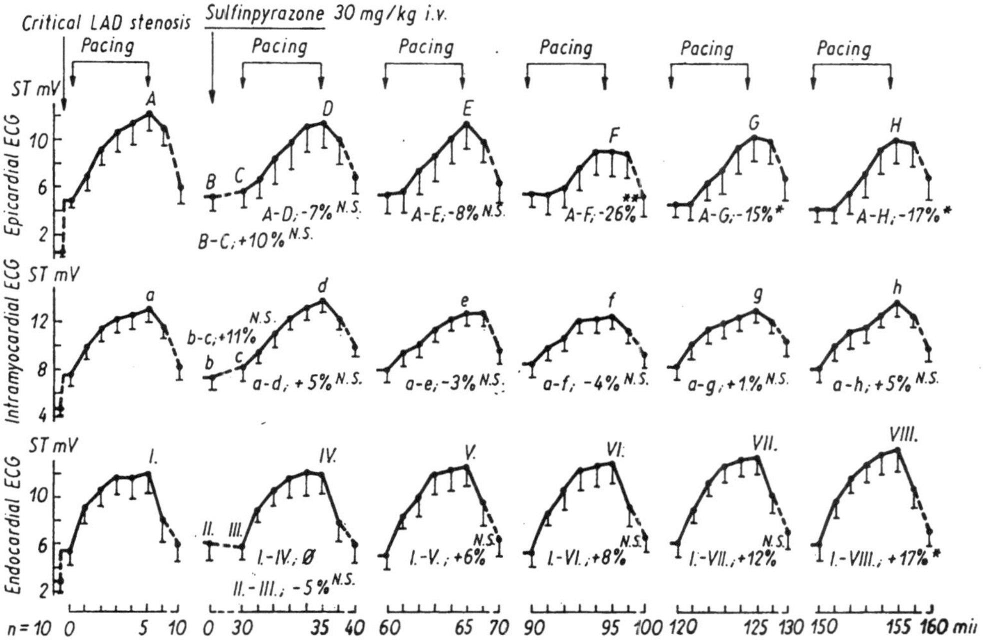

Fig. 3. Effect of sulfinpyrazone on pacing induced ST segment elevation in the area perfused by a critically constricted coronary artery in anesthetized, open-chest dogs.

that sulfinpyrazone was unable to prevent the ST segment elevation measured either on the intramyocardial or endocardial ECG.

The effect of sulfinpyrazone on the platelet aggregation was also determined. Sulfinpyrazone was administered intravenously to anesthetized dogs in a dose of 30 mg/kg. Venous blood was taken and the ADP-induced platelet aggregation was determined *ex vivo*. The time of maximal inhibition of platelet aggregation was found 90 minutes after the drug administration (Table 4), i.e. it coincides with the maximal protection by sulfinpyrazone against the ST segment elevation. From these data, it is suggested that the chance to prevent early postinfarction arrhythmias by this drug may be minimal provided that it is applied after the onset of myocardial infarction.

Table 4

Effect of sulfinpyrazone on ex vivo platelet aggregation induced by 36 μM ADP

Time after 30 mg/kg i.v. sulfinpyrazone administration (min.)	n	Platelet aggregation as % of the max. amplitude. (The difference between the platelet rich plasma and platelet poor plasma was taken as 100 %)	% difference from control
Control	4	74.7 ± 0.2	
30	4	65.7 ± 5.6	−12
60	4	60.2 ± 2.6	−19 $p < 0.01$
90	3	47.7 ± 2.4	−36 $p < 0.001$
120	5	61.2 ± 3.4	−18 $p < 0.01$
150	3	66.0 ± 7.4	−12

Results are given as mean ± S.E.
'p' value indicate statistically significant difference from control value

Theoretically all patients at high risk of acute myocardial infarction should receive a long term pretreatment assuring adequate drug level which protects against letal arrhythmias in case of myocardial infarction. A long term pretreatment, however, raises the problem of possible side effects. Therefore, preference should be given to those drugs which are found to be well tolerated by patients.

In Figure 4 we tried to summarize, without any claim to completeness, the metabolic, haemodynamic and vascular factors contributing to the transistory increase of the ischaemic area, also pointing to the possible mode of action of antiischaemic drugs. We would like to lay stress on the importance of those factors hitherto less taken into consideration. As a consequence of slowing of the blood flow and ischaemia an increase of the thromboxane (TXA_2): prostacyclin ratio may occur. Thus, transitory platelet aggregates could appear temporarily, obstructing blood flow, in the capillary bed. In addition, TXA_2 is a highly active vasoconstrictory substance contributing to the slowing of blood

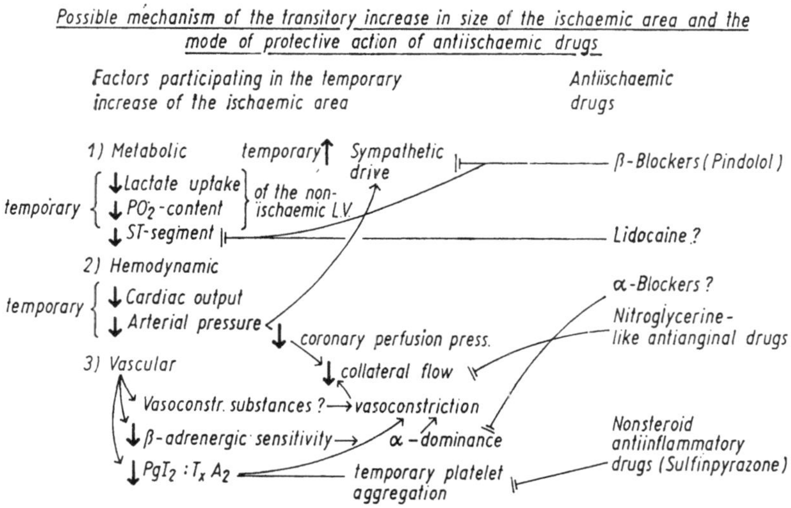

Fig. 4. Schematic diagram showing possible mechanism of the transitory increase in size of the ischaemic area and the mode of protective action of antiischaemic drugs.

flow and ischaemia [1, 7]. Probably, all non-steroid antiinflammatory drugs exert their protective antiischaemic action by inhibiting platelet aggregation.

As a conclusion it can be said that the period, when we were deemed to be helpless onlookers of the fatal sequence of postinfarction events leading to early sudden death, is over. We learn more and more about the pathomechanism of early arrhythmias developing to ventricular fibrillation. There are several promising measures at least in animal experiments capable of preventing or reducing the incidence of sudden death. Whether these new therapeutic trends will be useful in the clinical practice still remains an open question and requires extensive, well planned and controlled clinical trials.

References

[1] Coker, S. J., J. R. Parratt, J. McA. Ledingham and I. J. Zeitlin: Nature **291** (1981), 323–324

[2] Jennings, R. B., C. E. Ganote and K. A. Reiner: Amer. J. Pathol. **81** (1975), 179–198

[3] Leprán, I., M. Koltai and L. Szekeres: Eur. J. Pharmacol. **69** (1981), 235–238

[4] Leprán, I., W. Siegmund and L. Szekeres: Acta physiol. Acad. Sci. Hung. **53** (1979), 190

[5] Lie, K. I., H. J. Wellens, F. J. Van Capelle and D. Durrer: New Engl. J. Med. **291** (1974), 1324–1326

[6] Morgensen, L.: Proceedings of a Symposium held in Edinburgh in September 1970, (Ed.: Scott, D. B., Julian, D. G.), London, Livingstone (1971), 91–95

[7] Terashita, Z.-I., H. Fukui, K. Nishikawa, M. Hirata and S. Kikuchi: Eur. J. Pharmacol. **53** (1978), 49–56

[8] Szekeres, L.: Excerpta Medica. International Congress Series No. 470. Proceedings of the VIII. World Congress of Cardiology Tokyo 1978. (Ed.: Hayase, S., Murao, S.) Elsevier North Holland, (1979), 933–938

[9] Szekeres, L., É. Csordás Nagy and É. Udvary: Symposium on pharmacology of the heart, Budapest, Akadémiai Kiadó (1976), 29–37

Institut of General Pathology and Pathophysiology, Academy of Medical Sciences, USSR, Moscow

Stress Damages of the Heart: Pathogenesis, and Possibilities of Prevention and Removing

F. Z. Meerson

The idea of the stress-reaction key role in the pathogenesis of main human non-infectious diseases acquired an extreme popularity in the modern medicine. However during the evolution process stress-reaction undoubtly has formed not as a link of pathogenesis but on the contrary as a link of adaptation. In fact we can say that in natural conditions stress-reaction which naturally occures as a response to extremal and simply new situations is not at all an independent isolated event but it immediately becomes a link of more complex process that is the organism adaptation to the environment.

The scheme on the Figure 1 represents the concept formed in our laboratory on the mechanism of the organism individual phenotypic adaptation to the environment and shows the place of stress-reaction as a link of this mechanism. It can be seen that the environmental factor-induced disturbance of homeostasis activates systems responsible for adaptation via higher control levels. As a result the two following chains of events occure: first, presented in the top part of the scheme mobilization of the system specifically responsible for adaptation to a given concrete factor, for instance, to physical load, cold, oxygen shortage; second, an absolutely non-specific standard stress-reaction which arises under the action of any strong stimulator.

The enhanced physiological function subsequently activates the genetic apparatus in cells of the functional system specifically responsible for adaptation to activate the synthesis of nucleic acids and proteins which form the key cell structures, i.e. structures limited in their function. As a result of those key structures selective growth the so-called systemic structural trace forms which results in enhanced functional power of systems responsible for adaptation to make possible the transition of urgent but reliable adaptation to the stable long-term one. It is shown on the scheme that the systemic structural trace and stable adaptation are formed under the potentiating participation of stress-reaction which plays an especially important role precisely at the stage of the urgent adaptation transition to the long-term one.

It is secured, first, by the fact that stress-reaction provides not only mobilization of the organism energetic resources, but selectively directs them to the system responsible for adaptation where the structural trace forms. Second, it is secured by direct action of stress hormones which can induce the essential alterations in the membrane lipid bilayer, activate ionic transport and glycolysis and, when act more lengthly, the protein biosynthesis in cell of systems, responsible for adaptation.

After the systemic structural trace has completely formed and become a basis, for instance, of temporary connection, training to physical load or enhanced resistance to hypoxia stable adaptation eliminates the disturbances of homeostasis and, as a result, stress-reaction which has become unnecessary disappears.

In so-called hopeless situations when the factor which acts on the organism is too strong or the situation occured in the environment is too complex the effective functional system and systemic structural trace do not form. It results in retention of the initial disturbances of homeostasis and the stress-reaction stimulated by them achieves excessive intensity and duration. Precisely in this situation stress-reaction can turn from a general link of adaptation to a general link of the pathogenesis of various diseases.

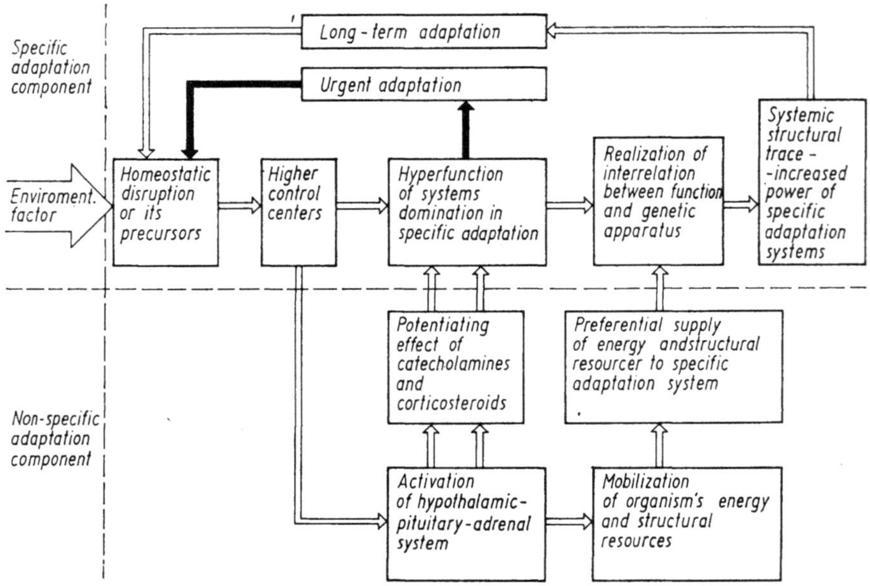

Fig. 1. The mechanism of phenotypic adaptation. Explanations in text.

In this work we should like to cite only one example of transition of the stress adaptive effect to the damaging one; this example regards the organ which is traditionally a subject of our investigations, namely the heart. The experiment in which the material have been obtained is the following; one series of rats was exposed to *a priori* short-term one-hour stress action according to the known Desiderato method (DESIDERATO and TESTA [2]) and the other series was exposed to long-term six-hour stress action. After the stress termination hearts were taken from animals and the isolated hearts were studied for the contractile function. The experiment was carried out under isovolumic conditions which allow the pressure inside the heart to reflect the real dynamics of the tension development and relaxation because the heart contracts around the hermetic capacity with constant volume.

The material of the Table 1 shows that under aerobic condition in hearts of animals exposed to short-term stress the contraction process occured in the same manner as in control and the relaxation process is essentially activated; its velocity is increased more than by 40%. The hearts of animals exposed to long-term stress on the contrary show a depression of developed pressure and to even more extent a depression of the relaxation process; relaxation velocity is reduced almost by one-third and the diastolic pressure is two-fold increased. Further the Table 1 shows that the heart hypoxic contracture, i.e. the disturbances of relaxation which shows in a great enhancement of the diastolic tension, a well-known phenomenon, which develops at the next stage of the experiment when the heart acts under hypoxic conditions. The main result of the experiment is in that this contracture which is known to depend on the disturbed functioning of the cardiomyocyte membrane Ca-pump was 2.5 fold less in hearts of animals exposed to short-term stress than that in control; correspondingly the values of developed tension and the velocity of its development during hypoxia were 1.5—2 fold less than in control.

Table 1

The influence of long and short emotional-painful stress on heart contractile function resistance to hypoxia and reoxygenation

	Groups of animals	Aerobic conditions	Hypoxia	Reoxygenation
Developed	I control	100.3 ± 4.1	22.9 ± 1.4	53.5 ± 5.1
tension	II EPS 1 hour	102.2 ± 3.9	38.6 ± 2.1*	100.9 ± 6.9*
mm Hg	III EPS 6 hours	68.4 ± 4.9	14.9 ± 1.2*	44.6 ± 3.8
Diastolic	I control	4.3 ± 1.3	40.3 ± 2.2	13.0 ± 1.3
pressure	II EPS 0.8 hour	4.4 ± 2.1	15.0 ± 2.4*	6.0 ± 1.3*
mm Hg	III EPS 6 hours	8.1 ± 8*	48.5 ± 2.5*	23.4 ± 3.0*
Maximal velocity of	I control	1.900 ± 89	400 ± 27	875 ± 69
pressure developing	II EPS 1 hour	2.150 ± 120	875 ± 92*	2016 ± 190
mm Hg/sec	III EPS 6 hours	1.380 ± 110*	286 ± 92*	586 ± 80*
Maximal velocity of	I control	1000 ± 84	188 ± 22	700 ± 49
relaxation	II EPS 1 hour	1.451 ± 45*	550 ± 44*	1100 ± 96*
mm Hg/sec	IIII EPS 6 hours	840 ± 45	162 ± 20	685 ± 99
Coronary	I control	8.0 ± 1.4	6.0 ± 0.8	6.5 ± 0.5
flux	II EPS 1 hour	11.0 ± 1.2	11.3 ± 1.1	11.2 ± 0.7
ml/min	III EPS 6 hours	7.5 ± 0.5	4.9 ± 0.3	6.5 ± 0.

Data in experimental groups in relation to the control are significant: * = $P < 0.05$

In the hearts of animals exposed to long-term stress the values of contracture and depression of the heart contractile function, on the contrary, were higher than in control. In other words the short-term stress resulted in some microstructural changes in the heart muscle which became a cause of the activation of the relaxation process and enhanced the heart resistance to hypoxia. The long-term stress, on the contrary, has an opposite effect: it potentiates the damaging effect of hypoxia. Further the attention should be concentrated not on the adaptive, but precisely damaging stress effect.

Facts evidence that stressful situations of the reality can cause or potentiate the development of the stomach and duodenum ulcerous disease, hypertension, atherosclerosis, ischaemic heart disease, diabetic, psychic, and dermatic diseases, and, as, it has been proved during the last decade, of the blastomatous growth. Thus excessively intensive stress-reaction and its transition from an adaptation link to a link of pathogenesis play an important and probably decisive role in the occurence of main non-infectious diseases, their prevention and therapy being the major unsettled problem of the contemporary medicine. Correspondingly the elaboration of methods for the stress damage prevention is a necessary stage in development of the problem concerning non-infectious disease prophylaxis which is one of the main issues of the contemporary pathophysiology in the whole, and of the heart pathophysiology in particular.

Apparently the popular impression concerning the role of stress in the pathology is far from sufficient for this problem solution; a progress in this area demands definition of such pathogenetic chain of damage and elucidation of concrete neuro-humoral cellular and molecular links of that chain which can be inhibited by certain anti-stress factors of the organism itself or by exogenous chemical substances.

In order to solve this problem the pathogenesis of stress damage would be studied with absolutely stable model by a complex analyzis of the dynamics of damages occuring in a given vitally important organ.

As such a model our laboratory and related institutes use emotional-painful stress (EPS), the so-called neurosis of anxiety induced according to the world-accepted Desiderato's method, the heart being the subject of investigations. Simultaneously rather wide researches of the brain neurotransmitter metabolism and also of other organ injuries under stress were carried out (see [4]).

The scheme in Figure 2 shows that in stress situations the excitation of higher vegetative centers determining stress — reaction results in a manyfold increase of the catecholamine concentration affecting the heart (the first link).

If results in an excessive activation of the adenylcyclase system and in enhanced Ca influx into cardiomyocytes (the second link). Subsequently two shifts develop which we suppose to form the third key link of the process. The first shift is shown on the scheme to be in the fact that the lipid triade of the cardiomyocyte biomembrane damage occures. It shows an excessive activation of lipid peroxidation, lipases, phospholipases and detergent action of fatty acids and lysophosphatides. The second event is in the fact that glycogen reserve decreases due to the excessive activation of glycolysis and glycogenolysis.

The lipid triade seems to form the basis of the lysosomic membrane damage which results in the proteolytic enzyme release from lysosomes (the fourth link).

The effect of lipid triad and lysosomic enzymes and the disturbances in the system of glycolysis result in the injuries of sarcolemmal and sarcoplasmic reticulum membranes responsible for calcium transport, in the cation pump disturbance, and in an increase of the sarcolemmal permeability for calcium (the fifth link). Simultaneously cleavages appear in the molecules of nuclear DNA; in most of nuclei these cleavages are eliminated by reparation and in some cases they lead to the DNA degradation and death of cells. Further the enhanced sarcolemma permeability for calcium and disturbances of the calcium pump work result in the progressing increase of calcium in the cardiomyocyte sarcoplasm (the sixth link). This important shift has two outcomes. First, it can activate the complex of processes constituting the lipid triade and thus close the vicious circle which redoubles the myocardial injury. Second, the excessive calcium has its own damaging effect, namely it induces development of the complex of shifts inside cells which has been designed before as calcium triade; it consists of myofibril contracture, disturbance of the calcium-overloaded mitochondria function, and activation of

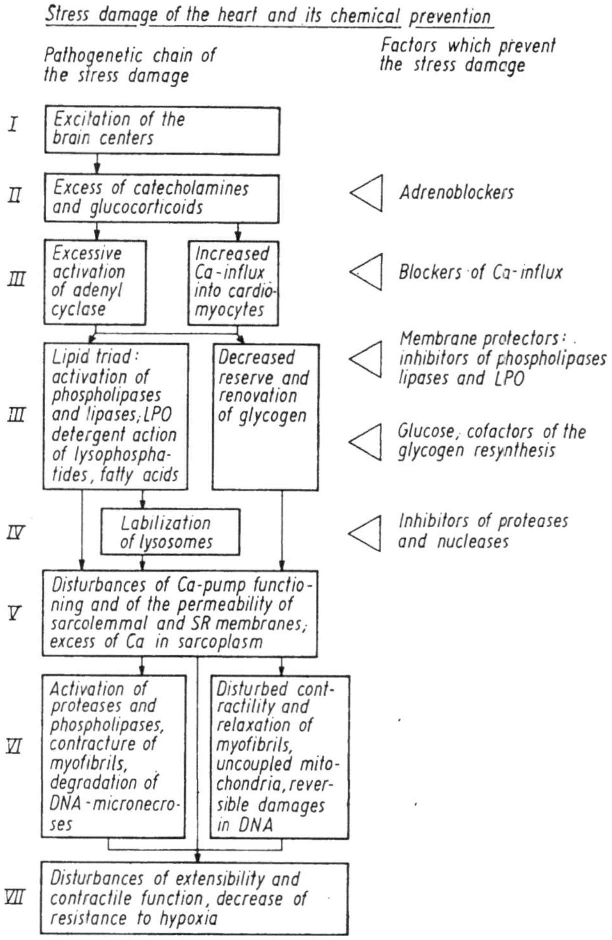

Fig. 2. Pathogenesis of stress damage of the heart. Explanations in text.

myofibrillar proteases and mitochondrial phospholipases to aggregate the damage (the seventh link).

As a result an irreversible contracture and necrobiosis of isolated cardiomyocyte groups appear to pronouncelly disturb the contractile function of the heart muscle as a whole.

The scheme examination permits at least two following outcomes: first, the revealed disturbances of metabolism, structure, and function were observed after the stress situation had passed, they appear to be not simply a response to stressor but a relatively stable sequences of the damage which had occured during stress. This fact together with expanded clinical data on the role of emotional stress in the ethiology of circulatory diseases give the ground to believe that precisely such relatively stable disruptions of metabolism and function which are retained after the stress itself has passed and accumulate from one stress episode to another can play a role in the gradual development of such forms of so-called primary non-coronarogenic cardiosclerosis and chronic cardiac insufficiency which non infrequently appear in humans who have not suffered from circulatory diseases before.

Second, there is many evidence that the represented pathogenetic chain occurs not only in cardiomyocytes but also in arterial and arteriolar myocytes to form a probable basis of the vessel stable spasm. Such an essentially contractural spasm now is shown to play a definite part in clinically typical stress states, disturbances of coronary, cerebral, and peripheric circulation, and also in the development the best of all studied by now stress damages, precisely ulcerous lesions of the stomach mucous coat.

So many things allow to believe that the just now examined pathogenetic chain plays a role in occurence of the coronarogenic ischaemic myocardium damages. These circumstances are essential for the cardiologic clinic.

The right part of the scheme shows anti-stress factors which can blockade links of the above-said pathogenetic chain and prevent the organism stress damages.

All those factors have been experimentally studied by our group of laboratories; they prevent or restrict the heart stress damages to different degrees. In this presentation we shall limit ourselves to some examples which evidence sufficiently effective action of antioxidants and factors restoring the glycogen reserve, i.e. the effect of factors adressed to the third that is to our mind key link of the pathogenetic chain of stress damage.

There are two possibilities by which the catecholamine excess and activation of its biosynthesis in stress can activate lipid peroxidation (LPO). First, the activated oxygen species are naturally formed at certain steps of catecholamine biosynthesis [1] and, second, epinephrine oxidation to adrenochrome drives rise to a semiquinone radical which can donate electron to oxygen, thus generating the superoxide radical, an important LPO inducer [3]. Prezisely those activated oxygen species are known to trigger LPO.

In full agreement with this assumption is the finding that the excitation of adrenergic regulation under emotional-painful stress reproduced in form of so-called "neurosis of anxiety" caused LPO activation in heart muscle and in other organs.

It can be seen from the Table 2 that in the myocardium of stress-exposed animals the content of intermediate and end-LPO-products is increased more than three-fold. It appears also that the stress-induced LPO activation can largely be prevented by injecting ionol, a synthetic free radical scavenger of a phenolic type prior to stress [7]. Further investigation have demonstrated that beside LPO activation prevention ionol and other LPO inhibitors prevent the stress damages of the heart and other organs [4].

Table 2

Effect of preliminary administration of ionol on LPO in the myocardium in stress

Series	Lipid hydroperoxides conv. units	Schiffs bases fluorescence conv. units
1. Control	1.08 ± 0.13	1.00 ± 0.33
2. Stress	2.53 ± 0.14	2.64 ± 0.40
3. Ionol	1.08 ± 0.10	1.01 ± 0.20
4. Ionol-stress	1.71 ± 0.14	1.26 ± 0.17
Significance of the differences	$P_{1-2} < 0.001$	$P_{1-2} < 0.001$
	P_{1-3} n.s.	P_{1-3} n.s.
	$P_{1-4} < 0.05$	$P_{1-4} < 0.5$

The results obtained in our laboratory allow to sum up that the stress-induced disturbances of metabolism such as decrease activity of sarcoplasmic reticulum Ca-pump [5], lower glycogen content [9], an uncoupling between oxidation and phosphorylation in mitochondria [8], and labilization of lysosomes [4], and reversible DNA damages [6] are partly or completely prevented by the LPO inhibitor ionol.

It was revealed then that in a similar way antioxidant prevents other stress damaging effect, namely the loss of enzymes by the myocardium [7], an appearance of small-focal contractural and necrotic lesions [5], a depression of the contractile function [10], and, finally, the post-stress decrease of heart resistance to calcium excess and hypoxia [7].

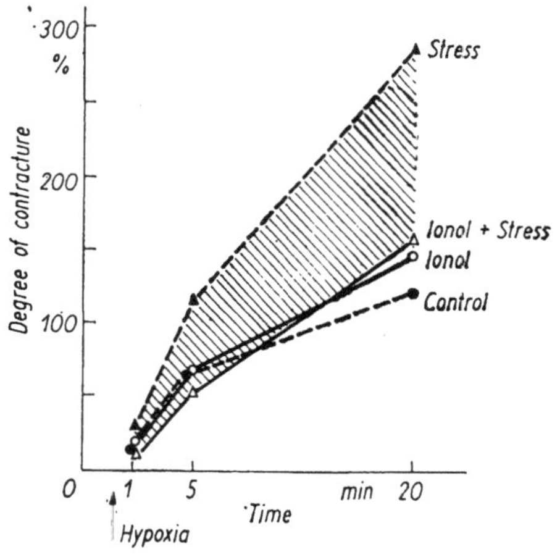

Fig. 3. Post-stress activation of hypoxic contracture and prevention of this phenomenon by antioxidant ionol.

The curves on the Figure 3 shows the dynamics of the well-known event that is hypoxic contracture of the myocardium. It can be seen that in the myocardium of stress-exposed rats the hypoxia-induced contracture is at least two times as high as in control. Preliminary injection of ionol completely prevents the post-stress decrease of myocardium resistance to hypoxia.

It may thus be concluded that LPO activation which naturally occurs in heart muscle in stress is a key link of the heart stress damage and can therefore be prevented by antioxidants.

In the further presentation it appears purposeful to examine an example of elimination of the stress-induced disturbances of the contractile function by factors which influence the glycogen reserve in the myocardium. As it was shown earlier, in hearts of stress-exposed animals glycogen concentration was reduced on 40 per cent and glycogen resynthesis measured by the labeled glucose incorporation, was disturbed [9]. A 4-fold increased glucose concentration in the incubation medium from 5.5 mM to 22 mM completely abolished the disturbances of myocardium extensibility and developed tension (data not shown). Figure 4 shows that the remove of the atrium contractile function post-stress disturbances can be achieved at 5.5 mM glucose by injection of glycogen resynthesis cofactor uridine in concentration of $2 \cdot 10^{-6}$ mM. Essentially those data mean, that disturbances in the system of glycolysis play a significant role in the developing of the post-stress depression of myocardium contractility.

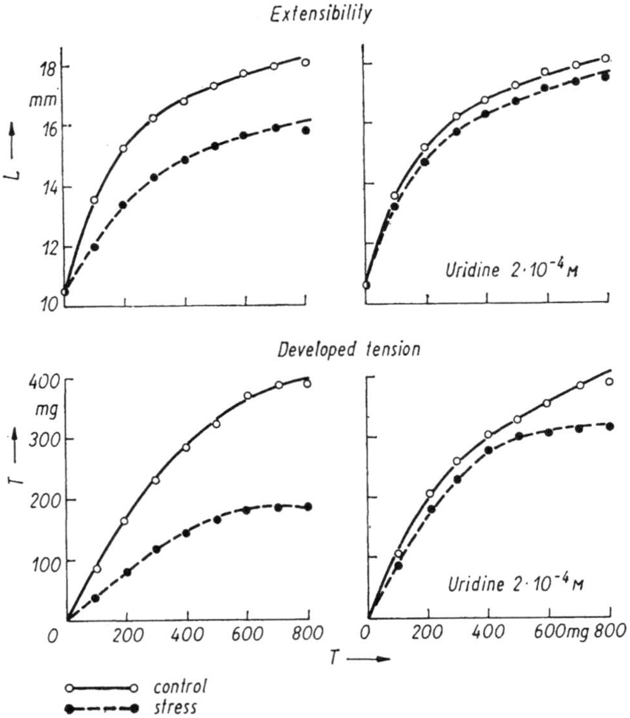

Fig. 4. Removing of post-stress disturbances of extensibility and developed tension of myocardium of the atrium by the injection of glycogen resynthesis cofactor uridine in the incubation medium.

To sum up the presentation it could be underlined that now physicians do not yet diagnose the "heart stress damage" and nevertheless this damage plays a tremendous role in human pathology, because stress not only preceedes the attacks of ischaemic disease but potentiates its development in the whole.

That's why it can be supposed that arsenal of drugs, which are elaborated by the theoretical cardiology for preventing and removing of stress damages of the heart today would find its application in the treatment of ischaemic disease tomorrow.

References

[1] BORS, W., C. MICHEL, M. SARAN and E. LENGFELDER: Biochim. Biophys. Acta **540** (1978), 162–172

[2] DESIDERATO, O. and M. TESTA: Physiol. and Behav. **16** (1976), 67–81

[3] DILIBERTO, E. J. and P. L. ALLEN: J. Biol. Chem. **256** (1981), 3385–3393

[4] MEERSON, F. Z.: Nauka (Moscow), 1981 (Russian)

[5] MEERSON, F. Z., J. B. ARHIPENKO, I. I. POZSHICKAYA and V. E. KAGAN: Bull. Exp. Biol. Med. (1981), 405–406

[6] MEERSON, F. Z. and B. K. VASILIEV: Voprosy Med. Khimii **27** (1982), 115–118

[7] MEERSON, F. Z., L. U. GOLUBEVA, V. E. KAGAN, M. V. SHIMKOVITCH and A. A. UGOLER: In: Fourth USA–USSR joint symposium on myocardium metabolism. Natl. Inst. Health Publication, Bethesda (1980), 217
[8] MEERSON, F. Z., V. V. MALISHEV, A. B. PETROVA and B. I. LIFANTIEV: Kardiologia (1982), 81–93
[9] MEERSON, F. Z., I. V. PAVLOVA, B. S. JAKUSHEV and E. X. KAMILOV: Kardiologia (1978), 52–59
[10] MEERSON, F. Z. and A. M. TRISHPOEVA: Bull. Exp. Biol. Med. (1980), 531–533

Science Institute, University of Iceland, Reykjavik, Iceland

Alterations in Fatty Acyl Chain Composition of Myocardial Phospholipids During Stress

S. Gudbjarnason, A. Emilsson and A. Gudmundsdóttir

Stress is considered one of the pathogenic factors in development of coronary artery disease. Increased sympathetic activity and elevated plasma levels of catecholamines influence markedly cardiac function and myocardial metabolism. The effects of exogenous or endogenous catecholamines on myocardial membranes and membrane lipids have received relatively little attention. The purpose of this study was to examine alterations in fatty acid composition of phospholipids in rat heart muscle in relation to various forms of stress.

The experimental animals were male Wistar rats fed ad libidum a standard rat chow. Rats were subjected to three types of stress.

I. *Catecholamine stress:* rats were injected s.c. daily for 15 days with increasing doses of norepinephrine bitartrate dissolved in water. During the first 3 days they received 1 mg/kg and then 2, 3, 4 and 5 mg/kg for subsequent three day periods.

II. *Emotional stress:* rats were subjected to the stress of daily handling and injection for 15 days with an inert substance, i.e. water.

III. *Neonatal stress:* hearts from newborn rats were studied in relation to age. The rats were killed on days 1, 7, 14, and 21 and at the age of 2 to six months.

I. Catecholamine stress

Rats subjected to daily injections of increasing amounts of norepinephrine (NE) had a mortality rate of 48 per cent during this period of severe stress. There were significant and partly reversible changes in the fatty acid composition of the two major myocardial phospholipids, phosphatidylcholine (PC) and phosphatidylethanolamine (PE). The changes were specific for each phospholipid class and were similar in nature to adaptation to increasing age. In PC the relative amount of arachidonic acid (20:4n6) increased during NE-administration in two weeks to levels similar to those expected in old rats [1]. When the NE-administration was stopped the arachidonic acid in PC returned to normal levels in one week [2], Figure 1.

The linoleic acid (18:2n6) level of PC decreased rapidly to less than half of normal during the period of NE-stress, to a level of linoleic acid expected in old rats [1, 2], Figure 2. During the recovery period linoleic acid returned to normal levels in one week.

In PE there were significant but opposite changes in linoleic acid and docosahexaenoic acid (22:6n3). After two weeks of NE-stress the levels of these fatty acids in PE resembled those observed in old rats. During the recovery period there was some reversal

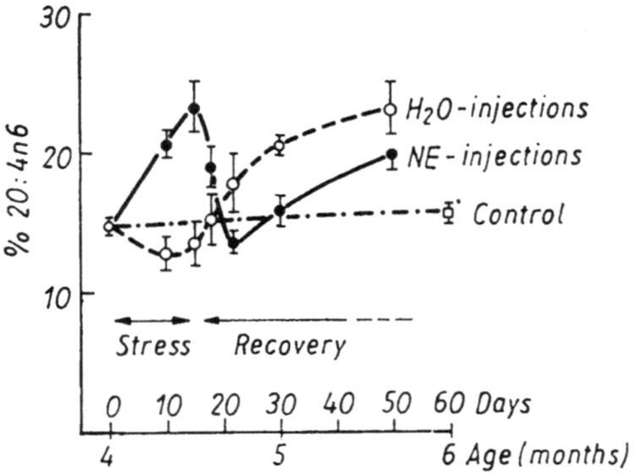

Fig. 1. Changes in arachidonic acid content of cardiac phosphatidylcholine during and after a period of daily injections with norepinephrine (NE) or water.

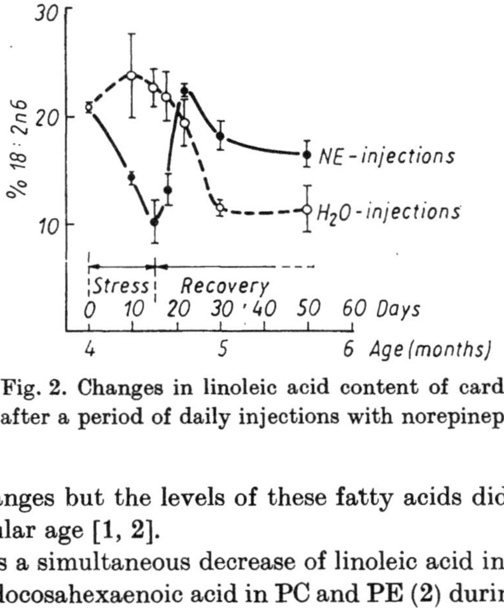

Fig. 2. Changes in linoleic acid content of cardiac phosphatidylcholine during and after a period of daily injections with norepinephrine (NE) or water.

of these changes but the levels of these fatty acids did not return to normal levels for that particular age [1, 2].

There was a simultaneous decrease of linoleic acid in both PC and PE, and a parallel increase in docosahexaenoic acid in PC and PE (2) during the period of NE-stress. There was, on the other hand, an inverse relationship between arachidonic acid levels in PC and Pe, 20:4n6 increased in PC and decreased in PE during the period of stress [2]. The inverse relationship between arachidonic acid content of PC and PE in our experiments suggests a specific methylation of PE, containing arachidonic acid, to PC.

The accumulation of arachidonic acid in phosphatidyl choline is of particular interest in light of its function as a precursor of prostaglandins. HIRATA and AXELROD [3] have postulated that catecholamine binding to β-adrenergic receptors on the cell surface activates methylation of PE to PC and that enzymatic methylation of phospholipids plays an important role in the transduction of receptor mediated signals through the membrane. Phospholipid methylation, i.e. conversion of PE to PC increases membrane fluidity and enhances the lateral mobility and rotation of the β-adrenergic receptor. This should unmask hidden receptors and facilitate the coupling of the receptor on the outer surface with adenylate cyclase facing the cytoplasmic side of the membrane

[3]. Our data are compatible with such a catecholamine induced conversion of PE, containing arachidonoyl chains, to PC.

This process is possibly coupled to desensitization of cells when they are exposed to excessive amounts of hormones or transmitters. The phospholipid methylation is coupled to activation of phospholipase A_2 which appears to be involved in the desensitization of β-adrenergic receptors. This desensitization is probably mediated by one or more products of phospholipase A_2 activity, such as lysophosphatidyl choline, arachidonic acid or its prostaglandin metabolites. Arachidonic acid may also play a role in inactivation of receptor-bound catecholamines and thus modulate the duration of cellular response to catecholamines.

II. Emotional stress

The nature of the stress is an important factor since different forms of stress induce different alterations in heart muscle. The emotional stress of handling the rats and daily injections of water also induced some alterations in myocardial PC during and after the period of stress. Figure 1 shows changes in arachidonic acid level of PC in rats receiving daily injections of NE or water. The alterations in the arachidonic acid level of PC during the recovery period were greater in rats subjected only to the emotional stress of daily handling and injection with water than in rats injected with large doses of NE. The alterations in linoleic acid content of myocardial PC were also greater during the recovery period in rats subjected to emotional stress (Fig. 2).

These data show that the nature and intensity of the stress affects the response and recovery of the heart muscle following cessation of stress.

III. Neonatal stress

One of the most stressful periods in life is probably the neonatal period, when the newborn animal or man must adjust to a new and very different environment and new conditions. During the first two to three weeks of life there were marked alterations in fatty acid composition of myocardial phospholipids in the newborn rat. These changes were partly reversed during the second month after birth.

The neonatal changes resembled the alterations observed during the period of NE-administration. Figure 3 shows the similarity in arachidonic acid response to postnatal stress and NE-stress in myocardial PC. In both cases there was a large increase in arachidonic acid during the period of severe stress. The arachidonic acid decreased again during adaptation of the young rat or cessation of stress in the adult animal. Figure 4 shows that linoleic acid in myocardial PC increased markedly during recovery from postnatal stress or NE-stress. Figure 5 shows the response of linoleic acid and docosahexaenoic acid to neonatal stress and NE-stress in myocardial PE. Certain similarities in response can be noted but the NE-induced alterations in fatty acid composition of myocardial PE were only partly reversible.

Activities of membrane bound enzymes and hormone receptors during these profound changes in membrane composition and microenvironment have not been studied thus far. Alterations in the microenvironment modify enzyme activities and should influence membrane structure and stability, i.e. myocardial resistance to tissue damage and necrosis.

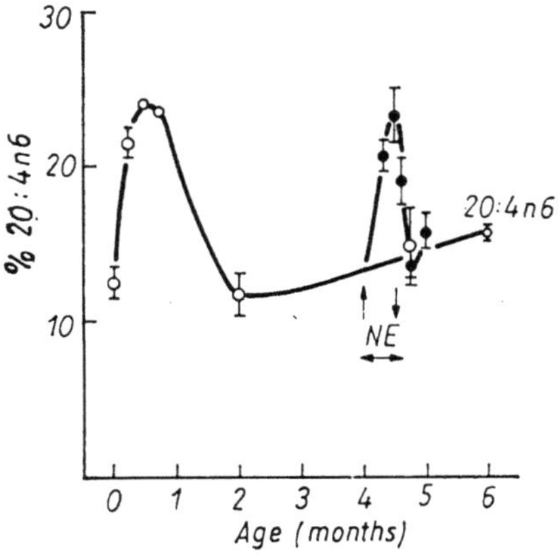

Fig. 3. Changes in arachidonic acid level of phosphatidylcholine in rat heart muscle after birth and during and following norepinephrine stress.

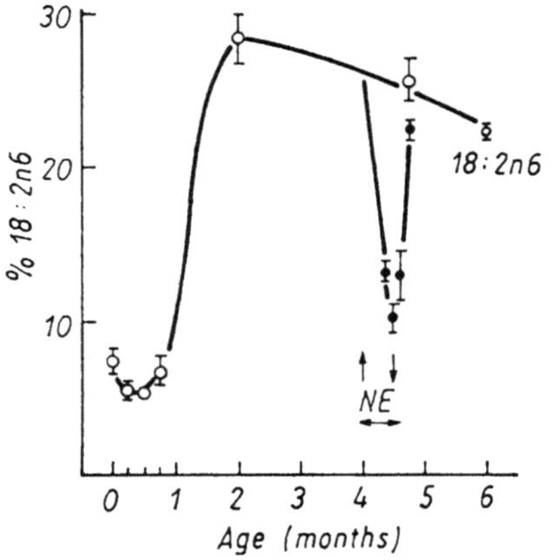

Fig. 4. Changes in linoleic acid level of phosphatidylcholine in rat heart muscle after birth and during and following norepinephrine stress.

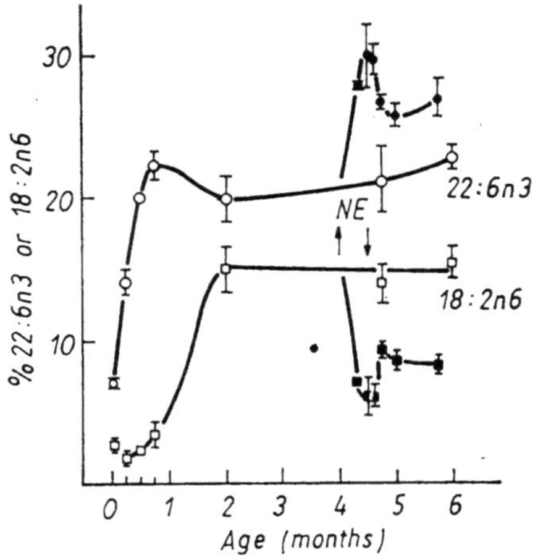

Fig. 5. Changes in docosahexaenoic acid and linoleic acid levels of phosphatidylethanolamine in rat heart muscle after birth and during and following norepinephrine stress.

References

[1] EMILSSON, A. and S. GUDBJARNASON: Biochim, Biophys. Acta **664** (1981), 82—88
[2] EMILSSON, A. and S. GUDBJARNASON: Biochim. Biophys. Acta, In Press.
[3] HIRATA, F. and I. AXELROD: Science **209** (1980), 1082—1090

Department of Pathology, Erasmus University, Rotterdam, The Netherlands

Molecular Species of Phosphatidylethanolamine in Rat and Mouse Heart

A. MONTFOORT, C. C. M. RUTTEN-VAN BEYSTERVELD and M. R. WORTELBOER

Introduction

Cell membranes in heart tissue are very dynamic structures and phospholipids play an important role in the structure and function of these membranes. In heart tissue the phospholipids of the cell membranes are rich in poly-unsaturated fatty acids. Membranes in heart tissue are very much susceptible to lipid peroxidation as the heart receives a supply of freshly oxygenated blood from the lungs. One of these poly-unsaturated fatty acids docosahexaenoic acid (22:6n3) is one of the more interesting fatty acids. It is mainly found in excitable tissues, like the retina of the eye, the brain and the heart [2, 8].

The major phospholipid class found in heart tissue is phosphatidylcholine.

One of the major risk factors in heart disease is stress. It was found by GUDBJARNASON et al. [8] that adaptation to catecholamine stress is accompanied by an extensive replacement of linoleic acid (18:2n6) by a more unsaturated fatty acid docosahexaenoic acid (22:6n3) in specific phospholids, e.g. phosphatidylethanolamine, which is the second major phospholipid class after phosphatidylcholine in heart [11, 16].

A similar shift in the fatty acid pattern in the phospholipids of the heart has been found during aging [8].

Changes in the fatty acid composition of the phospholipids found in biomembranes are reflected in the permeability [4, 16], membrane fluidity [1, 3, 12, 13] and the kinetic properties of the enzymes found in the membranes [10]. Therefore changes in the fatty acid composition of the phospholipids of heart tissue due to dietary influences, stress or age may have great implications for the proper functioning of the heart.

It was suggested by [8] that an inverse relationship exists between linoleic acid and both docosahexaenoic acid in heart tissue and the heart rate. Because of its high content of 22:6n3, phosphatidylethanolamine probably plays an important role in heart cell membrane function. Therefore we decided to analyze the molecular species of the diacyl fraction of phosphatidylethanolamine of heart tissue in two laboratory animals, the rat and the mouse.

Materials and methods

Animals: Normal laboratory animals were used (Wistar rats, 1 year old and BALB/c mice, 4 months old) of either sex. Standard laboratory mouse and rat food was given (Hope Farms, Woerden, Holland) and water was supplied ad libitum.

Lipid analyses: Lipid extraction of the heart tissue with 19 volumes of chloroform-methanol (2:1, by volume) was performed according to the method of [6]. Thin layer chromatography and fatty acid analysis were performed according to [14].

Results

The percentage distribution of the major phospholipids is given in Table 1. Phosphatidylcholine is the major phospholipid class as in most tissues but next to it phosphatidylethanolamine is quite abundant. Phosphatidylethanolamine represents 31—35% of the

Table 1

Percentage distribution of the major phospholipids in mouse and rat hearts[A]

	Mouse[B]	Rat[C]
Lysolecithin	0.4 ± 0.3	0.3 ± 0.3
Sphingomyelin	2.5 ± 0.5	2.6 ± 0.7
Phosphatidylinositol	4.2 ± 0.6	3.9 ± 0.7
Phosphatidylserine	2.0 ± 0.5	2.5 ± 0.4
Phosphatidylcholine	43.0 ± 2.2	40.4 ± 1.6
Phosphatidylethanolamine	31.5 ± 1.9	35.0 ± 1.7
Cardiolipin	15.9 ± 0.9	14.9 ± 1.0
Lysophosphatidylethanolamine	+	—
Others	0.5 ± 0.4	0.4 ± 0.2

A) Mean ± Standard error
B) 40 animals, 4 samples analyzed in duplicate
C) 30 animals, 4 samples analyzed in duplicate

Table 2

The fatty acid composition of diacylphosphatidyl ethanolamine from mouse and rat heart (%)

	Mouse Overall			Rat Overall		
Fatty acids	composition	1-position	2-position	composition	1-position	2-position
14:0	+	+	+	+	+	+
16:0	9.2 ± 0.2	19 2	2.0	13.5 ±2.7	24.8	3.1
16:1	0.2 ± 0.1	1.1	+	+	+	+
18:0	30.9 ± 1.6	58.1	1.1	31.2 ± 2.3	56.4	1.7
18:1	8.3 ± 0.3	18.5	3.1	8.1 ± 1.3	12.7	8.0
18:2n6	2.8 ± 0.4	3.1	2.7	7.9 ± 1.7	5.2	11.3
20:0/18:3	+	—	+	0.1 ± 0.1	—	0.1
20:1	0.2	—	—	+	0.1	—
20:4n6	7.5 ± 0.2	—	13.8	19.2 ± 1.4	0.5	36.4
20:5	+	—	0.1	0.1 ± 0.1	0.1	0.5
22:5n3 + n6	1.2	—	2.4	2.6 ± 1.4	0.1	5.1
22:6 n3	39.5 ± 0.9	—	74.5	15.0 ± 2.9	0.1	33.5
24:0	0.1	—	0.2	—	—	—
Others	0.1	—	0.1	1.4 ± 1.0	—	0.3

Table 3

Fatty acid composition of the subfractionated diglycerides derived from diacylphosphatidylethanolamine of mouse heart and the positional distribution of the fatty acids in each subfraction of diglycerides

Subfraction	1	2	3	4	5
weight percentages	70.5	19.0	4.4	4.2	1.9
fatty acid composition					
14:0	+	+	+	2.6	6.3
16:0	9.8	5.9	18.0	35.7	44.5
16:1	—	—	—	—	—
18:0	31.3	47.7	27.0	12.5	22.1
18:1	6.5	+	15.5	46.5	27.1
18:2n6	0.7	0.8	39.0	0.6	—
20:0/18:3	—	—	0.2	—	+
20:1	0.1	—	—	1.9	—
20:4n6	0.8	43.2	—	—	—
22:5 n3, n6	0.9	1.5	—	—	—
22:6n3	49.6	—	—	—	—
24:0	—	0.9	—	—	—
Others	0.3	—	0.3	0.2	—
Fatty acid composition of the 2-position					
14:0	+	+	+	5.0	6.9
16:0	3.4	4.8	18.3	19.4	39.1
16:1	—	—	—	—	—
18:0	4.3	5.4	14.0	8.0	30.1
18:1	2.9	3.1	12.9	64.5	22.4
18:2n6	0.2	0.6	54.8	0.6	1.5
20:0/18:3	—	0.7	—	—	—
20:1	0.1	—	—	2.2	—
20:4n6	1.5	82.4	—	—	—
22:5 n3, n6	1.9	1.8	—	—	—
22:6n3	85.7	—	—	—	—
24:0	—	1.1	—	—	—
Others	—	—	—	0.3	—

phospholipids in heart tissue of the rat and the mouse. In the mouse and rat, the phosphatidylethanolamine fraction of heart contained 25 and 40% plasmologens, respectively. The total amount of phospholipid in heart tissue is 15.7 ± 0.7 mg/g wet weight for the mouse and 19.1 ± 3.8 mg/g for the rat. Table 2 represents the fatty acid composition of diacylphosphatidylethanolamine from mouse and rat heart. The major saturated fatty acid is stearic acid in both animal species. The saturated fatty acids are almost exclusively found at the 1-position and the unsaturated fatty acids at the 2-position. In mouse heart docosahexaenoic acid (22:6n3) is the major poly-unsaturated fatty acid, while in diacylphosphatidylethanolamine of rat heart more arachidonic acid (20:4n6) than 22:6n3 is found. Table 3 represents the fatty acid composition of the subfractionated diglycerides derived from diacylphosphatidylethanolamine of mouse heart. The fraction containing 22:6n3 is the major fraction (70.5%). The fraction containing 4 double bonds contains almost exclusively 20:4 and the subfraction having 2 double bonds contains as well 18:2 as well as 18:1 molecular species. The saturated fraction is only a minor fraction and is contaminated with the fraction containing 1 double bond. The fatty acid composition of the diglycerides at the 2-position is given at the lower part of the table. The subfractionation of the diglycerides derived from diacylphosphatidylethanolamine of rat heart and the positional fatty acid distribution is given in Table 4. As can be seen from Table 3 and 4 some loss occured during the analysis procedure especially with the fraction containing docosahexaoenic acid. Subsequent analysis of the FFA's which were split off after pancreatic lipase degradation revealed that during this step of the analyses the 22:6n6 migrated from the 2-position of the 1,2-diclycerides to the 3-position of the molecule and was subsequently split off by the enzyme. About 5% of this fraction was lost due to oxidation. The molecular species that could be calculated from the analyzing data for diacylphosphatidylethanolamine are presented in the Figures 1 (rat) and 2 (mouse).

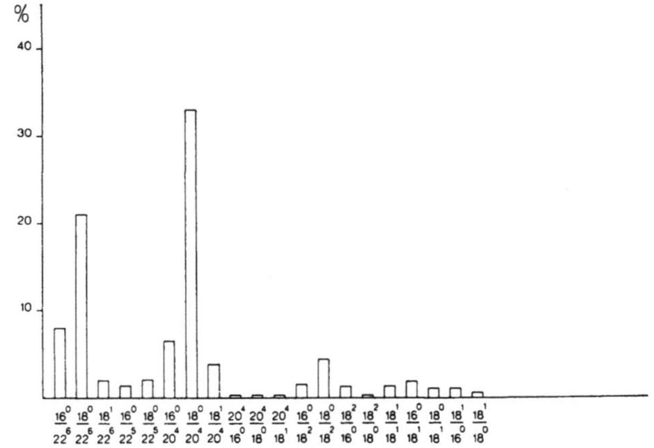

Fig. 1. Molecular species of diacylphosphatidylethanolamine in rat heart.

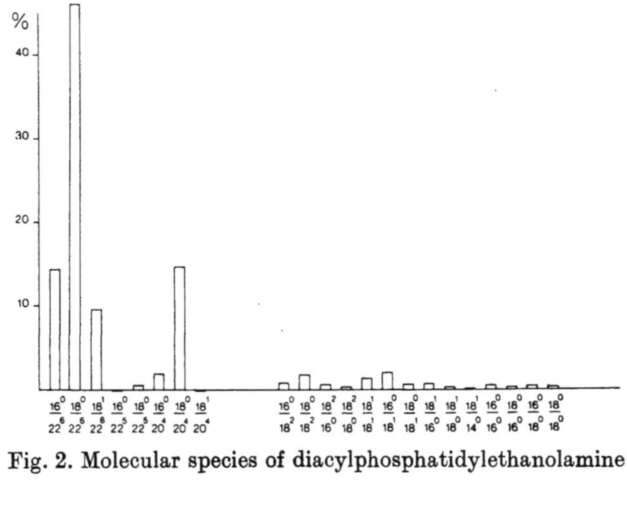

Fig. 2. Molecular species of diacylphosphatidylethanolamine in mouse heart.

Table 4

Fatty acid composition of the subfractionated diglycerides derived from diacyl phosphatidyl ethanolamine of rat heart and the positional distribution of the fatty acids in each subfraction of diglycerides

Subfraction	1	2	3	4	5
weight percentages	30.1	9.8	44.1	11.2	4.8
fatty acid composition					
14:0	+	+	+	+	+
16:0	12.4	14.5	7.6	13.3	32.5
18:0	33.5	27.5	37.0	24.5	17.2
18:1	3.1	8.0	5.2	14.9	45.0
18:2n6	0.7	5.1	0.3	41.8	3.3
20:0/18:3	0.9	—	1.3	1.7	0.7
20:4n6	0.3	17.4	46.0	0.9	—
22:5n3 + n6	+	27.5	—	—	—
22:6n3	48.6	—	—	—	—
Others	0.5	—	2.6	2.9	1.3
Fatty acid composition of the 2-position					
14:0	+	+	+	+	+
16:0	3.6	4.8	3.0	9.9	21.7
18:0	5.3	23.8	3.8	6.5	10.7
18:1	2.7	—	4.3	15.3	59.6
18:2n6	0.5	4.5	0.8	61.5	2.9
20:0/18:3	1.1	—	2.4	4.5	—
20:4n6	2.3	30.8	83.4	—	—
22:5n3 + d6	5.8	34.0	—	—	—
22:6n3	77.9	+	—	—	—
Others	0.8	2.1	2.4	2.3	5.5

Stearyl-arachidonoylphosphatidylethanolamine ($18^{\circ}/20^{4}$ PE) is the most abundant fraction in rat heart representing 33% of the molecules. Next $18^{\circ}/22^{6}$-PE is a major molecular species (21%) while $16^{\circ}/22^{6}$-PE represents 8% of diacylphosphatidylethanolamine. The molecular species containing linoleic acid are minor fractions ($16^{\circ}/18^{2}$-PE and $18^{\circ}/18^{2}$-PE resp. 1.5% and 4%). The most abundant molecular species of diacylphosphatidylethanolamine in mouse heart is $18^{\circ}/22^{6}$-PE (46%). Also very much abundant are $16^{\circ}/22^{6}$-PE (14%) and $18^{\circ}/20^{4}$-PE (15%). Even molecular species containing seven double bonds are found in reasonable amounts ($18^{1}/22^{6}$-PE, 10%). Species containing linoleic acid are present in just minor quantities.

Discussion

Molecular species of diacyl-PE containing four and six double bonds have been shown to be the major molecules. A preference for stearic acid to combine with docosahexaenoic acid has been demonstrated. Molecules containing seven double bonds were present in about 10% in mouse heart. So we can say that one of the major phospholipid classes of diacylphosphatidylethanolamine in mouse and rat heart consists of very unsaturated molecules. In the retina and other excitable tissues of some animal species, where more than 80% of the fatty acids in the lipids is represented by docosahexaenoic acid [2], molecules with this fatty acid on both positions must be present. Even during severe FFA-deficiency this percentage is kept at a constant level [2], indicating that these very unsaturated molecules are very important for proper functioning in excitable tissues. Phosphatidylethanolamine isolated from synaptic vesicles was demonstrated to contain 45% of docosahexaenoic acid [5]. From liposome experiments it has been demonstrated that molecules containing poly-unsaturated fatty acids give rise to fluid membrane structures [15]. Decrease in membrane fluidity can possibly lead to a greater chance of heart disease. We suggest that a fluid membrane, especially in the synaptosomal membranes, is necessary for a proper uptake of catecholamines.

During adaptation of stress there is a replacement of 18:2n6 by 22:6n3 in the phospholipids, which results in a fluidizing effect, most probably to keep the physico-chemical properties of the membranes within a very distinct fluid range. From experiments where animals were given diets rich in cholesterol, long chain saturated and mono-unsaturated fatty acids a magnification of the stress reaction was found [9]. Phospholipid molecules containing poly-unsaturated fatty acids in heart tissue are very much susceptible to lipid peroxidation, resulting in a decrease in membrane fluidity [7], decrease in permeability (A. MONTFOORT, unpublished results) and a breakdown of membrane functions. Increase in 22:6n3 is probably a protective adaptation to a maintainance of normal membrane function.

References

[1] ANDRICH, M. P. and J. M. VANDERKOOI: Biochemistry **15** (1976), 1257–1261
[2] AVELDAÑO, M. I. and N. G. BAZÁN: J. Neurochemistry **23** (1974), 1127–1135
[3] COGAN, U., M. SHINITZKY, G. WEBER and T. NISHIDA: Biochemistry **12** (1973), 521–528
[4] VAN DEENEN, L. L. M.: Progress in the Chemistry of Fats and Other Lipids **8** (1965), 56–60
[5] DEUTSCH, J. W. and R. B. KELLY: Biochemistry **20** (1981), 378–385
[6] FOLCH, J., M. LEES and G. H. SLOANE-STANLEY: J. Biol. Chem. **226** (1957), 497–500
[7] FUKUZAWA, K., H. CHIDA, A. TOKUMURA and H. TSUKATANI: Arch. Biochem. Biophys. **206** (1981), 173–180
[8] GUDBJARNASON, S., G. OSKARSDÓTTIR, B. DOELL and J. HALLGRIMSSON: Adv. Cardiol. **25** (1978), 130–144
[9] HÜLSMANN, W. C.: Mol. Cell. Endocrinol. **12** (1978), 1–8
[10] KIMELBERG, H. K.: Cell. surface reviews **3** (1977), 205–293
[11] KRAMER, J. K. G.: Lipids **15** (1980), 651–660
[12] LENTZ, B. R., Y. BARENHOLZ and T. E. THOMPSON: Biochemistry **15** (1976), 4521–4528
[13] LENTZ, B. R., Y. BARENHOLZ and T. E. THOMPSON: Biochemistry **15** (1976), 4529–4537
[14] MONTFOORT, A. and W. A. M. BOERE: Lipids **13** (1978), 580–587
[15] PAPAHADJOPOULOS, D.: In: Form and Function of Phospholipids (G. B. Ansell, J. N. Hawthorn and R. M. C. Dawson, Edits.) B. B. A. Library vol. **3** (1973), 143–169
[16] WHITE, D. A.: In: Form and Function of Phospholipids (G. B. Ansell, J. N. Hawthorn and R. M. C. Dawson, Edits.) B.B.A. Library vol **3** (1973), 441–482

V. Communication presented as posters

Institute of Physiology, Czechoslovak Academy of Sciences, Prague, Czechoslovakia

The Effect of Hypoxia on the Structural and Enzymatic Properties of Cardiac Myosin

V. PELOUCH, B. OŠTÁDAL and J. PROCHÁZKA

Contraction of the myocardium is brought about by the interaction of two contractile proteins-actin and myosin- and two regulatory proteins-tropomyosin and troponin, with the interplay of Ca^{2+} ions. Hypoxia significantly decrease myocardial contraction. According to KATZ [5] this can be explained in part by a decrease in the amount of calcium ions released during excitation-contraction coupling, and by displacement of Ca^{2+} ions from binding sites on troponin C by H^+. In Figure 1 there are summarized some further possible sites of the action of hypoxia on contractile protein in myocardium. The effect of hypoxia on myosin can possibly involve a change in the molecular structure and/or damage to the active centre (ATPase activity). Changes of the interaction in the thin part myofibres (I-zone) could also occur. The secondary effect of hypoxia may involve the breakdown of energy sources (such as ATP and CP). We have shown earlier that myosin aggregates with very low ATPase activity were formed in the parts of myocardium necrotically altered as the result of the administration of isoproterenol or ligation of the left coronary artery (PELOUCH et al. [11, 13]). In present communication we extended our interest towards solving the question whether similar changes would occur in the myocardium of rats exposed to intermittent high altitude hypoxia (IHA). We, therefore, compared structural and enzymatic changes myosin in the right and left ventricle [14].

Changes on the ATPase activity of cardiac myosin in the relation to the number of exposures to IHA (simulated in barochamber — adult male rats — McGRATH et al. [8]) are illustrated in Figure 2. No difference between the myosin ATPase activity of the right and left ventricle was found in controls. After the third exposure (2600 m), enzymatic activity in the left ventricle rose and a significant right-left difference appeared. After the 11th exposure (6000 m) ATPase activity fell down in both ventricles and the interventricular difference disappeared. After the 16th exposure (7000 m) enzymatic activity in both the right and left ventricles returned to the control values. The presence of polymers with low ATPase activity in both ventricles of animals exposed to IHA was demonstrated by independent chromatographic procedures [14]. In agreement with the localization of morphological changes [19] the proportion of polymers of myosin molecules was higher in the right ventricle. The conclusion about the structural changes of myosin was supported by a quite different methodological approach, i.e. by the investigation of isozymic composition of cardiac muscle [1, 3] using the native myosin from control and hypoxic animals (PELOUCH et al. [15]). Electrophoresis of myosin proteins under non-dissociating conditions has revealed two isozyme bands even in control animals; there were no differences between the right and left ventricles. The bands were, however, present in different proportions: whereas in control animals the band with higher ATPase activity was present predominantly, IHA induced synthesis of the isozyme with both lower mobility and ATPase activity. SDS polyacrylamide gel electrophoresis of different myosin preparation exhibits comparable subunit composition (Fig. 3).

It follows from our results that preferential synthesis of cardiac myosin with lower ATPase activity exists in hypoxic heart. Similar changes were also seen in the myocardium from animals in which cardiac work was increased by overloading [7, 17, 18]. At the moment it is impossible to decide whether the polymer is already formed *in vivo*, or whether a new type of myosin with lower ATPase activity isozyme with lower mobility on pyrophosphate gel is only transformed *in vivo* [16] and then polymerized *in vitro*. Supporting evidence for the later possibility is provided by our previous findings that a myosin preparation containing a polymeric fraction is more labile than the preparation from controls and the former's ATPase activity falls abruptly under *in vitro* conditions [12]. In agreement with the results of KATAGIRI and MORKIN [4] and SCHWARTZ et al. [17] we presume that tertiary structure of myosin is not modified even in hypoxic animals. The interference with the primary structure of light chains of myosin molecules [6] cannot be ruled out; finally changes can be also anticipated in HMM part of myosin [9]. The character of the struc-

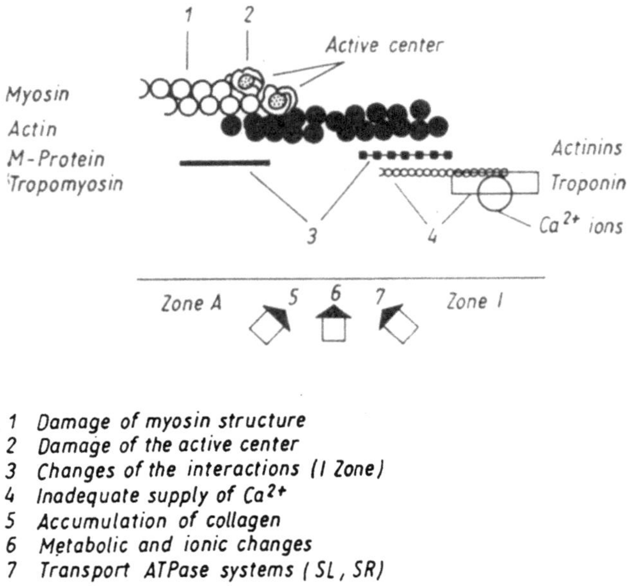

Fig. 1. Possible effect of hypoxia upon cardiac contractile proteins.

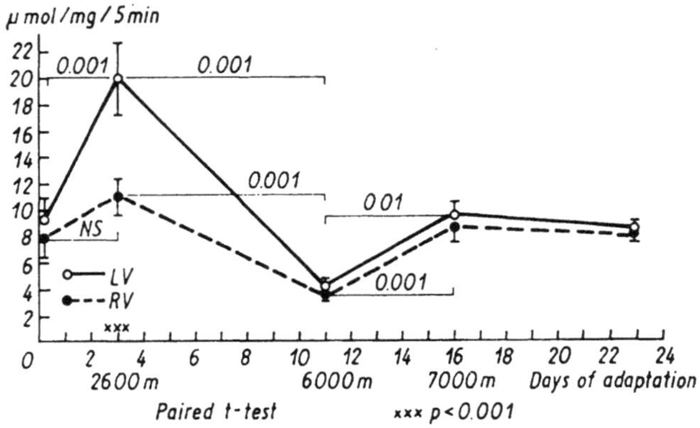

Fig. 2. Enzymatic activity of cardiac myosin during the exposure to intermittent high altitude hypoxia.
LV: left ventricle, RV: right ventricle

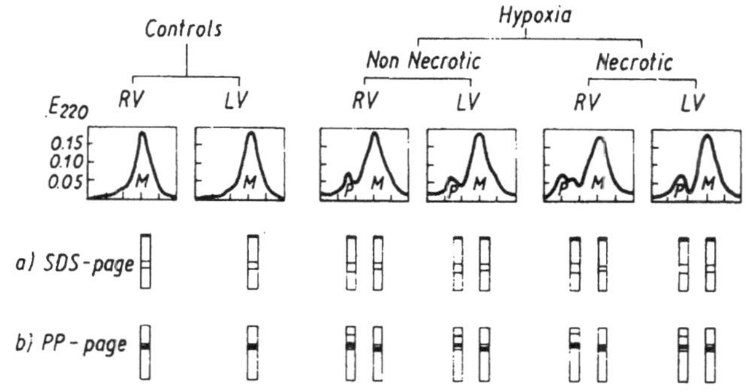

Fig. 3. Chromatographic and electrophoretic profile of cardiac myosin isolated from control and high altitude hypoxia animals. Myosin was isolated from both necrotic and intact parts of the right and left ventricular myocardium. The samples were analyzed by using a) column chromatography on DEAE-Sephadex A 50, b) electrophoresis of native myosin (pyrophosphate-PAGE) and after the dissociation of samples (SDS-PAGE).

tural and hence enzymatic changes of myosin described in the heart of animals exposed to IHA (chronic hypoxia) is similar to the changes observed after acute hypoxia. In any case the changes observed in myosin were associated with the areas of pathologically damaged myocardial fibres. The above results show that contractile properties in the hypoxic heart can be affected by the interference with the structure and enzymatic properties of the contractile proteins. IHA induced significant increase of the concentration of collagenous and non-collagenous proteins in both ventricles [10] as well as metabolic and ionic changes [2] can contribute to the final functional image of the heart muscle.

References

[1] D'ALBIS, A., C. PANTALONI and J. J. BECHET: Eur. J. Biochem. **99** (1979), 261–272
[2] HARRIS, P.: Myocardial Metabolism from Man at High Altitude (D. Heath, and D. R. Williams, eds.) II. edition, Churchill Livingstone, Edinburg London Melbourne and New York (1981)
[3] HOH, J., P. A. MCGRATH and P. T. HALE: J. Mol. Cell. Cardiol **10** (1978), 1053–1076
[4] KATAGIRI, T. and E. MORKIN: Life Sci. **16** (1974), 1079–1087
[5] KATZ, A. M.: Cardiol. **56** (1971/72), 276–283
[6] KLOTZ, C., J. C. LEGER and M. ELZINGA: Circul. Res. **50** (1982), 201–209
[7] LOMPRE, A. M., K. SCHWARTZ, A. D'ALBIS, G. LACOMBE, N. V. THIEM and B. SWYNGHEDAUW: Nature **282** (1979), 105–107
[8] MCGRATH, J. J., J. PROCHÀZKA, V. PELOUCH and B. OŠŤÀDAL: J. Appl. Physiol. **34** (1973), 289–293
[9] OGANESYAN, S., T. ZAMINIAN, N. BAY, V. PETROSIAN, A. KOSCHKARIAN, I. MARTIROSIAN and M. ELOYAN: J. Mol. Cell. Cardiol. **5** (1973), 1–24
[10] OŠŤÀDAL, B., E. MIREJOWSKA, J. HURYCH, V. PELOUCH and J. PROCHÀZKA: Cardiovasc. Res. **12** (1978), 303
[11] PELOUCH, V., Z. DEYL and O. POUPA: Physiol. Bohemoslov. **20** (1970), 9–13
[12] PELOUCH, V. and Z. DEYL: Physiol. Bohemoslov. **19** (1970), 341–342
[13] PELOUCH, V., B. OŠŤÀDAL and T. FIRST: Pflügers Arch. **364** (1976), 1–6

[14] PELOUCH, V., B. OŠTÀDAL, D. URBANOVÀ, J. PROCHÀZKA, J. RESSL and J. WIDIMSKY: Physiol. Bohemoslov. **29** (1980), 313–322

[15] PELOUCH, V., B. OŠTÀDAL and J. PROCHÀZKA: Physiol. Bohemoslov. **30** (1981), 449–450

[16] PERRY, S. V.: Progress in Biophys. Molec. Biol. **22** (1967), 328–381

[17] SCHWARTZ, K., P. BOUVERT, J. BERCOVICI and B. SWYNDHEDAUW: FEBS Lett. **93** (1978), 137–140

[18] SWYNGHEDAUW, B., C. DELCAYRE, J. M. MOALIC, Y. LECARPENTIER, A. RAY, J. J. MERCADIER, A. M. LOMPRE, C. AUMONT and K. SCHWARTZ: Eur. Heart. J. 3 (Suppl. A) (1982), 75–82

[19] URBANOVÀ, D., V. PELOUCH, B. OŠTÀDAL, J. WIDIMSKÝ, J. RESSL and J. PROCHÀZKA: Cor et Vasa **19** (1977), 246–250

Institute of Physiology Czechoslovak Academy of Sciences, Prague, Czechoslovakia and Central Institute of Heart and Circulation Research, Academy of Sciences, Berlin, GDR

A Possible Role of cAMP in the Cardiotoxicity of Catecholamines During Embryonic Life

B. Oštàdal, T. Janatová, V. Pelouch and E. G. Krause

It has previously been reported that intraamnial administration of necrogenic doses of isoprenaline (IPRO) to chick embryos induces serious disturbances of myocardial and hepatic development [2, 4, 7]. The most powerful embryo toxic effect was observed between the 5th and 14th embryonic day (ed) which corresponds to the period of development of coronary vascularization. At this stage malformations of great vessels, cardiomegaly, blockade of the development of coronary vascularization related to deffects in cardiac myoarchitecture and cardiac and hepatic necroses have been observed.

Myocardial β-adrenergic stimulation has been ordinarily accompanied by an increase in cAMP levels in the myocardium including that of the chick embryo [10, 11]. It was, therefore, of interest to determine whether the period of high sensitivity of the chick embryonic heart to IPRO was associated with the corresponding stimulation of cAMP levels in the myocardium [8].

The results demonstrated that the administration of IPRO at its period of high toxicity i.e. on the 7th ed significantly increased the cAMP content in the myocardium. At a later developmental stage, characterized by a considerably lower sensitivity to IPRO, the myocardial cAMP response was significantly lower. Intraamnial administration of dibutyryl cAMP increased the mortality of chick embryos and induced pathological changes in the myocardium. In comparison with IPRO, however, the effect of cAMP was significantly less pronounced [5].

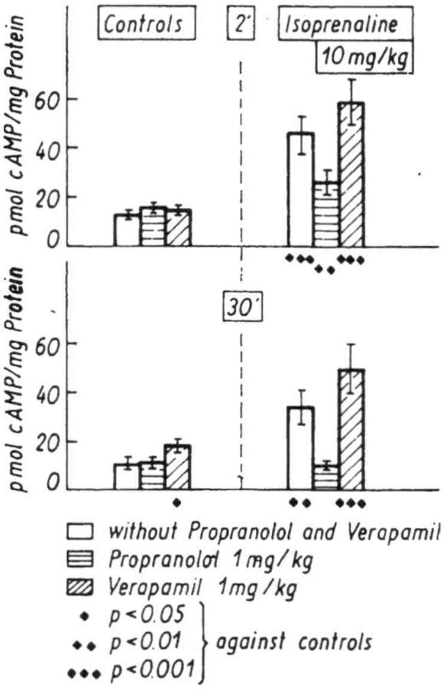

Fig. 1. The effect of propranolol and verapamil on the cardiac cAMP level in control and isoprenaline treated animals. Chick embryos, the 10th embryonic day, 2 and 30 minutes after intraamnial administration.

The cardiotoxic effect of β-mimetic catecholamines can be significantly reduced in adult animals either by β-blockade [6] or by calcium antagonists [3]. Our investigations should have determined whether these drugs as well had a protective effect on the development of IPRO-induced pathological changes in the embryonic heart tissue [9]. It was found, that propranolol in a dose of 1 mg/kg completely blocked the cardiotoxic effect of IPRO. On the other hand, Ca antagonist verapamil was found to have no protective effect in any dose used. It, furthermore, induced disturbances of the development of coronary vascularization and even significantly increased the mortality of experimental animals. Similar results were obtained in our experiments with stimulation of cAMP level in the embryonic myocardium. Whereas the administration of propranolol significantly reduced the cAMP level after IPRO, verapamil was without any effect (Fig. 1).

These results suggest, but do not prove that cAMP may constitute an important factor in the cardiotoxicity of IPRO as was the case in adult animals [1]. The fact, that the Ca antagonists, in comparison with adult mammals are not capable to reduce the IPRO induced myocardial lesions as in the young, supports the hypothesis that the sensitivity of myocardial membrane to catecholamines and calcium may differ during ontogenetic development. Our results, furthermore, draw attention to the possible embryotoxic effect of chronic administration of beta mimetic catecholamines in clinical practice, particularly during the prenatal life.

References

[1] BHAGAT, B., J. M. SULLIVAN, V. W. FISCHER, E. M. NADEL and N. S. DHALLA: Recent Adv. Stud. Card. Struct. Metab. **12** (1978), 465–470

[2] DUSEK, J. and B. OŠTÀDAL: Physiol. Bohemoslov. **27** (1978), 558

[3] FLECKENSTEIN, A.: In: Calcium and the Heart (P. Harris and L. H. Opie eds.) Academic Press, London and New York (1971), 135–188

[4] HODACH, R. J., E. A. HODACH, J. F. FALLON, J. D. FOLTS, J. H. BRUYERE and E. F. GILBERT: Teratology **12** (1975), 33–46

[5] JANATOVÀ, T., B. OŠTÀDAL and J. DUŠEK: Physiol. Bohemoslov. **30** (1981), 422

[6] MRÀZ, M., E. FALTOVÀ, J. SEDIVỲ, J. PROTIVOVÀ and J. PILNỲ: Physiol. Bohemoslov. **29** (1980), 323–331

[7] OŠTÀDAL, B., Z. RYCHTER and V. RYCHTEROVÀ: J. Mol. Cell. Cardiol. **8** (1976), 533–544

[8] OŠTÀDAL, B., E. G. KRAUSE, I. BEYERDÖRFER, V. PELOUCH and A. WOLLENBERGER: J. Mol. Cell. Cardiol. **11** (1979), 1183–1187

[9] OŠTÀDAL, B., T. JANATOVÀ and J. DUŠEK: Physiol. Bohemoslov. **30** (1981), 447–448

[10] POLSON, J. B., N. D. GOLDBERG and F. E. SHIDEMAN: J. Pharmacol. Exp. Therapeut. **200** (1977), 630

[11] RENAUD, J. F., N. SPERELAKIS and G. LEDOUARIN: J. Mol. Cell. Cardiol. **10** (1977), 281–286

Department of Pharmacology, University of Bern, Bern, Switzerland

Properties and Regulation of β-Adrenoceptors in Living Cardiac Cells

H. Porzig, C. Becker and H. Reuter

The properties of the β-adrenoceptor adenylate cyclase system of mammalian tissues have been studied predominantly in cell homogenates. Little is known of the dynamic interaction between specific ligands and the β-adrenergic system in intact cells. Moreover, the mechanisms responsible for regulatory changes in the strength of a cell's adrenergic response remain controversial. In the present study we have used beating tissue cultured rat cardiac cells to investigate acute and chronic interactions of various ligands with β-adrenoceptors and receptor mediated adenylate cyclase activation. We have also studied the role of intracellular cAMP in regulating β-adrenergic responses in normal and desensitized cells.

Primary cultures of newborn rat heart cells were prepared combining several established methods [1, 2, 4]. Rat heart ventricles were first dissociated with trypsin. Myocardial cells and fibroblasts were than separated by a differential attachment technique. Finally heart cells were seeded onto glass coverslips. The coverslip cultures were maintained at 5% CO_2/95% air and 37 °C for 5—8 days in DMEM-medium supplemented with 10—20% fetal calf serum. Binding assays and measurement of cAMP accumulation were performed in culture medium using intact coverslip cultures as described by [6] without removing the cells from the growth surface. ^{3}H-(±)-carazolol and ^{3}H-(±)-CGP 12177 (4-(3-tert. butyl-amino-2 hydroxypropoxy]-benzimidazol-2-on-hydrochloride, [3]) a lipophilic and a hydrophilic adrenergic antagonist respectively, were used for specific β-adrenoceptor radio-labelling. Unspecific binding was always defined as that fraction of total binding that could be displaced by 1 μM (—)-timolol. β-Receptor mediated cAMP formation was measured in the presence of a phosphodiesterase inhibitor by stimulating coverslip cultures for 1 min with (—) isoprenaline. After heat inactivation cAMP was measured according to [7].

Competitive and noncompetitive interactions of β-adrenoceptors and specific labels in intact cells

Carazolol (K_D = 40 M) and CGP (K_D = 352 μM) labelled a homogeneous class of ~ 5,000 β-adrenoceptor sites per cell. In short term experiments both compounds could be displaced competitively by non-radioactive β-adrenoceptor antagonists. After prolonged pretreatment (180 min — 5 days) the fraction of carazolol that could be displaced competitively by agonists or antagonists decreased progressively to less than 20% of the initial value even though total binding remained unchanged. Upon removal of carazolol from the culture medium, the ligand dissociated in a monoexponential fashion from its binding sites. Normal receptor binding properties recovered with a half time of 2 hours. By contrast, at least 80% of specifically bound CGP remained displaceable after chronic exposure. These results suggested that β-adrenoceptor antagonists can interact with receptors in a specific but non-competitive way to reduce agonist-mediated receptor activation. A second form of non-competitive inhibition of the β-receptor adenylate cyclase system was observed when we measured isoprenaline stimulated cAMP accumulation in intact cells in the presence of various antagonists ((±) carazolol, (±) CGR 12177, (±) propranolol, (−) timolol). Except for timolol the antagonists reduced the maximal rate of cAMP formation by 50−70%. The effect was observed both after short term or chronic exposure to antagonists and was not correlated to changes in receptor density or displaceability of the ligands. We interpret this finding as an antagonist-induced decoupling between receptor occupation and cyclase activation.

Effect of cellular cAMP on β-adrenoceptor density in intact cells

Receptor density decreased by about 70% if tissue cultured cardiac cells were exposed for 5 days to 10^{-6} M (−) isoprenaline. The effect was half maximal after 24 hours. This desensitization on the receptor level was preceded by a rapid loss in β-receptor-mediated adenylate cyclase stimulation down to 8% of the control values. This effect was half maximal within ~ 4 hours. To test whether the accumulation of cellular cAMP was involved in the desensitization processes we exposed heart cell cultures for 6 to 120 hours to 10^{-4} M 8-bromo-cAMP. In part of the cultures 10^{-4} M 8-bromo-cAMP and 10^{-6} M isoprenaline were present simultanously. Chronic exposure to 8-bromo-cAMP *increased* mean receptor density from 138 ± 8.5 to 190 ± 5 fmol/mg protein. However, agonist binding constants and dose-response curves for β-receptor-mediated adenylate cyclase stimulation remained unchanged. These findings suggest that cAMP-induced receptors were not coupled to adenylate cyclase. Thesame conclusion can be drawn from the fact that cAMP induced β-receptors were resistent to isoprenaline-mediated desensitization. In the presence of isoprenaline, 8-bromo-cAMP prolonged the half time for half maximal loss of β-receptor coupled adenylate cyclase activity from 4 hours to 18 hours. However, the induction of new receptors and the inhibition of cyclase desensitization followed completely different time courses. Therefore, the two effects are probably not causally related. We conclude from the results with 8-bromo-cAMP that a pronounced cAMP-mediated feed-back regulation exists in the β-adrenergic system of living cardiac cells. Such functions of cellular cAMP have as yet not been observed in other tissues.

Acknowledgments

We thank Prof. STÄHELIN, Friedrich-Miescher-Institut, Basel, Switzerland for a gift of ^{3}H−(±)−CGP 12177 and the Roche Animal Farm, Füllinsdorf/Switzerland for the gift of pregnant rats. Our work was supported by the Swiss National Science Foundation grant No. 3.154−0.81]

References

[1] BLONDEL, B., I. ROIJEU and J. P. CHENEVAL: Experientia **27** (1971) 356−358
[2] MARK, G. E. and F. F. STRASSER: Exptl. Cell Res. **44** (1966), 217−233
[3] MEIER, M., A. G. TRUOG and K. A. JAEGGI: Proc. VIII World Congress of Cardiology (1978) Abstract 969
[4] PAUL, J.: Cell and Tissue Culture, 5th ed. Churchill Livingstone, Edinburgh London New York
[5] PERKINS, J. P., T. K. HARDEN and J. F. HARPER: In: Handb. exp. Pharm. Vol. **58**/I, (J. A. Nathanson and J. W. Kebabian, eds.) Springer, Berlin, Heidelberg, New York (1982), 185−224
[6] PORZIG, H., C. BECKER and H. REUTER: Naunyn-Schmiedeberg's Arch. Pharmacol. **321** (1982), 89−99
[7] TOVEY, K. C., K. G. OLDHAM and J. A. M. WHELAN: Clin. Chim. Acta **56** (1974), 221−234

Central Institute of Heart and Circulation Research, Academy of Sciences of the GDR, 1115 Berlin-Buch, German Democratic Republic

Ischaemia-Induced Changes of the Cardiac Adenylate Cyclase System. I. Cytochemical Studies of Adenylate Cyclase Activity

W. SCHULZE

It is known that the depletion of ATP during ischaemia leads to a loss of cyclic nucleotides in the cardiac muscle. But the reaction of the adenylate cyclase (AC) is not clear. DRUMMOND and SORDAHL [1] reported a progressive decline in the stimulation of AC by catecholamines in dog heart after 20 to 60 min of total ischaemia, whereas an opposite effect was observed by MORI [3].

The aim of this study was to examine the activity and the localization of the receptor-coupled AC cytochemically minutes after the onset of a total ischaemia. The results were compared with quantitative biochemical analysis of homogenates from tissue of the same rat hearts (WILL-SHAHAB in these proceedings) and they are discussed in connection with structural damages of the sarcolemma under ischaemia.

Material and methods

Rat hearts quickly excised after ether anesthesia were placed in ice-cold tyrode solution containing 250 IU/ml heparin. The test tubes with the hearts were flushed with nitrogen. After 10 and 20 min the hearts were cannulated via the aorta and fixed by perfusion with 2% cacodylate buffered glutaraldehyde (pH 7.4). The pretreatment was finished by washing and dissecting of small parts (smaller than 1 mm in diameter) of the left ventricle. The cytochemical methods were carried out according to WAGNER and BITENSKY [5] with AMP-PNP as the substrate, lead nitrate as the capture reagent and maleate buffer for keeping the free lead concentration at a nontoxic level [4].

Results and discussion

Biochemical analysis showed a time-dependent depletion of ATP in the hearts of this *in-vitro* model of ischaemia [2]. The loss of ATP is less rapid than in electrically active totally ischaemic hearts. The ultrastructural changes, however, are similar. But they are not developed in all cells simultaneously. JENNINGS and HAWKINS [2] described the irreversible injury in a few cells only after 20 min of total ischaemia of dog hearts. Under our conditions we saw characteristic structural features after 10 min of ischaemia. These changes can be defined in a mitochondrial alterationg, glycogen depletion, margination of nuclear chromatin and relaxation of myofibrils with prominent I-bands. The affected myocytes appeared to be swollen. In many cells the sarcolemma is lifted off and formed discontinuities and vesiculations. The prolongation of ischaemia to 20 min enhanced all structural damages. In the ischaemic heart tissue there are no changes in the localization of AC activity in comparison to normal controls. The enzyme is localized at the sarcolemma and its vesicle, at the T-tubule membranes and at some parts of the sarcoplasmic reticulum (Fig. 1). But the number of cells with positive reaction is decreased. This tendency is more pronounced after the 20 min period of ischaemia. Adjacent to cells which show nearly normal localization are myocytes without any reaction products. There is no remarkable change in the intensity of the reaction after incubation with sodium fluoride or isoproterenol in the presence of Gpp(NH)p. But it seems that more junctional SR membranes are marked by lead precipitates (Fig. 2.) Usually cells which have prominent features of structural damages showed less markers of the AC activity.

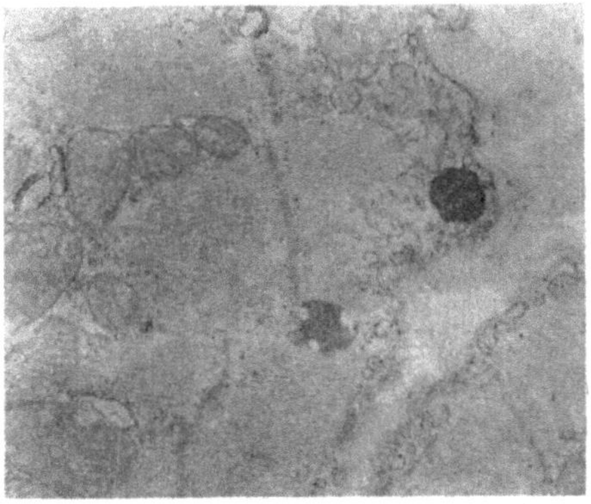

Fig. 1. Localization of adenylate cyclase in rat heart myocyte after 10 min of total ischaemia. Reaction products are localized at the plasmamembrane of the sarcolemma and its vesicles and at the junctional sarcoplasmatic reticulum (20000×).

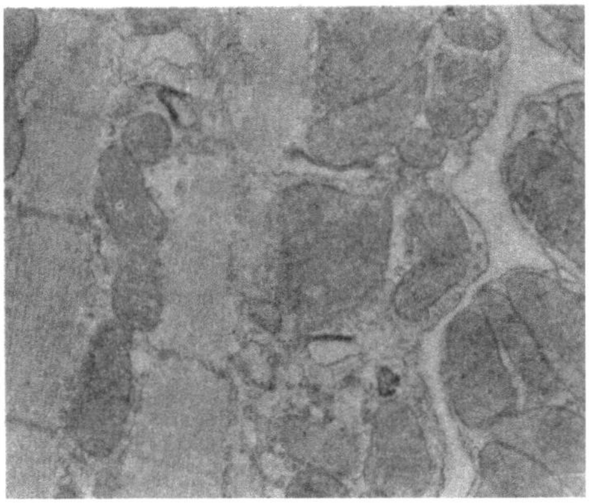

Fig. 2. After 20 min of ischaemia the localization of the adenylate cyclase is not changed. A loss of the enzyme activity of the sarcolemma can be seen. But the intensity of the localization on the junctional SR is not influenced (20000×).

Although there were structural changes of the myocytes including the sarcolemma the localization of the AC activity is not changed. However, the number of cells with reactions are decreased. Future studies need to examine whether [1] all parts of the heart likewise involved in the loss of the enzyme activity and [2] the reversibility of the cytochemically changes found are combined with the structural regeneration.

References

[1] Drummond, R. W. and L. A. Sordahl: J. Mol. Cell. Cardiol. **13** (1981), 323–330
[2] Jennings, R. B. and H. K. Hawkins: In: Wildenthal (Ed.) Degradation Processes in Heart and Skeletal Muscle. Elsevier/North-Holland Biomedical Press, 1980, 295–346
[3] Mori, K.: Nagoya J. med. Sci. **39** (1976), 9–14
[4] Schulze, W.: Histochemistry **74** (1982), 133–143
[5] Wágner, R. C. and M. W. Bitensky: In: Hayat, M. A. (Ed.) Electron Microscopy of Enzymes. Principles and Methods, vol. **2**, Van Nostrand, New York, 1974, 110–131

Central Institute of Heart and Circulation Research, Academy of Sciences of the GDR, 1115 Berlin, GDR

Ischaemia-induced Changes of Cardiac Adenylate Cyclase Activity. II. Reversible Inhibition of Adenylate Cyclase

L. WILL-SHAHAB and I. KÜTTNER

The ability of cells to modulate its response to endogenous hormones or exogenous effectors may be of major physiologic importance in many circumstances, including myocardial ischaemia. The functional effects of the hormones result from their primary interaction with a specific membrane-associated receptor site on the sarcolemma, which then initiates activation of adenylate cyclase at the inner side of the membrane.

In contrast to MORI [5], DRUMMOND and SORDAHL [3] observed a decline in adenylate cyclase activation 20 minutes following coronary artery occlusion in the canine heart. Changes in β-adrenergic receptor properties have been shown as well in the ischaemic [6] and non ischaemic myocardium [1], although it seems to be a slower and long-persisting process. Changes in receptor number have been not detected earlier than 45 minutes after onset of ischaemia. Recently KRAUSE and ENGLAND [4] reported that acute ischaemia leads to loss of cyclic AMP accumulation induced by isoproterenol in the isolated rat heart.

The purpose of our investigation was to clear up whether adenylate cyclase activation becomes affected by acute ischaemia.

Global ischaemia has been used by keeping isolated rat hearts unperfused in metabolic shakers at 37 °C containing Tyrode-solution equilibrated by N_2/CO_2 (95/5 vol%). After 5, 10, 15, 20, 30, and 45 min of incubation adenylate cyclase activation by NaF, guanylyl imidodiphosphate and isoprenaline has been measured in homogenate and a 30000 × g particulate fraction of ischaemic hearts. As controls served isolated aerobically perfused rat hearts.

As could be seen from Figure 1, acute ischaemia is accompanied by a progressive decline in the stimulation of adenylate cyclase by isoprenaline. Likewise the same decline has been observed

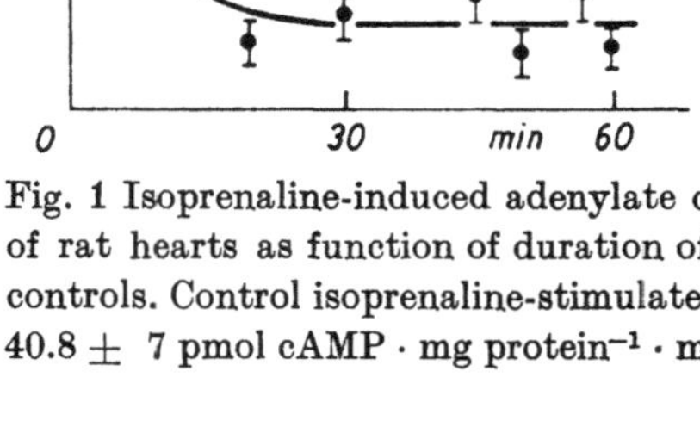

Fig. 1 Isoprenaline-induced adenylate cyclase activity (10^{-4} M) in crude homogenate of rat hearts as function of duration of ischaemia. All values are expressed as % of controls. Control isoprenaline-stimulate activity was
40.8 ± 7 pmol cAMP · mg protein^{-1} · min^{-1}; n = 3

with NaF and guanylyl imidodiphosphate. Activation of the enzyme was completely restored when ischaemic hearts were aerobically reperfused for 10 min. It was excluded that adenylate cyclase was released from sarcolemma. Since not only receptor-coupled AC was inhibited but also stimulation by NaF and Gpp(NH)p was markedly reduced, one has to suggest that the catalytic subunit of the enzyme is primarily altered in function. In contrast to the ischaemic dog heart [3], where no changes of AC in ischaemic myocardium following 10 min of coronary artery occlusion has been observed, global ischaemic rat hearts revealed marked decreases in ischaemic heart AC activity from 5—10 min after onset of ischaemia. There was a close correlation between lactate accumulation in the ischaemic myocardium and the decreased AC function.

The reduced responsiveness of AC in the acute ischaemic myocardium might indicate an initial damage of sarcolemma. It might of phyiological relevance by protecting the myocardium from high catecholamine concentrations which have been found in ischaemic hearts.

References

[1] BAUMANN, G., G. RIESS, W. D. ERHARDT, S. B. FELIX, L. LUDWIG, G. BLUMEL and H. BLOMER: Amer. Heart J. **101** (1981), 569—581
[2] BERSOHN, M. M., K. D. PHILIPSON and J. Y. FUKUSHIMA: Amer. J. Physiol. **242** (1982), C288 to C295
[3] DRUMMOND, R. W. and L. A. SORDAHL: J. Molec. Cell. Cardiol. **13** (1981), 323—330
[4] KRAUSE, E.-G. and P. J. ENGLAND: J. Molec. Cell. Cardiol. **14** (1982), 611—613
[5] MORI, K. and J. NAGOYA: Med. Sci. **39** (1976), 9—14
[6] MUKHERJEE, A., L. R. BUSH, K. E. MCCOY, R. J. DUKE, H. HAGLER, L. M. BUJA and J. T. WILLERSON: Circul. Res. **50** (1982), 735—741

Intstitute of Pharmacology, Faculty of General Medicine, Charles University, Prague 2, Czechoslovakia

Adenylate Cyclase Activity in the Heart and Some Other Tissues Treated by α-Chymotrypsin

S. Hynie

Recent experimental findings contributed substantially to our knowledge concerning the molecular structure and function of adenylate cyclase complex. In spite of this fact site of action of some nonspecific activators of adenylate cyclase as fluoride ion, guanine nucleotides, vanadate or forskolin is not yet exactly known [4, 7, 8, 12]. One of the possible approaches for the determination of the site of action of the activators of adenylate cyclase is the following of their differential response after the mild proteolytic digestion of adenylate cyclase preparations or after the addition of agents which increase the fluidity of plasma membranes [5, 6, 10, 11, 1, 3].

Materials and methods

Forskolin was from Calbiochem AG, vanadate was used as $Na_3VO_4 \cdot 14H_2O$ (Poole, U.K.), guanylyl imidodiphosphate (GPP/NH/P) was a product of Boehringer Mannheim GmbH, FRG, and α-chymotrypsin was from Worthington, USA. All other chemicals used were from sources described earlier [3].

Adenylate cyclase preparations from rat liver and heart were prepared as described earlier [3]. The preparation of adenylate cyclase from turkey erythrocyte ghosts was prepared by a new procedure [2]. In experiments with preincubation, plasma membrane fractions were incubated for 5 min with appropriate additions at 37 °C. Then the preparations were cooled, centrifuged and two times washed [3].

Adenylate cyclase activity was determined as described earlier [3]. Typical experiments performed in duplicate or triplicate are presented.

Results and discussion

Rat hepatic and myocardial adenylate cyclase preparations as well as adenylate cyclase from turkey erythrocyte ghosts responded to all activators with a typical manner (Table 1). The addition of α-chymotrypsin (5—10 μg/ml) to the assay system potentiated the activity of adenylate cyclase. In dependence on tissue preparation and the activator used there was 2—10 fold increase of adenylate cyclase activity. The highest activation was observed in preparation from turkey erythrocyte ghosts stimulated by isoproterenol or GPP/NH/P alone. Very small increase of adenylate cyclase activity was observed in the preparation from rat heart. In this preparation the effect of vanadate or forskolin was as potent as that of sodium fluoride, however, their effects were essentially unaffected by the addition of α-chymotrypsin.

In the following experiment (dada not shown) with the heart adenylate cyclase we tested the percentual change in adenylate cyclase activity due to the addition of GPP/NH/P, isoproterenol, sodium fluoride, forskolin or vanadate, both in the presence and absence of increasing concentrations of α-chymotrypsin (5–20 μg/ml) or n-propanol (0.2–0.8 mol/l). The first three mentioned activators were substantially potentiated by the addition of α-chymotrypsin, while the effects of vanadate and forskolin were unaffected. The addition of n-propanol to the assay strongly potentiated the activation by GPP/NH/P and sodium fluoride while the effects due to vanadate and

Table 1

Adenylate cyclase activity in three preparations treated by α-chymotrypsin

Adenylate cyclase preparation	Turkey erythrocyte ghosts		Rat liver homogenate		Rat myocard homogenate	
Additions	Adenylate cyclase activity					
	RV[1])	CHYM[2])	RV[1])	CHYM[2])	RV[1])	CHYM[2])
None	1[3])	< 2–3x	1[4])	3x	1[5])	1.7x
Isoproterenol, 0.1 mM	2–3	5–10x	—	—	2	1.4x
GPP/NH/P, 10 μM	8–10x	5–10x	5–7	2–3x	2–3	1.6x
Iso + GPP/NH/P	> 40	2–3x	—	—	—	—
Vanadate, 3 mM	—	—	4–5	2x	9–10	1.1x
Forskolin, 1–100 μM	2–5	< 2–3x	9–10	2x	9–10	1.0x
Fluoride, 10 mM	> 40	< 2–3x	9–10	3x	9–10	1.6x

1) R.V. = relative values of adenylate cyclase activity

2) CHYM = x fold increase of R.V. due to treatment by α-chymotrypsin (5 to 10 μg/ml)

3) Specific activity 20–100 pmol · mg^{-1} · 20 min^{-1} (n = 5)

4) Specific activity 83 pmol · mg^{-1} · 10 min^{-1} (n = 2)

5) Specific activity 79 pmol · mg^{-1} · 10 min^{-1} (n = 2)

Table 2

The effect of α-chymotrypsin on the activity of rat liver adenylate cyclase preparation preincubated with and without this enzyme

Preincubation[1])	Control	α-chymotrypsin (10 μg/ml)
Additions	Adenylate cyclase activity[3]) (pmol · mg protein^{-1} · 10 min^{-1})	
None	13 ± 1	10 ± 1
None + CHYMO[2])	39 ± 2	12 ± 1
GPP/NH/P, 10 μM	82 ± 6	60 ± 4
GPP/NH/P + CHYMO	198 ± 8	54 ± 2
Forskolin, 10 μM	129 ± 4	37 ± 1
Forskolin + CHYMO	180 ± 8	31 ± 3
Vanadate, 3.2 mM	57 ± 4	21 ± 1
Vanadate + CHYMO	113 ± 9	22 ± 2
Fluoride, 10 mM	142 ± 9	111 ± 8
Fluoride ± CHYMO	457 ± 9	113 ± 6

1) Adenylate cyclase preparations were preincubated as described in methods

2) α-chymotrypsin added to assay at conc. 10 μg/ml

2) Average from triplicates ± S.E.M.

forskolin were strongly reduced. This differential influence of α-chymotrypsin and n-propanol on the activation by sodium fluoride, vanadate and forskolin exclude the possibility of their effect on the identical site, i.e. the same site on N-regulatory protein.

The experiment with the preincubation of adenylate cyclase preparation with α-chymotrypsin was performed on the preparation from rat liver (Table 2). The addition of α-chymotrypsin to the adenylate cyclase assay substantially increased the activity of this preparation stimulated by all agents with the exception of forskolin and vanadate which were increased very little. The most interesting finding is the lack of the stimulatory effect of α-chymotrypsin in the preparations preincubated with this enzyme. In addition to that, these preparations were only very slightly sensitive to the activating effect of vanadate and forskolin.

The disappearance of the stimulatory effect of α-chymotrypsin in preparations pretreated with this enzyme suggests the existence of a component which may restrict adenylate cyclase activity and which may be removed from adenylate cyclase preparations by their pretreatment with α-chymotrypsin. Finally, the attenuation of the effect of vanadate and forskolin in the α-chymotrypsin-preincubated preparations, with the concomitant preserved effect of sodium fluoride and GPPNH/P, excludes the possibility of their direct effect on the catalytic unit of adenylate cyclase, as it was suggested for forskolin [12].

Acknowledgment

The author would like to express his gratitude to Dr. H. Metzger, Hoechst AG, Pharma Biochemie, Frankfurt, for providing a sample of forskolin.

References

[1] Harper, J. F. and G. Brooker: J. Cycl. Nucleot. Res. **6** (1980), 51–62

[2] Hynie, S.: Association des Physiologistes, Réunion, Commune, Comptes Rendus, 13.–17. 9. 1982, Praha

[3] Hynie, S. and V. Klenerová: Naunyn-Schiedeberg's Arch. Pharmacol. **310** (1980), 231–236

[4] Krawietz, W., R. W. Downs, Jr., A. M. Spiegel and G. D. Aurbach: Biochem. Pharmacol. **31** (1982), 843–848

[5] Lacombe, M.-L., D. Stengel and J. Hanoune: FEBS Lett. **77** (1977), 159–163

[6] Pinkett, M. O., C. J. Jaworski, D. Evain and W. B. Anderson: J. Biol. Chem. **255** (1980), 7716–7721

[7] Rodbell, M., P. M. Lad, T. B. Nielsen, D. M. F. Cooper, W. Schlegel, M. S. Preston, C. Londos and E. S. Kempner: Adv. Cyclic. Nucl. Res. **14** (1981), 3–14

[8] Seamon, K. and J. W. Daly: J. Biol. Chem. **256** (1981), 9799–9801

[9] Seamon, K. B. and J. W. Daly: J. Cycl. Nucl. Res. **7** (1981), 201–224

[10] Stengel, D. and J. Hanoune: Adv. Cyclic. Nucl. Res. **14** (1981), 657

[11] Stengel, D., M.-L. Labombe, M.-C. Billon and J. Hanoune: FEBS Lett. **107** (1979), 105–109

[12] Sternweis, P. C., J. K. Northup, E. Hanski, L. S. Schleifer, M. D. Smigel and A. G. Gilman: Adv. Cyclic Nucl. Res. **14** (1981), 23–36

Central Institute of Heart and Circulation Research, Academy of Sciences of the GDR, Berlin-Buch, GDR

Supersensitivity to Isoprenaline in Cultured Rat Myocardial Cells Exposed to L(+)-Lactate and Pyruvate

G. Wallukat, L. Will-Shahab and A. Wollenberger

Introduction

As was recently reported [7], neonatal rat myocardial cells are more sensitive to β-adrenoceptor stimulation in stationary culture than they are in nonstationary (rocker) culture. The higher sensitivity correlated with a higher cellular lactate content. The present study (see also 10) is concerned with the influence of lactate and other metabolites on the chronotropic response of rat myocardial cells to isoprenaline in 4- to 8-day rocker cultures.

Materials and methods

As described in detail [2], single cells were dissociated from the minced heart ventricles of neonatal Wistar rats with a 0.2% solution of trypsin and were cultured for 4 to 8 days at 37 °C in air as monolayer in Müller flasks.

The flasks were continuously moved on a rocker platform at a speed of 2 cycles of 2×30 degrees each per min (rocker culture). Halle medium [3] was used containing 10% heat inactivated calf serum and 2×10^{-6} M fluorodeoxyuridine, the latter to prevent an overgrowth of the myocardial cells by the non-muscle cells [4]. On the last day the cells were washed and the medium was replaced by fresh medium free of serum. The cells were incubated for 2 hours in the presence or absence of metabolites. The number of pulsations was counted on the warm stage (37 °C) of an inverted Zeiss-Jena contrast microscope. Dose response curves were obtained by cumulative addition of isoprenaline. Cell protein was determined by the method of Lowry et al. [5] using ovalbumin as standard. The cyclic AMP content was measured by the method of Gilman [1] after purification of the cell extracts as described in detail by Wollenberger and Irmler [9].

Results and discussion

The results indicate that incubation of rocker-cultured neonatal rat myocardial cells with 3 mM l(+)-lactate or 1 mM pyruvate for a minimum of 45 to 60 min resulted in a lowering of the threshold concentration and the EC_{50} for the chronotropic response to isoprenaline by 3 to 4 orders of magnitude (Tab. 1 and Fig. 1). This effect was not impeded by the protein synthesis inhibitor puromycin (10^{-4} M), suggesting that the sensitization of the cells to isoprenaline after pretreatment with l(+)-lactate or pyruvate was unrelated to the process of protein synthesis. Phosphoenolpyruvate (3 mM) and

Table 1

Potency of chronotropic action of isoprenaline on cultured neonatal rat hearts cells exposed to various metabolites. 2-hour preincubation with metabolites

Metabolite	Threshold concentration (M)	EC_{50} (M)
8-day cultures		
Control	$10^{-8}-10^{-7}$	1.0×10^{-6}
L-(+)-Lactate, 1 mM	$10^{-11}-10^{-10}$	3.2×10^{-7}
L-(+)-Lactate, 3 mM	$10^{-13}-10^{-12}$	4.3×10^{-9}
Pyruvate, 1 mM	$10^{-13}-10^{-12}$	1.1×10^{-9}
Phosphoenolpyruvate, 3 mM	10^{-11}	5.9×10^{-9}
Malate, 3 mM	$10^{-13}-10^{-12}$	1.3×10^{-10}
D-(−) Lactate, 3 mM	$10^{-9}-10^{-8}$	4.1×10^{-7}
β-Hydroxybutyrate, 3 mM	$10^{-9}-10^{-8}$	3.3×10^{-7}
Oxalacetate, 3 mM	$10^{-8}-10^{-7}$	8.3×10^{-7}
Acetate, 3 mM	$10^{-7}-10^{-6}$	—
3 to 4 day cultures		
Control	$10^{-10}-10^{-9}$	4.9×10^{-8}
Pyruvate, 1 mM	$10^{-13}-10^{-12}$	1.5×10^{-9}
Citrate, 3 mM	10^{-9}	6.8×10^{-8}

malate (3 mM) caused changes similar to those observed with l(+)-lactate and pyruvate, while 3 mM d(−)-lactate, acetate, oxaloacetate, citrate, and β-hydroxybutyrate were ineffective (Tab. 1). The sensitization of the cultured cells to isoprenaline by pyruvate was abolished by 10^{-8} M (−)-propranolol (Fig. 1), indicating that β-adrenergic receptors probably were involved in this phenomenon. Indeed, the number of β-adrenergic receptors, as revealed by the specific binding of [^{3}H]dihydroalprenolol[8], increased 2-fold following exposure to 1 mM pyruvate.

Positive chronotropic responses to dibutyryl cyclic AMP (10^{-6} to 10^{-4} M) and to the phosphodiesterase inhibitor 1-methyl-3-isobutylxanthine in a concentration (10^{-4} M) causing a significant increase in the cyclic AMP content of cultured neonatal heart cells [9] were not affected by pyruvate (not shown). This finding suggests that if the potentiation of the chronotropic effect of isoprenaline by pyruvate involves cyclic AMP, the action of pyruvate must be exerted on a step leading to the formation of the cyclic nucleotide. As suggested by the binding data, this step could be the activation of β-adrenergic receptors.

An increase in the number of measurable β-adrenergic receptors has been observed [6] 1 hour following coronary artery ligation in the ischaemic region of the heart. Conceivably lactate, which is known to accumulate in ischaemic myocardium, may be a factor responsible for this effect and may render the ischaemic myocardial tissue more sensitive to arrhythmogenic effects of β-receptor stimulation.

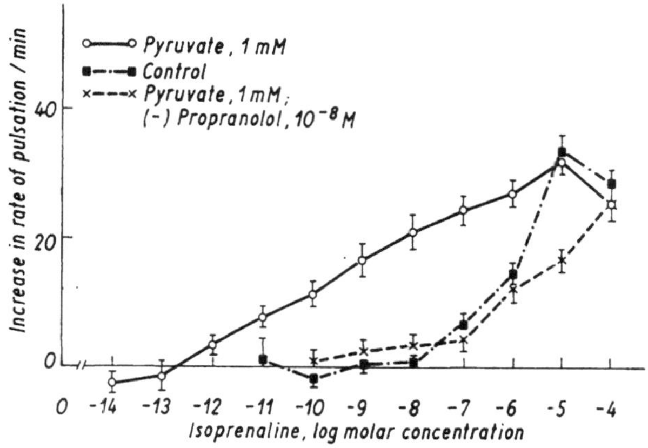

Fig. 1. Effect of pyruvate on the chronotropic response of cultured neonatal rat heart ventricle cells to isoprenaline and abolition of the pyruvate effect by (—)-propranolol.

References

[1] GILMAN, A. G.: Proc. Nat. Acad. Sci. USA **67** (1970), 305—312

[2] HALLE, W. and A. WOLLENBERGER: Myocardial and other cell cultures, in Methods in Pharmacology, Vol. 1 (A. SCHWARTZ, Ed.) (1971), 191—245

[3] HALLE, W. and A. WOLLENBERGER: Am. J. Cardiol. **25** (1970), 292—299

[4] KÖSSLER, A.: Acta biol. med. germ. **29** (1972), 119—134

[5] LOWRY, O. H., N. J. ROSEBROUGH, D. L. FARR and R. J. RANDALL: J. Biol. Chem. **193** (1951), 265—275

[6] MUKHERJEE, A., T. M. WONG, M. BUJA, R. J. LEFKOWITZ and J. T. WILLERSON: J. Clin. Invest. **64** (1979), 1423—1428

[7] WALLUKAT, G. and A. WOLLENBERGER: Acta biol. med. germ. **39** (1980), K7—K13

[8] WALLUKAT, G., L. WILL-SHAHAB and A. WOLLENBERGER: Abstr. IX World Congr. Cardiol., Vol. I (1982), No. 1039

[9] WOLLENBERGER, A. and R. IRMLER: Recent Adv. Stud. Cardiac Struct. Metab. **12** (1978), 689—695

[10] WOLLENBERGER, A. and G. WALLUKAT: In Advances in Studies on Heart Metabolism (C. M. CALDARERA and P. HARRIS, Eds.), CLUEB, Bologna (1982), 133—137

Central Institute of Heart and Circulation Research and Central Institute of Molecular Biology, Academy of Sciences of the GDR, Berlin-Buch, GDR

Activation of Cyclic AMP-dependent Protein kinase in the Ischaemic Myocardium

S. Bartel, E.-G. Krause and J. G. Reich

The activation of cyclic AMP-dependent protein kinase(s) (cA-PK) includes a dissociation of the inactive holoenzyme complex in the active catalytic and the regulatory subunit induced by cyclic AMP binding to the regulatory moiety [1, 9]. Although this dissociation may be influenced by Mg · ATP, iones as well as substrates of the enzyme *in vitro* [6] a satisfactory correlation was found between increased levels of cyclic AMP and the degree of cA-PK activation in various tissues *in vivo* [7] after external hormone administration.

Following acute ischaemia the cyclic AMP levels and the activation of cA-PK was found to be increased in heart muscle [5]. This study describes the relationship between the level of cyclic AMP and the activation of cA-PK in the myocardium followed coronary artery ligation. Employing a mathematical model the calculated K_a values for cyclic AMP markedly differ from those determined under *in vitro* conditions.

Methods

For the experiments anaesthetized dogs were maintained on artifical respiration. After thoracotomy the left coronary artery was ligated (CAL). Tissue samples were freeze clamped from the left ventricular muscle at 0, 2 and 20 min after CAL.

Cyclic AMP was measured in chromatographically purified extracts according to [4]. The cA-PK activity was estimated in tissue homogenates in the absence and presence of 2×10^{-6} M cyclic AMP in a modification as recently described (1,2). The enzyme activity is expressed as the protein kinase activity ratio (−cAMP/+cAMP).

Results and discussion

As a consequence of cyclic AMP accumulation in the heart muscle after 2 and 20 min CAL a rise in the cA-PK activity ratio occurs from 0,11 ± 0,02 to 0,26 ± 0,02 (Fig. 1). The rise in myocardial cyclic AMP levels and the activation of cA-PK could be prevented by 2 mg/kg d, l propranolol [5], supporting the hypothesis [8] that these processes are probably induced by release of catecholamines from sympathetic nerve terminals in the heart. The obtained relationship between the assayed levels of cyclic AMP and the activity ratio of cA-PK in the individual tissue samples is given in Figure 2. As shown the postulated linear correlation between both parameters seems to be inadaquate for the cardiac muscle *in vivo*. Therefore a mathematical model was used for describing the apparent non-linear correlation between the studied parameters. This model includes i) a binding site for cyclic AMP at the regulatory subunit which is related to the dissociation process of the subunits (C and R) and ii) a second, high affinity binding site (P) for cyclic AMP not related to the activation of this enzyme. Such a functional compartmentalization of the intracellular cyclic AMP probably explains the observed low activity ratio of cA-PK in the pre-

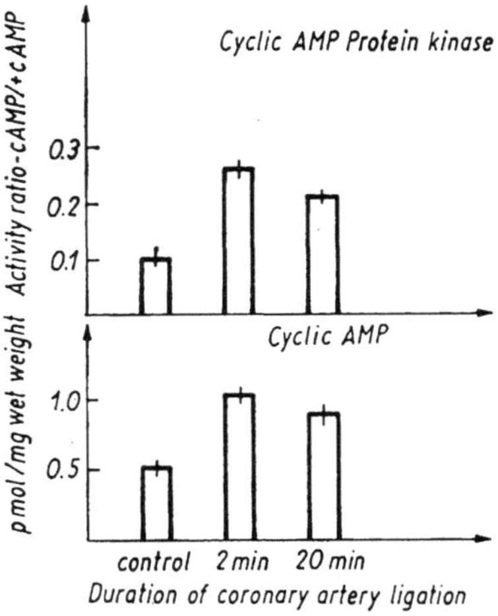

Fig. 1. Changes in cyclic AMP levels and cyclic AMP-dependent protein kinase activity ratio in dependence of ischaemic time.

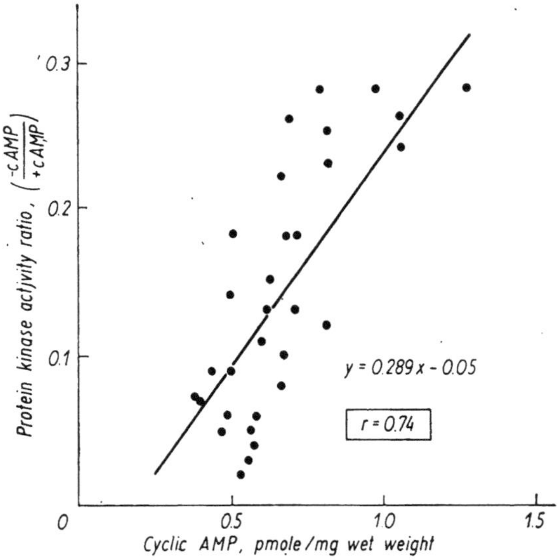

Fig. 2. Correlation between cyclic AMP-dependent protein kinase activity ratio and cyclic AMP in aerobic and ischaemic heart.

sence of a relative high concentration of this nucleotide in the cell. By the aim of the obtained equation (see Fig. 3 inset) the concentration of cyclic AMP for the half-maximal activation dependents on the expected total activation of this enzyme (Table 1), and was calculated in a range of 0,2 to $0{,}9 \times 10^{-6}$ M, which is several times higher than the K_a value for the isolated enzyme in salt solution. In spite of the validy of the proposed model it seems of interest, that DOKHUAC [3] calculated a K_a-value for cyclic AMP of $0{,}33 \times 10^{-6}$ M for the intact skeletal muscle using a titration technique for measuring the amount free R-subunits.

$$\text{I)}\quad RC + A \rightleftharpoons C + RA \qquad \frac{[C]\cdot[RA]}{[A]\cdot[RC]} = K$$

$$\text{II)}\quad A + P \rightleftharpoons PA \qquad \frac{[A]\cdot[P]}{[PA]} = I$$

$$A_0 = RA + A + PA;\quad R_0 = C + RC;\quad C = RA$$

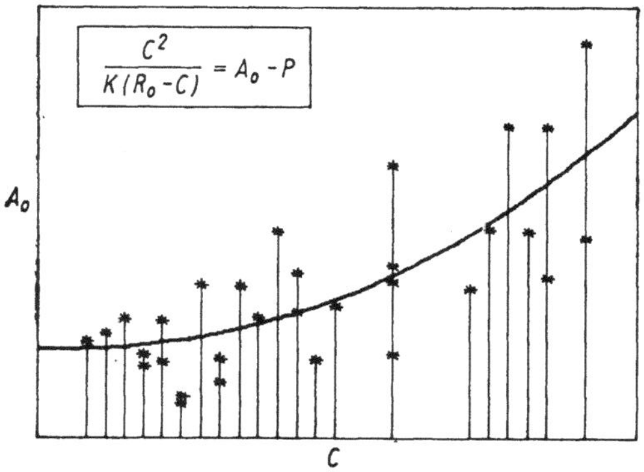

Fig. 3. Model of cyclic AMP compartmentalization and its relationship to cyclic AMP-dependent protein kinase in the myocardium *in vivo*.
A_0 = cyclic AMP_{total}; C = catalytic subunit (active) (both parameters are given in relative values). Stars represent experimentally obtained data.

Table 1

Apparent constant (K_a) for cyclic AMP-dependent protein kinase activation in dog myocardium

Conditions	R_0', Relative unit[1])	K_a 10^{-6} M	Range of var., %
in vivo	0.45	0.25	16.2
	0.50	0.35	16.1
	0.75	0.94	15.9
tissue homogenate	1.00	0.05	8

R_0' = expected maximal enzyme activation presumably equal to the extent of enzyme dissociation
$K_a = A_{0.5}$ equal to $R_0'/2K + P$

References

[1] Corbin, J. D. and S. L. Keely: J. Biol. Chem. **252** (1977), 910—918
[2] Dobson, J. G.: Am. J. Physiol. **234** (1978), 638—645
[3] DoKhuac, L., S. Harbon and H. J. Clauser: Eur. J. Biochem. **40** (1973), 177—185
[4] Gilman, A.: Proc. Natl. Acad. Sci. USA **67** (1970), 305—312
[5] Krause, E.-G., S. Bartel, P. Karczewski and K.-F. Lindenau: Advances in Myocardiology Vol. **4**, (1982), 521—530
[6] Rannels, S. R. and J. D. Corbin: J. Biol. Chem. **255** (1980), 7085—7088
[7] Sengupta, K., K. J. Long and D. O. Allen: J. Pharmacol. Exp. Ther. **218** (1981), 128—133
[8] Shahab, L., M. Haase, U. Schiller and A. Wollenberger: Acta biol. med. germ. **22** (1969), 135—143
[9] Yücel, M. and I. Özer: FEBS Lett. **125** (1981), 120—122

Institute of Drug Research, Academy of Sciences of GDR, Berlin, GDR

Myocardial Protection in Vitro by o-(β-Hydroxyethyl)-Rutoside, a Flavone Derivative and by Mannitol

H. Löwe, I. E. Blasig, C. Hennig and B. Oczko

During a hypoxia of myocardial tissue it comes more or less quickly to disturbances of biological membrane, demonstrable by swollen and disrupted mitochondria, by swollen endothelial cells of the capillaries with narrowing the lumen, and by extracapillary edema. Parallel to those morphological changes, it can be shown *in vitro* an increase of the release of cell enzymes-LDH for instance-and an increase of the coronary resistance of retrograd perfused isolated hearts. Reoxygenation after a hypoxia results in a drastical enhancement of the tissue lesions. There are some directions in the literature of the last years that the cause of those more or less reversible (dependent from the time of hypoxia) disturbances in biological membranes during a hypoxia, and in an extensive manner during a following reoxygenation is the reaction of oxygen radicals, with unsaturated fatty acids of phospholipids in the biological membranes. The reduction of molecular oxygen in one-electron steps runs every time parallely to the reduction catalysed by cytochrome oxidases, and results in the formation of the oxygen radicals — superoxide, peroxide, and the hydroxyl radical. There are some physiological pathways to scavenge the radicals by superoxide-dismutase, by catalase/peroxidase, by tocopherol, and by glutathion. During a hypoxia those physiological protecting mechanisms seem to be diminished. Therefore it must be possible to protect the hypoxic tissue by applicating substances with radical scavening activities.

We tested two substances with those activities: The first of them was the 0-(β-hydroxyethyl)-rutoside, a water soluble flavonoid from the Zyma-GmbH/München, called Venoruton. Siegers and Younes [2] have shown the radical scavenging activities of some flavonoids. The second substance, tested by us, was mannitol. Mannitol ist also known as an OH/-scavenger [1], and was already formerly used in experimental myocardial protection.

Our testing model was a retrograde perfused isolated rabbit heart with registration of the perfusion resistance and other physiological parameters (amplitude of contration, frequency, perfusion flow). The perfusion medium (Krebs-Ringer-medium) was gassed with oxygen or nitrogen and was substituted with the substances to be tested. In the effluent we determined the release of lactatedehydrogenase (LDH). After a period of about 30 min. of oxygenated perfusion (pO_2 ca. 65 kPa; fixed perfusion rate of 25 ml/min) to stabilize the heart actions, we started to perfuse the heart hypoxically without substrate in the perfusion medium. The flow per minute was decreased to 2.5 ml and the oxygen pressure in the perfusion medium was diminished to 6.7 kPa.

The duration of the hypoxic period was in most cases 180 min. followed by a period of 30 min. reoxygenation and substrate supply (11 mM glucose). It can be shown in Figure 1 that there was an increase of the LDH release during the first 120 min of hypoxia ,showing the tissue injury. In this time the rutoside-perfused hearts showed a significant diminished release of LDH. Mannitol-perfused hearts released LDH also in a decreased ratio, but significantly only in the first 800 min rof hypoxia. After 120 min there are no more differences between the three tested groups. The teoxygenation resulted in a drastical increase of LDH-release, but without significant differences between the groups, caused by the high scattering between the individual hearts, too.

In Figure 2 it can be shown an increase of the resistance of the coronary system of the isolated

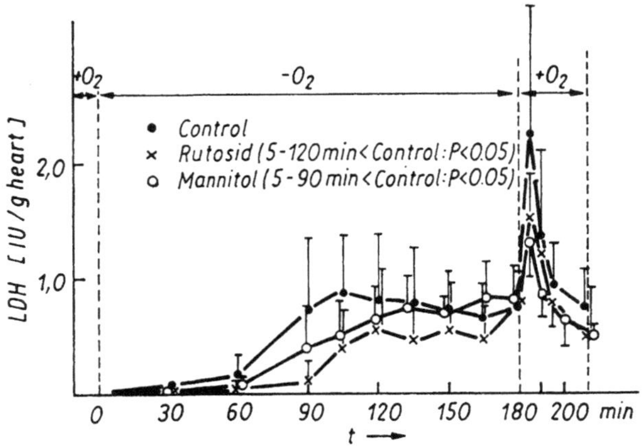

Fig. 1. Release of LDH from hearts during hypoxia and reoxygenation.

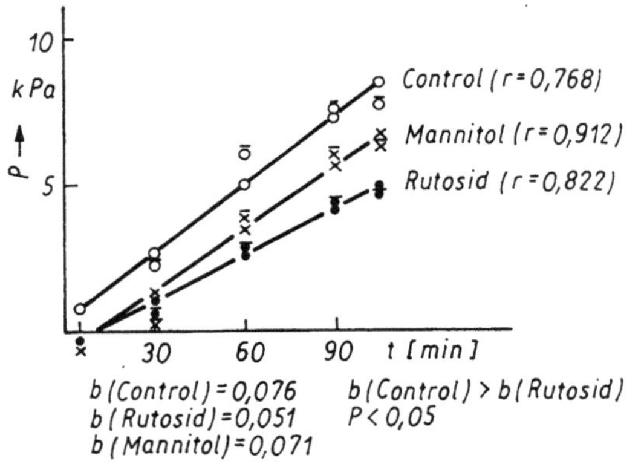

Fig. 2. Regression of the flow resistance in hypoxia.

hearts during the first 90 min of hypoxia. This increase of the resistance of the coronaries was significant in all three groups, but this increase of the coronary resistance is significant lower in the rutoside treated group than in the control group. The increase in the mannitol-treated group was statistically not different from the controls.

Since there was a remarkable relation between the release of LDH during the hypoxia and the increase of the coronary resistance we tested the correlation of these two parameters. We found a high significant correlation with a coefficient by Spearman of 0.8445 ± 0.114. This shows that both parameters are likewise parameters of the injury of the myocard.

References

[1] Marklund, St.: J. Biol. Chem. **251** (1976), 7504—7507
[2] M. Younes and C. P. Siegers: J. Med. Plant Res. **43** (1981), 240—244

Institute of Drug Research, Academy of Sciences of GDR, Berlin, GDR

Can Blood Flow Reduction after Isoproterenol Overdosage Induce Myocardial Ischaemia?

I. E. Blasig, P. Muschick, E. Rohde, R. Richter, D. Modersohn and H. Löwe

Since Rona's work in 1959 [6] it has been known that isoproterenol overdosage, > 0.02 mg/kg, induces infarct-like necroses in myocardium. Recently, Blasig et al. [1, 3] found a decrease of local myocardial blood flow (MBF) following application of 50 mg/kg. To investigate the question whether the lesions are preceded by an ischaemia initial time course and dose dependence of metabolic and hemodynamic parameters and the influence by cardioprotective drugs were investigated.

Male adult Wistar rats received a single dose of isoproterenol i.p. 60 min afterwards, heart excision was performed about 5 s after the begin of thoracotomy. Slight anaesthesia was caused by 1250 mg/kg urethan i.p. Immediately after preparation, membrane potential was intracellularly estimated *in vitro* in tissue pieces. The content of lactate, pyruvate, phosphocreatine and inorganic phosphate was determined after deep freezing by the Wollenberger technique. The combination narcosis of 90 mg/kg α-chloralose and 850 mg/kg urethan i.p. was used during the measurements of arterial blood pressure (BP), heart rate, and local MBF, latter done by the hydrogen clearance, in open chest rats during artificial respiration. Local parameters were measured in left

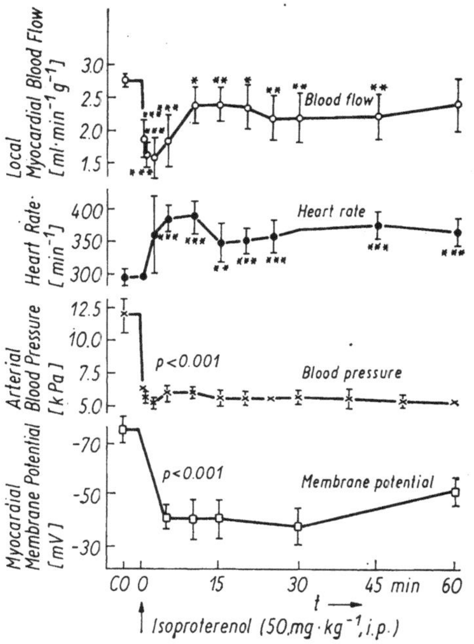

Fig. 1. Initial time course of some hemodynamic and electrophysiological changes, compared to control conditions (CO), after i.p. injection of 50 mg/kg isoproterenol.
Data represent means ± S. D. *,**,*** —p < 0.05, 0.01, and 0.001

ventricular myocardium. L-propranolol, verapamil, and nitroglycerine were given for a period of 15, 30 and 0.5 min, respectively.

The injection of 50 mg/kg isoproterenol immediately leads to a strong decrease of local MBF correlated to strong depression of mean arterial BP and increase of heart frequency within the first 45 min (Fig. 1). The observed flow reduction is assumed to be at least partially caused by the fall of BP below 9 kPa (70 mm Hg). According to [7] and [4] lower levels result in myocardial underperfusion. Moreover, the tachycardia could diminish the blood flow in subendocardium main-

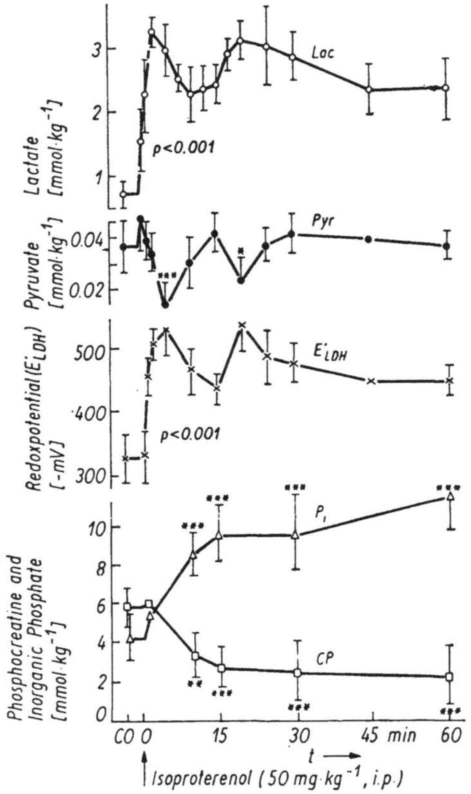

Fig. 2. Initial time course of some metabolic alterations in myocardium, compared to the control (CO), following i.p. application of 50 mg/kg isoproterenol. Statistics see Fig. 1.

ly perfused during diastole because of the shorter diastolic time interval. The time course of flow diminution is related to increased anaerobiosis and breakdown of energy-rich phosphate (Fig. 2) characteristically for ischaemic conditions. Especially, the similarity of the biphasic changes in MBF, heart rate, content of lactate, and pyruvate including the corresponding redoxpotential is evident. Also the measured drop in resting membrane potential (Fig. 1) is comparable to observations of [4] during experimental coronary artery ligation.

The dose dependence studies (Fig. 3) exhibit a MBF reduction after injection of more than 0.1 mg/kg isoproterenol. The well known perfusion stimulating action can be reproduced between 0.01 and 0.1 mg/kg. By doses of about 0.01 mg/kg, a fall of lactate content is shown. Smaller dosage is ineffective probably depending on the used i.p. application and 25 min exposure time. The flow reducing doses, > 0.1 mg/kg, cause myocardial lactate accumulation further indicating ischaemic conditions. Enrichment of the product of anaerobic glycolysis also occurs during the increased flow seen by about 0.1 mg/kg. It is assumed that the higher MBF insufficiently

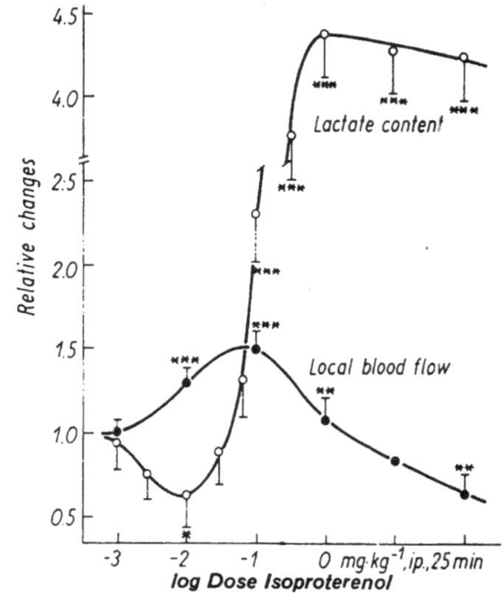

Fig. 3. Dose response curves of local bloodflow and lactate content in myocardium 25 min after i.p. administration of isoproterenol. Statistics see Fig. 1.

supplies the much more stimulated myocardial function. Concluding the data, the mode of action of isoproterenol on myocardium can be divided depending on the used dosage as follows:

1. Up to 0.05 mg/kg, isoproterenol improves myocardial function accompanied by an adequate metabolic and hemodynamic supply.
2. The application of 0.05 to 0.1 mg/kg leads to an acute hypoxia or relative ischaemia with increased but not sufficient blood supply, compared to the stronger increased demand, resulting in metabolic and hemodynamic defects.
3. Mg-doses induce the same, only stronger disturbances as in 2. but reduce MBF showing absolute ischaemic conditions.

Different effects are also demonstrated at different isoproterenol doses by interventions with drugs being well effective in the therapy of ischaemic heart disease. During the improved status, the MBF increased by isoproterenol, ~ 0.01 mg/kg, is not affected by verapamil and nitroglycerin.

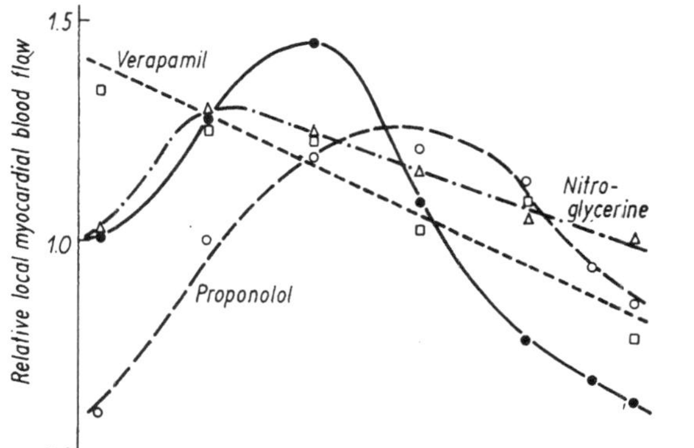

Fig. 4. Effect of pretreatment with L-propranolol (— —), verapamil (— — — —), both 10 mg/kg i.p., and nitroglycerine (—·—), 0.01 mg/kg i.v., on dose response curve of myocardial blood flow 25 min after i.p. injection of isoproterenol (———).

Only the β-adrenergic antagonist l-propranolol develops its own flow decreasing effect. However, all the flow alterations accompanied by metabolic disturbances, > 0.01 mg/kg isoproterenol, are reduced by all used pharmaca (Fig. 4). The beneficial drug effects are also shown in the dose dependent reduction of isoproterenol-induced lactate accumulation (data not shown). Both indirectly support the concept of ischaemic conditions in myocardium. The unexpected effect of the nitrobody leeds to the assumption of a further pathomechanism included in the disturbances in addition to the known β-adrenergic and Ca^{2+} inflow overstimulation. Also no explanation can be given concerning the increased myocardial content of free arachidonic acid (C 20:4) contrary to all other detected free fatty acids found earlier by [2]. It is speculated that these deteriorations could be associated with alterations in membrane lipids. The observed acute ischaemia-like changes in myocardium induced by isoproterenol overdosage can be accepted as an additional model for testing drugs against ischaemia.

References

[1] BLASIG, I. E., P. MUSCHICK, D. MODERSOHN and H. LÖWE: International symposium of socialist contries on "Pathomechanism and Prevention of Sudden Cardiac Death due to Coronary Insufficiency". Szeged (1981), Abstracts 26
[2] BLASIG, I. E., R. BLASIG, S. KEDOR, K. JANOWSKI and H. LÖWE: 6th joint symposium of the biochemical societies of the GDR and USSR "Regulation in Metabolism and Bioenergetics". Tallin (1981), Abstracts 143
[3] BLASIG, I. E., P. MUSCHICK, G. HARTMANN and H. LÖWE: Proceed. IX. World Congr. of Cardiol. Moscow (1982), Abstract vol. II 37
[4] DOWNAR, E., M. J. JANSE and D. DURRER: Circul. **56** (1977), 217–224
[5] MOIR, T. W. and D. W. DE BRA: Circ. Res. **21** (1967), 65–74
[6] RONA, G., C. I. CHAPPEL, T. BALAZS and R. GAUDRY: Arch. Pathol. **67** (1959), 443–445
[7] SALISBURY, P. F., C. E. CROSS and P. A. RIEBEN: Amer. Heart J. **66** (1963), 650–656

Charité Hospital of Humboldt University, Berlin and Central Institute of Heart and Circulation Research, Academy of Sciences of GDR, Berlin-Buch, GDR

The Influence of Prostacyclin on Experimental Myocardial Infarction in Dogs

H. Goos, K.-F. Lindenau, E.-G. Krause, J. Nöhring, S. Gehlhar, J. Schinke, C. Wagenknecht, H. David, J. Liebetruth, B. Jonas and P. A. Parsi

Recently prostacyclin (PGI_2), a metabolite of arachidonic acid, has become of interest because of its physiological actions and its possible therapeutic value. PGI_2 has some cardiovascular effects [1, 5, 7, 12]. Investigations during acute myocardial ischaemia have shown that PGI_2 may protect ischaemic myocardial cells. The protective effect was shown by the prevention of ST segment changes [4], by reduced release of lysosomal cathepsin D [9] or creatine kinase [3, 10].

We studied the influence of PGI_2 alone or in combination with intraaortic balloon pumping (IABP) on the tissue contents of energy-rich phosphates and lactate. Furthermore the release of cathepsin D into serum as well as morphological changes in the ischaemic heart were investigated following coronary artery occlusion.

Material and methods

The experiments were carried out in 40 mongrel dogs of both sexes. After left thoracotomy the left anterior descending coronary artery was ligated for 3 hours. In control dogs the same procedure was performed exept the occlusion of coronary artery. 1 hour after coronary artery occlusion the infusion of PGI_2 (0.1 μmol/kg body weight/min) was started. PGI_2 application was done via intravenous infusion with or without IABP or electronically triggered via precoronary catheter directly into the aortic root combined with IABP.

Duration of therapeutic interventions was 2 hours. Tissue from the ischaemic and non-ischaemic region of the left ventricle were then freeze-stopped in situ with a Wollenberger-clamp [13]. Before freeze-stop ischaemic and non-ischaemic tissue were taken for electron microscopy. Cathepsin D activity was measured in the sinus coronarius blood every hour.

The experiments were made in 5 groups.

1. control group	7 dogs
coronary occlusion groups	
2. without therapeutic procedure	14 dogs
3. PGI_2 i.v.	6 dogs
4. PGI_2 i.v. and IABP	5 dogs
5. precoronary and IABP	7 dogs

Creatine phosphate and ATP content were enzymatically measured in a 0.5 n perchloric acid extract after neutralization with KOH [8]. Lactate was estimated in the same tissue according to [6]. Cathepsin D was measured by a modified method according to [2].

All values are reported in terms of means ± S.E.M. Changes were analysed statistically by the Students-t-test for paired values. A p value less than 0.05 was considered to be significant.

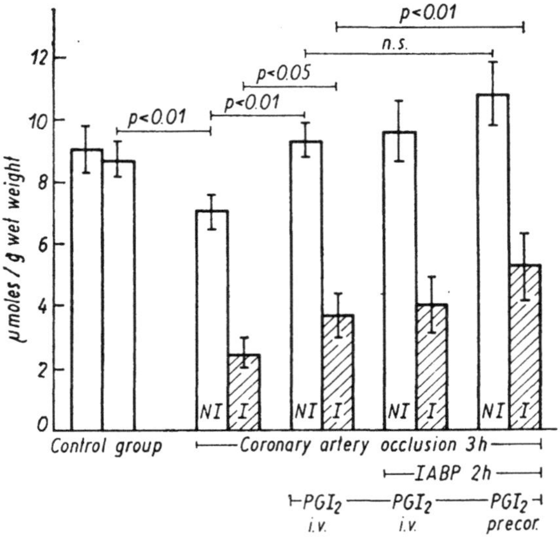

Fig. 1. Changes in creatine phosphate content in the ischaemic and non-ischaemic left ventricular myocardium following coronary artery ligation with and without protective intervention.
Mean ± S.E.M. are given.
NI: non-ischaemic tissue
I: ischaemic tissue
precor: precoronary

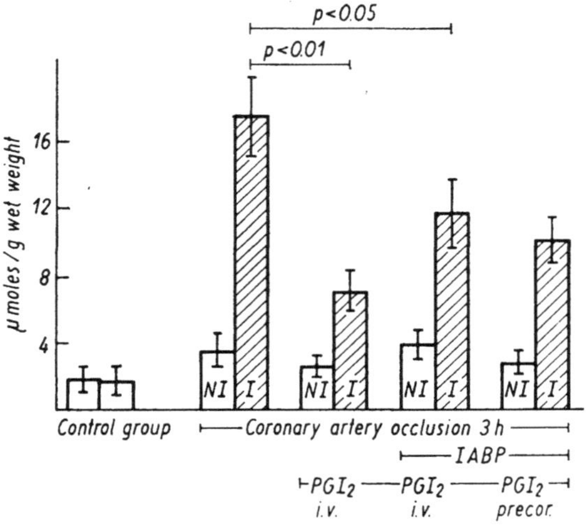

Fig. 2. Changes in lactate content in the ischaemic and non-ischaemic left ventricular myocardium following coronary artery ligation with and without protective intervention.
Mean ± S.E.M. are given.
NI: non-ischaemic tissue
I: ischaemic tissue
precor: precoronary

Results and discussion

The myocardial level of ATP was significantly decreased in the ischaemic myocardium. We found no significant ATP content changes in any of the coronary artery occlusion groups.

Changes in the levels of creatine phosphate, lactate and of cathepsin D activity are demonstrated in the Figures 1 to 3.

In accordance with the results of RÖSEN et al. [11] also in our experiments PGI_2 prevented an increase in lactate and the lactate pyruvate ratio (data not shown). In contrast to those authors we found that PGI_2 is able to protect the creatine phosphate content in the ischaemic myocardium which was significantly higher compared to the non-treated group. The protective effect of PGI_2 was most effective in the case of electronically triggered precoronary application into the aortic root combined with IABP.

PGI_2 significantly reduces the cathepsin D release, which may be due to a stabilizing effect on lysosomal membranes in the ischaemic heart [9]. These results support the findings of other authors [3, 4, 9, 10]. First electron microscopic measurements support our biochemical findings.

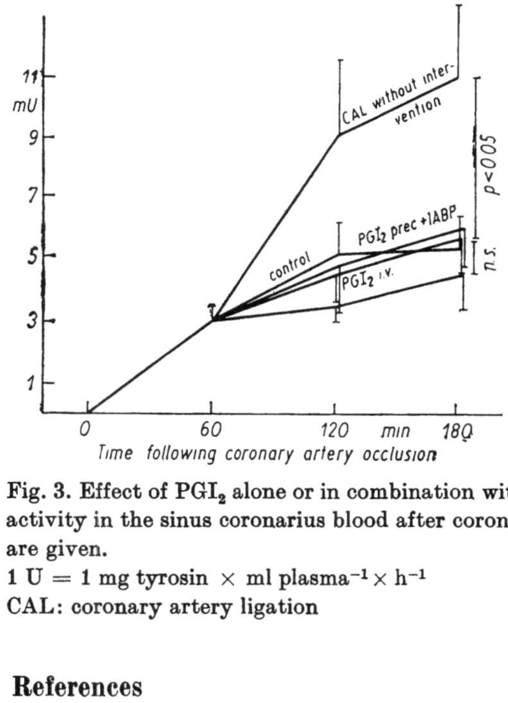

Fig. 3. Effect of PGI_2 alone or in combination with IABP on the plasma cathepsin D activity in the sinus coronarius blood after coronary artery ligation. Mean ± S.E.M. are given.
1 U = 1 mg tyrosin × ml $plasma^{-1} \times h^{-1}$
CAL: coronary artery ligation

References

[1] ALLAN, G. and R. LEVI: J. Pharmacol. Exp. Ther. **214** (1980), 45–49
[2] ANSON, M. L.: J. Gen. Physiol. **22** (1939), 79–81
[3] ARAKI, H. and A. M. LEFER: Circ. Res. **48** (1980), 757–763
[4] COKER, S. J. and J. R. PARRATT: Basic. Res. Cardiol. **76** (1981), 457–462
[5] DUSTING, G. J. and J. R. VANE: Circ. Res. 46 Suppl. I (1980), 183–187
[6] HOHORST, H. J.: In: Methoden der enzymatischen Analyse (ed.: H. U. Bergmeyer) Akademie Verlag Berlin 1970, 1425–1429
[7] KARMAZYN, M., B. S. TUANA and N. S. DHALLA: Can. J. Physiol. Pharmacol. **59** (1981), 1122–1127

[8] Lamprecht, W., P. Stein, F. Heinz and H. Weisser: In: Methoden der enzymatischen Analyse (ed.: H. U. Bergmeyer) Akademie Verlag Berlin 1970, 1734–1737

[9] Lefer, A. M. and E. F. Smith: In: Prostacyclin (ed.: J. R. Vane and S. Bergström) Raven Press New York 1979, 339–347

[10] Ogletree, M. L., A. M. Lefer, J. B. Smith and K. C. Nicolaou: Europ. J. Pharmacol. **56** (1979), 95–103

[11] Rösen, R., P. Rösen, R. Ohlendorf and K. Schrör: Europ. J. Pharmacol. **69** (1981), 489–491

[12] Schrör, K.: Basic. Res. Cardiol. **76** (1981) 239–249

[13] Wollenberger, A., O. Ristau and G. Schoffa: Pflügers Arch. ges. Physiol. **270** (1960), 399–412

Central Institute of Heart and Circulation Research of the Academy of Sciences of GDR, Berlin; Surgical Clinic and Clinic of Internal Medicine of the Charité, Humboldt-University of Berlin, GDR

Glycogen Phosphorylase b Activity in Human Serum after Acute Myocardial Infarction and Coronary Bypass Surgery

G. RABITZSCH, H. GOOS, J. NÖHRING, J. LEMBCKE, K.-F. LINDENAU, E.-G. KRAUSE, R.-A. PARSI and H. HEINE

Introduction

Glycogen phosphorylase **b** (GP_b; EC 2.4.1.1.) is present as a constituent of the sarcoplasmic reticulum-glycogenolytic complex [4] in the heart muscle cells. The special importance of GP for glycogenolysis and the observed GP_b release into the circulation under the conditions of ischaemic heart damage seem to be causally related to its expected diagnostic significance for acute myocardial infarction [3, 7, 8].

Continuing earlier investigations [2] the diagnostic validity of GP_b was proved in this study in view of a differentiation between acute myocardial infarction (AMI) and chronic ischaemic heart diseases (CIHD). Furthermore preliminary data are presented concerning pre- and postoperative changes in serum enzyme activities of GP_b, as well as creatine kinase (CK) and its isoenzyme MB (CK-MB) before and after coronary artery bypass surgery in connection with acute evolving myocardial infarction (AEMI).

Methods

Serum GP_b activity was assayed in the direction of phosphorylysis using an enzymic UV test [8] or its adaptation to fluorometry [10]. Serum CK and its isoenzyme CK-MB were assayed with the test combinations "monotest CPK activated" (Boehringer, Mannheim) and "Merck-l-Test CK-MB" (E Merck, Darmstadt), respectively.

Results and discussion

Acute myocardial infarction

GP_b was found to be a sensitive serological parameter for indicating the early phase of AMI with a first appearance of about two hours and a peak time of 15 hours after the onset of infarction [9]. On the basis of the reference value with $\leqq 0.12$ U/l $=$ (n $=$ 216) (11), the discrimination point was calculated to be $\geqq 0.18$ U/l. In AMI the average peak value was found to be 0.80 ± 1.15 U/l (range 0.1–10 U/l; n $=$ 79) (Fig. 1).

Proving the diagnostical parameters of the enzyme for a differentiation between acute and chronic ischaemic heart diseases the maximal activities of serum GP_b were compared of 79 patients with AMI (characterized according to WHO criteria), 92 patients with CIHD (severe angina pectoris syndrom with and without arrhythmias) and 216 healthy persons, respectively (Fig. 1). In the differentiation of the two pathological groups the parameters of the diagnostical sensitivity and specificity, the positive predictive value, and the negative predictive value of GP_b have been calculated to be 91.1%, 93.5%, 92.3%, and 92.5%, respectively. These results are in correspondence to our earlier data [2], which, however, have not been confirmed by [5].

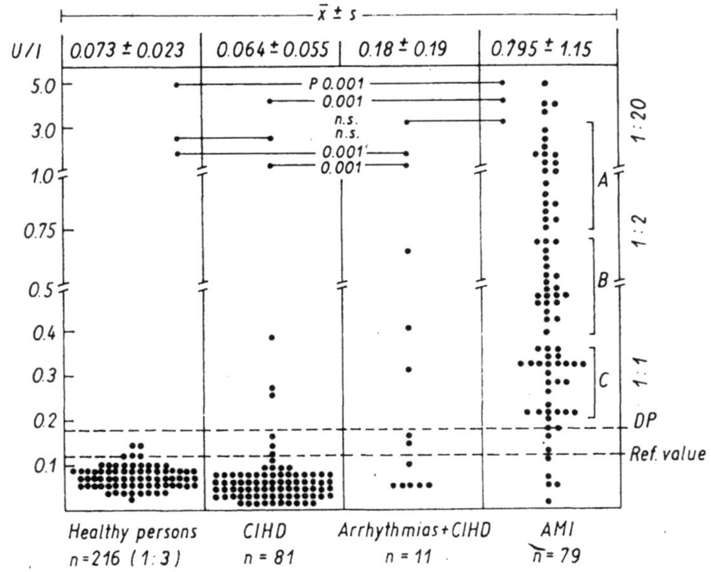

Fig. 1. Comparison of the maximal serum GP_b activities of patients with acute myocardial infarction (AMI), chronic ischaemic heart disease (CIHD), and healthy persons.
Reference value: ≦ 0.12 U/l; DP: discrimination point (≧ 0.18 U/l) [11]

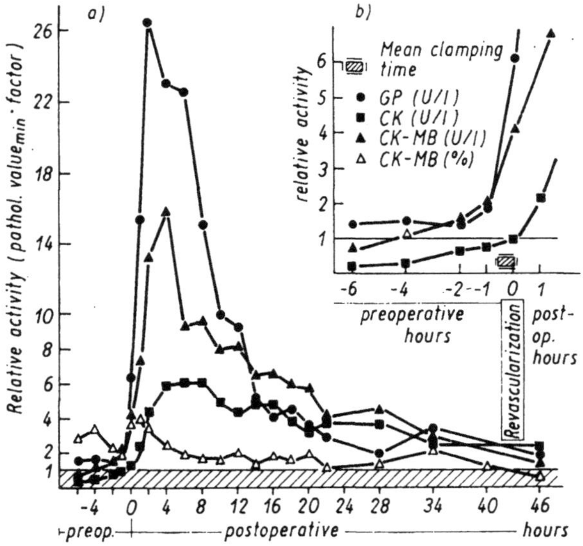

Fig. 2. Comparison of pre- (b), intra-, and postoperative serum GP_b, CK and GK-MB isoenzyme activities before and after coronary artery bypass surgery (mean; n = 7). Pathological value: GP_b 0.18 U/l; CK 160 U/l; CK-MB 10 U/l; $CK\text{-}MB/CK_{total}$ 6%

Coronary artery bypass surgery for acute evolving myocardial infarction (AEMI)

Seven male patients (mean age 50 years) with AEMI underwent revascularization by coronary artery bypass grafting ([6] (mean of grafts: 1.7; range: single to threefold) with a mean aortic clamping time of 36 ± 18 minutes, on average, 15 hours after onset of pain and increased ST segment. 3 patients underwent cardiogenic shock in the preoperative acute ischaemic period.

The pre- and postoperative cardiac enzyme release was characterized by serological activities of GP_b, CK, and CK-MB isoenzyme. These enzymes showed a remarkable increase in their serum activities up to the 6- to 25-fold discrimination value 1 to 15 hours after revascularization, demonstrating an additional removal of the enzymes released during the ischaemia and the reflow (Fig. 2), described as the washout phenomenon (1). The enzyme activities immediately respond on the aortic crossclamping with rapid increasing in the serum (Fig. 2/b). GP_b activity increased to peak values up to 9 U/l two hours after revascularization. Although a correlation between enzyme activities and different surgery variables (data not shown) was not observed the studied patients are possibly divided according to the intensity of enzyme release into two groups, which should be studied in more detail in future.

References

[1] Berg, R., Jr., S. L. Selinger, J. J. Leonard, R. P. Grunwald and W. P. O'Grady: J. Thorac. Cardiovasc. Surg. **81** (1981), 493–497

[2] Böhm, M., G. Rabitzsch, E.-G. Krause, J. Läuter, M. Koschel, J. Lembcke, R. A. Parsi, H.-G. Heinrich, A. Wollenberger and R. Baumann: Dt. Gesundh.-Wesen **33** (1978), 159–166

[3] Entman, M. L., T. Futch, J. M. Wood and A. Schwartz: Circulation 51/52 Suppl. II (1975), 65

[4] Entman, M. L., K. Kaniike, M. A. Goldstein, T. E. Nelson, E. P. Bornet, T. W. Futch and A. Schwartz: J. Biol. Chem. **251** (1976), 3140–3146

[5] Liese, W., K.-D. Boguschewski, R. Reppin, S. Päge, J. E. Peters and H. Urbahn: Dt. Gesundh.-Wesen **36** (1981), 704–709

[6] Lindenau, K.-F., H. Warnke, J. Bohm, L. Dressler, D. Olthoff, H. David and P. Romaniuk: Dt. Gesundh.-Wesen **36** (1981), 1452–1457

[7] Krause, E.-G., M. Böhm, H. Will and A. Wollenberger: Dt. Gesundh.-Wesen **27** (1972), 903–904

[8] Krause, E.-G., H. Will, M. Böhm and A. Wollenberger: Clin. Chim. Acta **58** (1975), 145–154

[9] Rabitzsch, G., M. Böhm and E.-G. Krause: FEBS Special Meeting on Enzymes, Dubrovnik/ISFRJ, 17.–21. 4. 79, Abstract 55–48

[10] Rabitzsch, G., J. Schache, S. Schache and K. Onnen: In preparation

[11] Schache, S. and J. Schache: Diplomarbeit, Humboldt-Univ. Berlin, 1981

Department Pharmacology and Toxicology, Martin Luther University Halle-Wittenberg, Halle, GDR

Influence of β-Receptor Blocking Drugs on Prostacyclin and Thromboxane Synthesis

W. Förster, I. Heinroth, H.-U. Block, P. Mentz and K. Pönicke

The β-receptor blocking drugs with potent antianginal, antiarrhythmic and antihypertensive effects were in the first line considered as β-adrenergic blocking agents though in experiments on animals also membrane stabilizing and local anesthetic properties were seen. Relations to the arachidonic acid metabolism were firstly suggested by [2, 5]. In 1979 we could demonstrate that propranolol evoked an enhanced transformation of PGH_2 to PGI_2 under the influence of the microsomal fraction of pig aorta [3]. In Langendorff heart preparations of guinea pigs propranolol and pindolol enhance the liberation of PGI_2 in a dose having a negative inotropic effect (Fig. 1). Considering the AA-induced aggregation in rabbit and human PRP propranolol (0.1—1.0 mmol/l) inhibited dose dependently the aggregation whereas the TXA_2-biosynthesis (bioassay) was not influenced (Fig. 2). Only higher concentrations up to 5 mmol/l — not shown in the Figure — inhibited partly also the TXA_2 formation. Our results are in good agreement with results with washed platelets from normal volunteers [4]. In hypertensive patients Campbell et al. [1] found an inhibition of the platelet TXA_2 only with the very high dose of 640 mg/day. Contrary to propranolol pindolol inhibited the AA-induced aggregation as well as the TXA_2 synthesis in a dose dependent manner (Fig. 3). Effective concentrations were 0.1 mmol/l or more of both the (—) or (+) isomeres. The cause of the inhibition of TXA_2 by pindolol may be found in its relatively potent inhibition

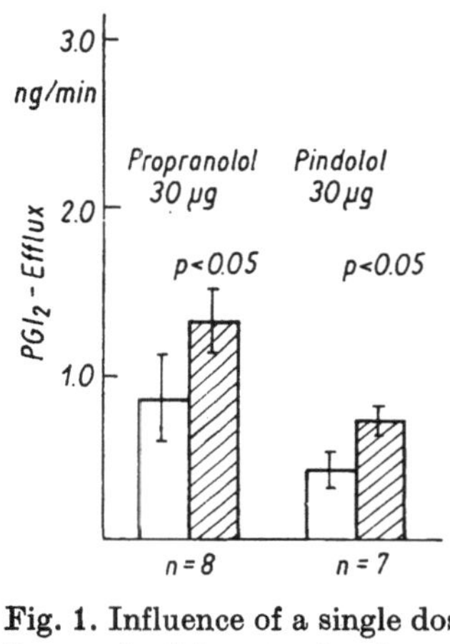

Fig. 1. Influence of a single dose of propranolol and pindolol on the PGI_2 efflux from Langendorff hearts of guinea pigs (O_2 gassed Tyrode solution, 37 °C, 8 kPa, strain gauge transducers, photoelectrical drop counting). PGI_2 was extracted with redestilled ether at pH 5.6 and 5 °C after short lasting addition of a NaH_2PO_4 solution and determined by inhibition of ADP (5 µmol/l)-induced platelet aggregation in comparison with a PGI_2 standard.

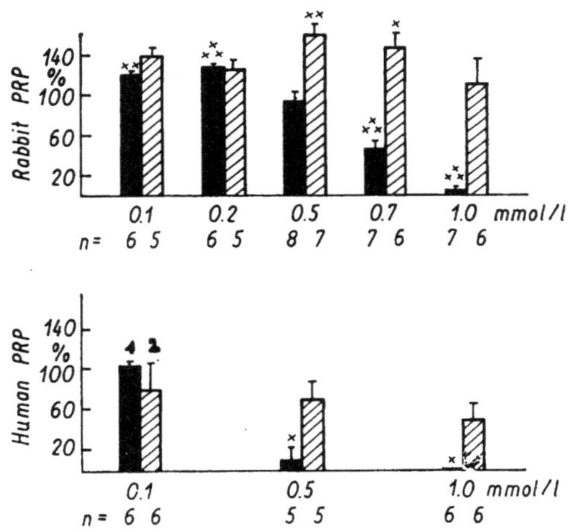

Fig. 2. Influence of (±)-propranolol on AA-induced aggregation and TXA_2 formation in rabbit PRP (at the top) and in human PRP (at the bottom).
(Aggregation and TXA_2 formation measured 90 s after addition of AA to the PRP; TXA_2 content measured by bioassay; significance of difference from control values: *$p < 0.05$; **$p < 0.01$; ***$p < 0.001$; ▇ AA-induced aggregation. ▨ TXA_2 formation).

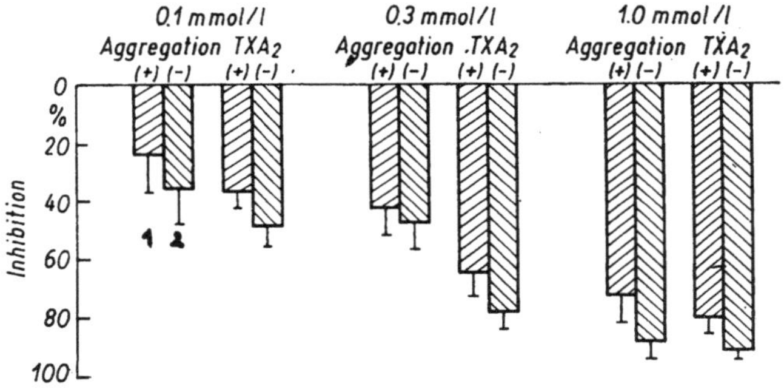

Fig. 3. Influence of pindolol isomers on AA-induced aggregation and TXA_2 formation in rabbit PRP
(▨ (+)-pindolol, ▧ (−)-pindolol; aggregation and TXA_2 formation measured 90 s after addition of AA to the PRP; TXA_2 content measured by bioassay; n = 7).

of the cyclooxygenase (Fig. 4): 10 μM inhibits it by about 60% and 200 μM by 76—83%. By comparison, indomethacin was about one power of ten more potent. The inhibiting effects on the platelet aggregation and the cyclooxygenase were more potent by the (−) isomere than the (+) isomere. In contrast to pindolol propranolol even in the high concentration of 200 μM did not significantly inhibit the cyclooxygenase and showed with 1 mM only a slight inhibition.

Another difference of pindolol and propranolol was seen in different influences on platelet aggregation induced with the PG endoperoxide analogue U 46619 (Fig. 5). Propranolol exerted an inhibition one power of ten more potent than pindolol. One possible hypothesis of this effect is a better direct antagonistic action of propranolol to TXA_2.

We compared also the effects of propranolol and pindolol with those of practolol. Up to more than 1 mmol/l practolol did not influence the platelet aggregation and the TXA_2 formation or the U 46619 induced aggregation.

Thus one part of the mechanism of action of some — but not all — β-adrenergic blocking drugs can be explained via their β-adrenolytic effects. The antihypertensive and the antiplatelet action is induced independently of their adrenolytic action, because both isomeres have a nearly equipotent influence on the synthesis of AA metabolites and the platelet aggregation. These effects are different between substances of this group. Pindolol could be a prototyp with a potent TXA_2 synthesis inhibiting effect due to a relatively potent cyclooxygenase inhibition. Propranolol on the other side has a more potent antagonistic effect on „TXA_2-receptors" than on the TXA_2 synthesis. Practolol seems to be a prototyp of a third group without significant influences on both effects.

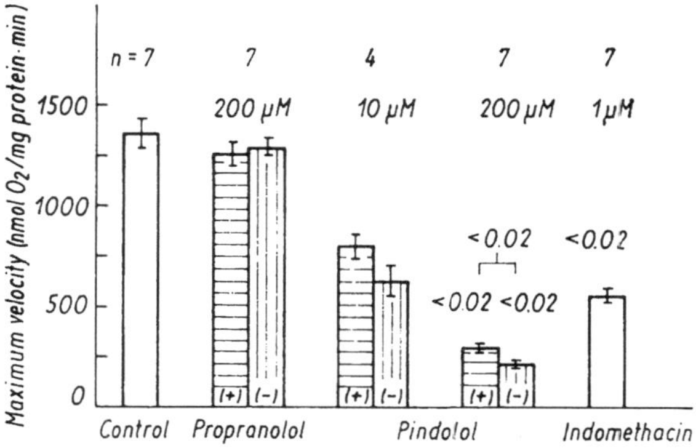

Fig. 4. Influence of propranolol and pindolol isomers on the cyclooxygenase activity of rat seminal vesicle microsomes.

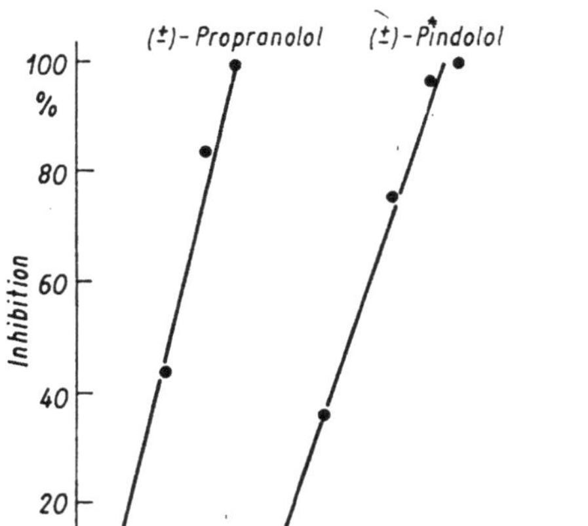

Fig. 5. Dose-effect-curves of (±)-propranolol and (±)-pindolol on the U-46619-induced aggregation in human PRP
(U-46619 = 15(S)hydroxy-11a, 9a-epoxymethanoprosta-5Z, 13E-dienoic acid; concentration of U-46619: 1 µmol/l; n = 6).

Possibly these differences can be correlated with differing membrane stabilizing properties of the β-blocking drugs. The blockade of adrenergic receptors combined with an anti-TXA_2 effect and a PGI_2 enhancement could be a new explanation for the superior effects of β-adrenoceptor blocking drugs in long term trials for a secondary prevention of myocardial infarction [6].

References

[1] CAMPBELL, W. B., K. S. CALLAHAN, A. R. JOHNSON and R. M. GRAHAM: Lancet II (1981), 1382–1384
[2] DURAO, V., and G. T. RICO: Europ. J. Pharmacol. **43** (1977), 377–383
[3] FÖRSTER, W.: Beiträge zur Wirkstofforschung, Heft 6, Institut für Wirkstofforschung, Akademie der Wissenschaften der DDR, Berlin.
[4] LUDERER, J. R., L. DEMERS, R. SCHNAARS, K. MILLER and A. H. HAYES: Clin. Pharmacol. Ther. **29** (1981), 263
[5] LOPEZ-OVEJERO, J. A., M. A. WEBER, J. I. DRAYER, J. E. SEALEY and J. H. LARAGH: Clin. Sci. mol. Med. **55** (1978), 203–207
[6] MAY, G. S., K. A. EBERLEIN, C. D. FURBERG, E. R. PASSAMANI and D. L. DEMETS: Progr. Cardiovas. Dis. **24** (1982), 331–352

Central Institute of Heart and Circulation Research, Academy of Sciences of GDR, Berlin-Buch, GDR

In Vivo Experiments on Phospholipid Metabolism in Rat Heart

B. Schirpke

Phospholipids play an important role in maintaining cardiac structures and biochemical processes. Contrary to more recently paid attention to fatty acid composition — among others Gudbjarnason, Montfoort, this symposium — their metabolism as a whole has not gained adequate inteest. Thus metabolic characteristics are rarely to be found in the literature [1]. To obtain more insight in this subject, a series of experiments was performed on *in vivo* labeling of rat heart lipids, the results of which are outlined in this poster.

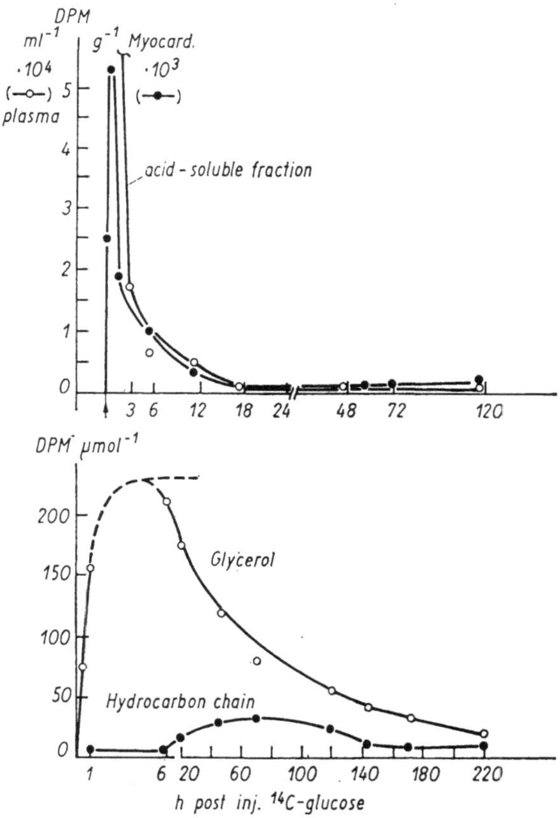

Fig. 1. Time course of radioactivity from ^{14}C-glucose in acid soluble fractions (upper part), and in cardiac phospholipids (lower part).

Following intravenous shot-injection into rats of ^{14}C-glucose and ^{14}C-acetate, degree and time course of radioactivities in neutral and polar lipids of blood plasma as well as neutral fat in myocardium exclude a major role in labeling heart phospholipids. The same is true for glycogen (^{14}C-glucose experiments). Phospholipid synthesis was predominantly supplied with radiocarbon from initially highly labeled "acid-soluble metabolites" in blood plasma, thence in heart muscle. Here, the availability of ^{14}C was restricted to the early 10 to 15 h following tracer injection (Fig. 1, 2 upper halfes), best reflected from the decay of label in the key metabolite diglyceride. The similarity of time courses allows a direct comparison of phospholipid labeling. Incorporation of glucose-^{14}C in the glycerol moity was by fat the most active process (t/2 of ^{14}C invasion 35 min, Fig. 1 lower part). In union with the fast elimination of radiocarbon, this pointed towards a relatively rapid exchange of the carbohydrate backbone (turnover 2 per cent bulk-labeled glycerol · h^{-1}).

Incorporation of acetate-^{14}C in the fatty chains — 85 per cent ester —, 15 per cent ether linkage — exhibited less activity (approached t/2 2.5 h). With the moderate decrease of label (Fig. 2 lower part) it typified a much slower turnover, approximately 0.2 per cent · h^{-1}, but recycling of labeled fatty side chains could not be ruled out.

The decrease of radioactivity in the "primarily" labeled phospholipid constituent seemed to be ocunteracted by an increase in "secondarily" labeled components. With regard to the obvious lack

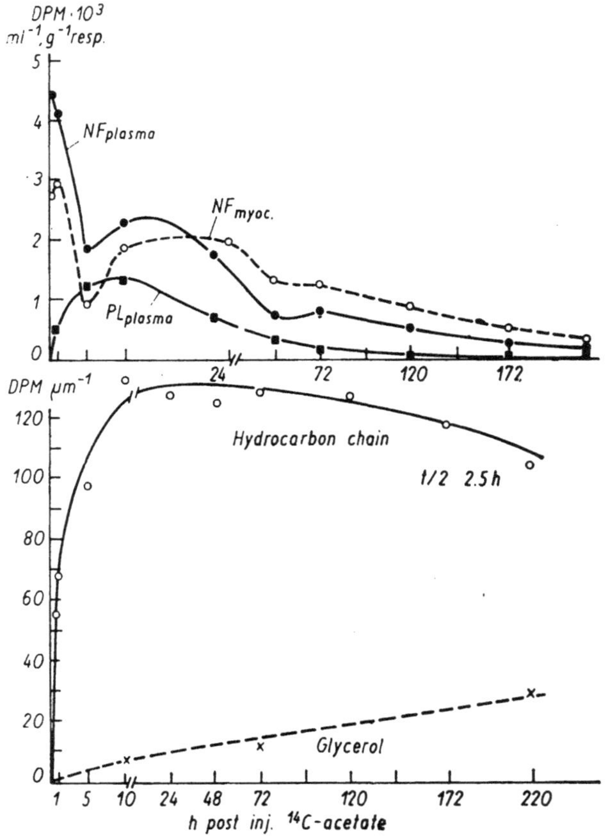

Fig. 2. Time course of radioactivity from ^{14}C-acetate in neutral fat (NF, upper part) and in cardiac phospholipids (lower part).

of other tracerkinetic precursor: substrate relationships, this "intramolecular" shift of ^{14}C is suspicious for a reincorporation of carbon units within a (compartimented) phospholipid breakdown — resynthesis cycle: approximated reutilization of glycerol carbon 40 per cent (72 h), fatty chain carbon 20 per cent (220 h).

The biphasic manner of incorporation of ^{32}P in total phospholipids had to be connected causally to a similar biphasic availability of radiocarbon in P_γ of myocardial ATP (Fig. 3). Moreover, the close parallelism (semilog plot) evidences a relatively unbuffered passage of original P_γ from ATP to the lipid position via the multiple phosphate group exchanges within ATP → CTP transfer and "Kennedy" pathway of phospholipid synthesis (availability = 0→24 h DPM μgatom^{-1} P_γ; increment = DPM $t_2 - t_1$ (24 h) μgatom^{-1} lipid-P).

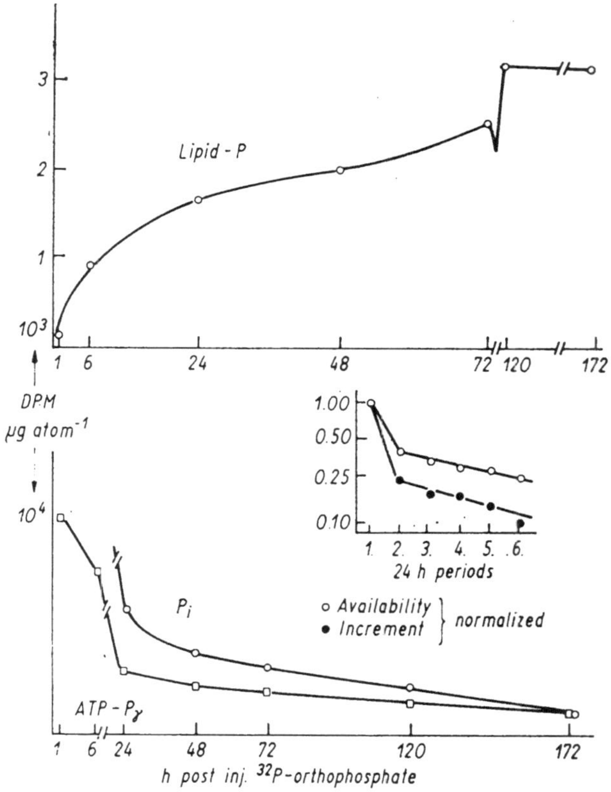

Fig. 3. Progress of ^{32}P incorporation in cardiac phospholipids (upper part); decline of label in P_i and P_γ from ATP in heart muscle (lower part).

Labeling of individual phospholipids is shown in Fig. 4. Movement of bulk radioactivities as the sum of singular processes was predominantly determined by phosphatidyl ethanolamine (PE, 37.5 per cent of total lipid P), phosphatidyl choline (PC, 37 per cent), cardiolipin (CL, 15 per cent) and sphingomyelin (SM, 3.5 per cent). Incorporation of glucose-^{14}C — not discriminated in glycerol and hydrocarbon moities — was rather similar for the main phosphatides PE and PC. In SM the radioactivity decreased readily and was extraordinarily low in CL. With ^{14}C-acetate as precursor labeling next active to PC was observed for SM. It was remarkably low in PE and even less in CL. Incorporation of ^{32}P did not show gross differences between PE and PC. As with tracer glucose a relatively low level of radioactivity was seen in CL and SM. The findings manifest a certain metabolic inertness of the more specifically membrane-sited SM (plasma membrane) and before all CL (mitochondrial membrane). For the latter phospholipid this seems to agree with the relative stability of its fatty acid pattern under a variety of experimental conditions (GUDBJARNASON, personal.communication).

References

[1] KATZ, A. M.: Circul. Res. 48 (1981), 1—16
[2] GUDBJARNASON, S.: Personal communication
[3] MONTFOORT, S.: Personal communication

Medical Clinic and Radiological Clinic of the Karl-Marx-University Leipzig and Central Institute of Isotopes and Radiation Research, Acad. Sci. GDR, Berlin, GDR

Influence of Drugs, Hormones and Ischaemia on Glucose Uptake, CK Release and Energy Potential of Langendorff-Rabbit Hearts

TITLBACH, O., H. MAREK, P. FEYER, L. BÖLKE and R. FIEBER

Glucose-insulin-potassium infusion is difficult to evaluate in respect to its myocardial protective effect. The isolated, retrograde perfused rabbit heart is a suitable model to study different stages of ischaemic damage in dependence on time and in dependence on oxigenation of Tyrode-solution. According to OPIE [2], the infarcted area of the myocardium is not homogenous. In accordance with energy metabolism one can distinguish between central infarct (zone 1), peripheral infarct (zone 2), periinfarct border (zone 3), and nonischaemic myocardium (zone 4). A similar classification has been proposed by JENNINGS [1]. The subject of our interest was the border zone, since myocardial cells of this region can survive at favourable conditions or perish at unfavourable conditions.

Ischaemic damage was induced either by reducing coronary flow to 10% of the normal flow or by interruption of perfusion. In respect to the energy potential this damage corresponds to that of zone 1 and zone 2. Glucose uptake, lactate formation, creatin kinase (CK) release, and energy-rich phosphates have been estimated. Thyroid hormones (T_3, T_4), glucocorticoids, adrenaline, insulin, the β-blockers talinolol and propranolol, and ouabain have been tested to their ability to reduce ischaemic damage. Insulin increased cellular glucose uptake. This effect was more pronounced at low glucose concentration. Thus, at glucose concentration of 0.55 mmol/l, glucose uptake increased from 13.6 μmol/g heart to 28.7 μmol/g heart. CK release was diminished when ischaemic hearts were perfused in presence of 5.55 mmol/l glucose + insulin. T_3 increased glucose uptake by more than 100% at physiological doses. T_4 failed to show this effect. As has to be expected, adrenaline exerted the strongest effect on glucose uptake. On the contrary, talinolol, propranolol and ouabain decreased glucose uptake of myocardial cells.

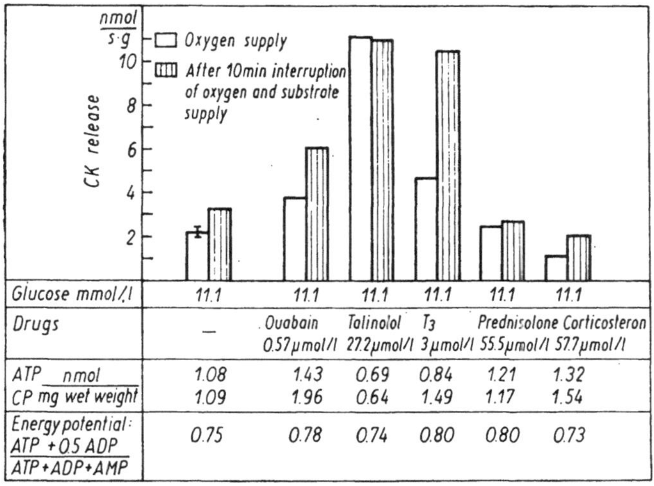

Glucose mmol/l	11.1	11.1	11.1	11.1	11.1	11.1
Drugs	—	Ouabain 0.57 μmol/l	Talinolol 27.2 μmol/l	T_3 3 μmol/l	Prednisolone 55.5 μmol/l	Corticosteron 57.7 μmol/l
ATP nmol/mg wet weight	1.08	1.43	0.69	0.84	1.21	1.32
CP nmol/mg wet weight	1.09	1.96	0.64	1.49	1.17	1.54
Energy potential: $\frac{ATP + 0.5\,ADP}{ATP + ADP + AMP}$	0.75	0.78	0.74	0.80	0.80	0.73

Taking CK release as a basis for myocardial damage, glucose-insulin and glucocorticoids exhibited a beneficial effect on ischaemic damaged but still viable myocardial cells. Increase of glucose uptake per se does not guarantee salvage of ischaemic cells, especially not when the increased glucose uptake is accompanied by an increased lactate accumulation in the myocardium.

References

[1] JENNINGS, R. B. and K. A. REIMER: Amer. J. Pathol. **102** (1981), 241–255
[2] OPIE, L. H. and P. OWEN: Amer. J. Cardiol. **38** (1976), 310–321

Institute of Pathology, Humboldt University, Berlin, GDR

Biochemical and Electron Microscopic Findings on the Myocardium of Trained and Untrained Rats after Infarction

H. BRASELMANN, W. KRAUSE and H. GUSKI

After a moderate swim training the numerical and volume density of heart muscle mitochondria of young rats is elevated (Fig. 1). This may be a reaction to increased physical work [3]. The question arises: What is the significance of these mitochondrial alterations for pathological states of myocardium?

In connection with ischaemic heart disease it is of interest to know the response of mitochondria in non-ischaemic myocardium (close to the ischaemic area) to coronary occlusion.

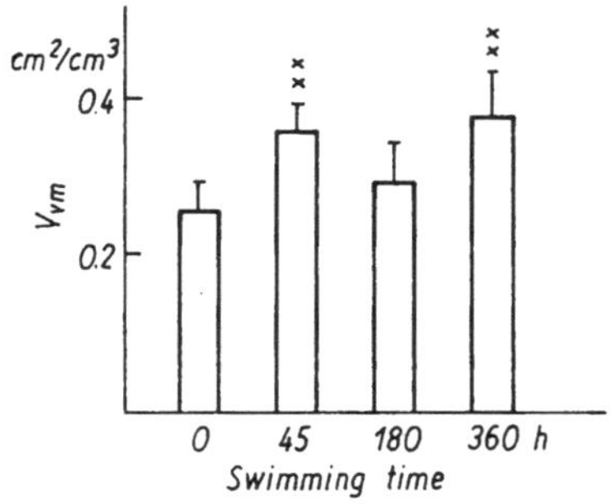

Fig. 1. Volume density (V_{vm}) of heart muscle mitochondria depending on total swimming time of rats [3].

A statistical significance of $p > 99\%$ against the control group (0 h) was indicated by $\overset{x}{x}$

Methods

Male Wistar rats (one month of age) were subjected to a moderate swim training of increasing daily duration (up to 90 minutes/day). At the end of the training period (after 45 h total swimming time) all rats reached an age of 3 month. For the detailed training schedule and the determination of morphometrical data on electron micrographs see [3].

24 h after coronary artery occlusion rats were killed by vertebral luxation. Heart mitochondria of the non-ischaemic area were isolated according to [7]. Determinations of SDH-activity and of respiratory data were carried out according to [8] and[2], respectively. ^{14}C-leucine was incorporated into isolated mitochondria in a medium described by [5]. The reaction was started by addition of 3.7 10^4 Bq ^{14}C-leucine (specific activity 8810 Bq/nmol). Initial values of ^{14}C-leucine incorporation rates into mitochondrial proteins were calculated by assuming zero initiation rate for

peptides. The starting concentration of the prebuilt receptor protein may be z_0, then the rate of ^{14}C-leucine incorporation is

$$dy/dt = k_1(z_0 - y) \quad (1)$$

assuming first order kinetics. The total radioactivity y incorporated after a time t is given by

$$y = z_0 - k_2 \exp(-k_1 t) \quad (2)$$

The first derivative of (2) gives the initial rate $(dy/dt)_0$ of ^{14}C-leucine incorporation by setting $t = 0$ (Fig. 2). Equation 2 was fitted to the experimental points by means of a HP 9825 A computer using least square approximation. The statistical significance of results was calculated by Student's t-test method.

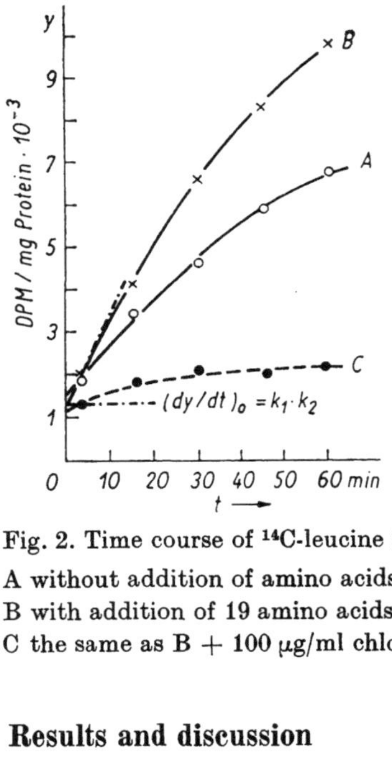

Fig. 2. Time course of ^{14}C-leucine incorporation into mitochondrial proteins.
A without addition of amino acids
B with addition of 19 amino acids (20 μM each, without leucine)
C the same as B + 100 μg/ml chloramphenicol

Results and discussion

After coronary occlusion a significant stimulation of SDH-activity in heart mitochondria of trained and untrained rats was seen (Table 1). The specific SDH-activity in mitochondria of trained rats were significantly lower than in mitochondria of controls (in both cases, sham operated hearts and hearts with coronary occlusion). Nevertheless the total SDH-activity was higher in hearts of trained rats due to the increase of the numerical and volume density of mitochondria compared to control hearts [3]. The behaviour of state 3 respiration was similar to that of SDH-activity. Respiratory control ratios with glutamate as substrate were not significantly different in all groups.

By accepting *in vitro* incorporation of ^{14}C-leucine as reflection of *in vivo* protein synthesis in some way, the lower rate of leucine incorporation into mitochondrial proteins of group IV in relation to group II may be explained by the hypothesis of MEERSON and POMOINITSKY [6], who have stated that decreasing ATP levels might initiate mitochondrial protein synthesis. In hearts of trained rats the decrease of ATP in non-ischaemic myocardium [4] may be lower than in untrained rat hearts due to 1. the higher numerical and volume density of mitochondria, 2. the possibly smaller area of infarction.

Table 1

Biochemical data of rat heart mitochondria

I Untrained group, sham operated
II Untrained group, with coronary occlusion
III Trained group, sham operated
IV Trained group, with coronary occlusion

	SDH¹)	State 3²) respiration	Initial rate of³) ^{14}C-leucine incorporation
I	0.33 ± 0.04 (6)	251 ± 31 (6)	138 ± 24 (7)
II	0.50 ± 0.07 (6)	291 ± 13 (6)	153 ± 30 (6)
III	0.26 ± 0.04 (9)	229 ± 16 (9)	120 ± 34 (9)
IV	0.40 ± 0.06 (7)	271 ± 10 (7)	90 ± 18 (7)

1) μmoles succinate min^{-1} mg^{-1}
2) ng atomes 0 min^{-1} mg^{-1}
3) DPM min^{-1} mg^{-1}
Means ± S.D. are given; (number of animals)

We suppose that a smaller infarction area results in a lower ATP decrease of the non-ischaemic myocardium. The last expectation may also influence the significance of our results owing to the great variability of infarction area after coronary artery occlusion [1].

References

[1] Braselmann, H., U. Osswald, K. Wenzelides and E. Seidler: Experientia **34** (1978), 1478–1479
[2] Buffa, P., I. Pasquali-Ronchetti, A. Barasa and G. Godina: Cell Tiss. Res. **183** (1977), 1–23
[3] Guski, H.: Zelluläre Grundlagen der Adaptation des Myokards. Dissertation (Dr. sc. med.) 1982
[4] Jones, C. E., J. X. Thomas, J. C. Parker and R. E. Parker: Cardiovasc. Res. **10** (1976), 275–282
[5] Kuzela, S., K. Luciakova and J. Lakota: FEBS letters **114** (1980), 197–201
[6] Meerson, F. Z. and V. D. Pomoinitsky: J. Mol. Cell. Cardiol. **4** (1972), 571–597
[7] Sordahl, L. A., H. R. Besch, J. C. Allen, C. Crow, G. E. Lindenmayer and A. Schwartz: Meth. Achievm. exper. Pathol. **5** (1971), 287–346
[8] Wooten, W. L. and J. Cascarano: J. Bioenerg. Biomembr. **12** (1980), 1–12

National Institute of Cardiology, Diagnostic and Research Department, Budapest, Hungary

The Role of Altered Diabetic Coronary Reactivity in Myocardial Ischaemia

G. POGÁTSA and M. Z. KOLTAI

It is well known that in diabetes the risk factors for ischaemic heart diseases consists primarilly of accelerated and severe coronary atherosclerosis, of cardiovascular manifestations of diabetic autonomic neuropathy, and of diabetic microangiopathy in coronary arteries. In 1978 *Dandona* et al. demonstrated an altered vascular reactivity in diabetic cerebral arteries. Therefore it seemed worth to elucidate whether does any alteration exist in coronary reactivity during diabetes, and its possible role in ischaemic heart diseases.

Methods

Diabetes was induced in mongrel dogs of both sexes, 2–3 years of age by 560 mmol/kg alloxan tetrahydrate iv. Plasma glucose [1] and urea nitrogen [2], plasma disappearance rate of glucose [3], body weight and glucose [1] as well as acetone [4] content of urine collected over 24 hours were determined at the beginning and during the observation at least once weekly. Hemodynamic investigations were carried out 3 months after the induction of diabetes under pentobarbital (133 μmol/kg) narcosis. In 12 animals cardiac plexus was stimulated by a Disa stimulator 13G04 with 5 minutes long trains of square pulses of 1 ms duration, 8 volt amplitude and increasing frequency. Arterial blood pressure was recorded in the thoracic aorta with a Statham gauge p23Db and blood flow of left anterior descending coronary artery was measured by an electromagnetic flowmeter (Statham SP 2202). In further 53 animals the following groups were performed: 1. control, norepinephrine 2 hours after coronary exploration (n = 6). 2. control, saline 2 hours after coronary ligation (n = 6), 3. control, norepinephrine 2 hours after coronary ligation (n = 6), 4. control, norepinephrine 48 hours after coronary ligation (n = 6), 5. diabetic, norepinephrine 2 hours after coronary exploration (n = 11), 6. diabetic, saline 2 hours after coronary ligation (n = 6), 7. diabetic, norepinephrine 2 hours after coronary ligation (n = 6) and 8. diabetic, norepinephrine 48 hours after coronary ligation (n = 6). Ligations or explorations were performed always just proximal to the first major oblique branch of left descending coronary artery. Norepinephrine was infused in 3 ml/kg saline for 10 minutes at a rate of 6 nmol/kg iv. Immediatelly before and 30 minutes after completion of infusion cardiac output was measured by thermodilution method [5], left ventricular end-diastolic and arterial carotid blood pressure by a Statham gauge p23Db, and left ventricular passive elastic modulus – characteristic of global diastolic wall stiffness – by the modified [6] method of DIAMOND and FORRESTER [7]. Left ventricular tissue thiocyanate space – characteristic of extracellular water content – was measured by the modified [8] method of CRANDALL and ANDERSON [9], and the size of necrotic myocardial area was determined in the groups studied 48 hours after coronary ligation at the end of the experiment.

Results

Alloxan caused a clinically manifested diabetes but without ketosis (Fig. 1). Sympathetic stimulation of the cardiac plexus induces vasoconstriction in diabetic coronary arteries, while it evokes vasodilatation in metabolically healthy ones (Fig. 2). Accordingly the vascular reactivity in diabetic coronary arteries is altered.

A previous experiment [6] demonstrated that myocardial water content augments significantly in the para-ischaemic zone when 60 nmol/kg norepinephrine was infused during a 10 minutes long period, 2 or 48 hours after the ligation of left anterior descending coronary artery just proximal to its first major oblique branch, and it was suggested that this myocardial edema is a consequence of enhanced collateral blood flow. The present experiment confirms that myocardial water content

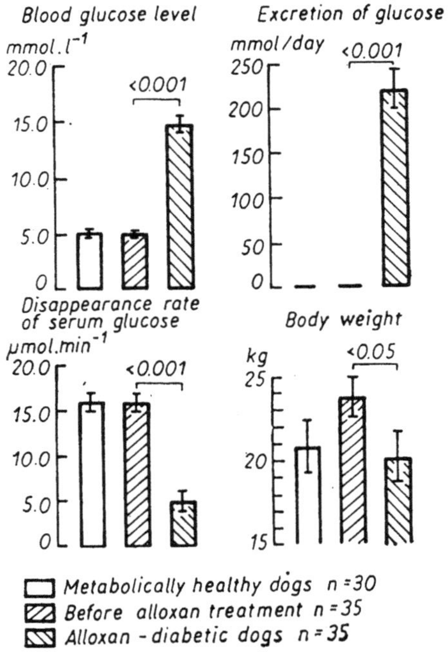

Fig. 1. Metabolic variables of the experimental groups.

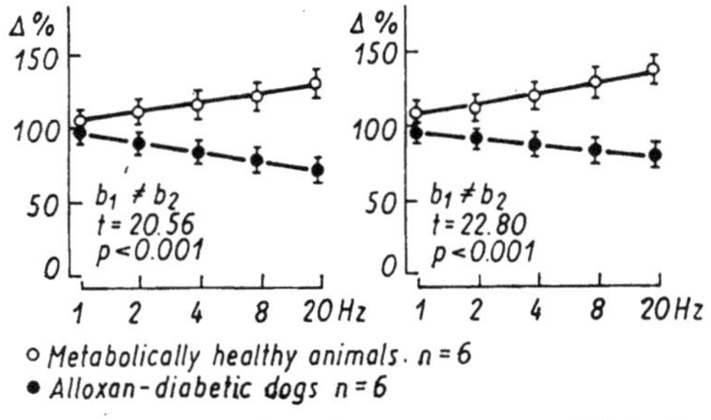

Fig. 2. Conductivity of coronary arterial bed under the electrical stimulation of the cardiac plexus in alloxan-diabetic dogs.

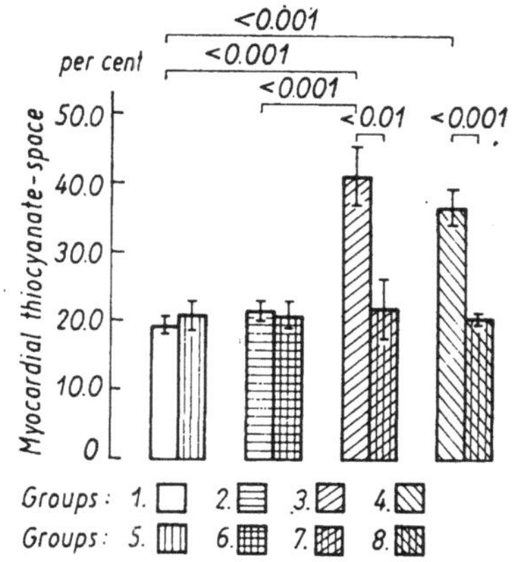

Fig. 3. Myocardial thiocyanate-space in left ventricular wall.

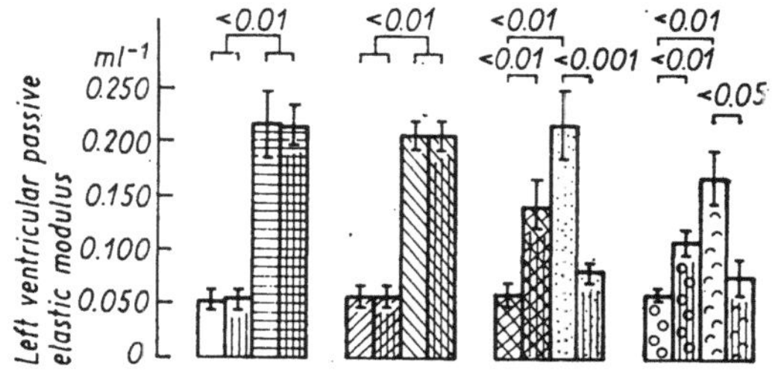

Fig. 4. Diastolic stiffness of the left ventricular wall.
Symbols: see Fig. 3

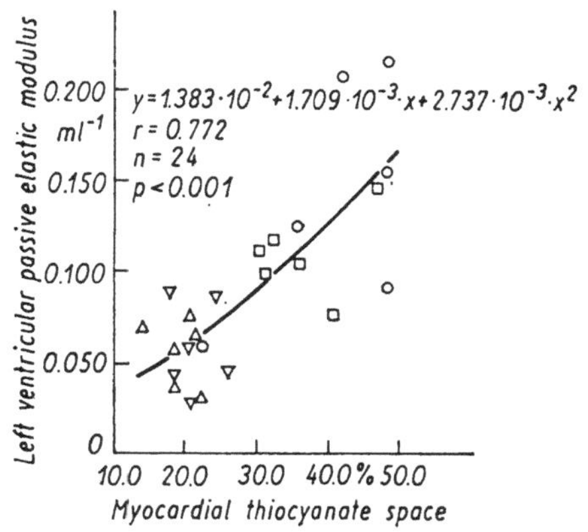

Fig. 5. Correlation between diastolic stiffness and myocardial edema in left ventricular wall.
Groups: 3 △ 4 ▽ 7 ○ 8 □

increases in the nonischaemic part of ventricular wall only in the metabolically healthy animals, when norepinephrine is administered 2 or 48 hours after coronary ligation. In alloxan diabetic animals myocardial edema does not develop under such circumstances. (Fig. 3). Left ventricular diastolic stiffness, characterised by the values of passive elastic modulus, enhances in metabolically healthy animals parallely to the development of myocardial edema. In diabetic dogs left

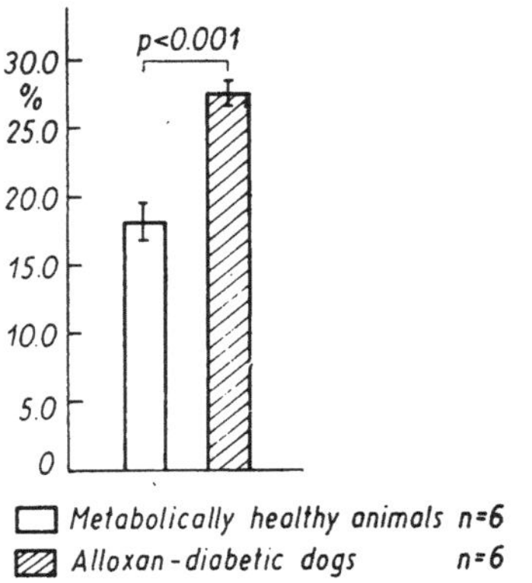

Fig. 6. Size of necrotic area related to the total myocardium of left ventricle.

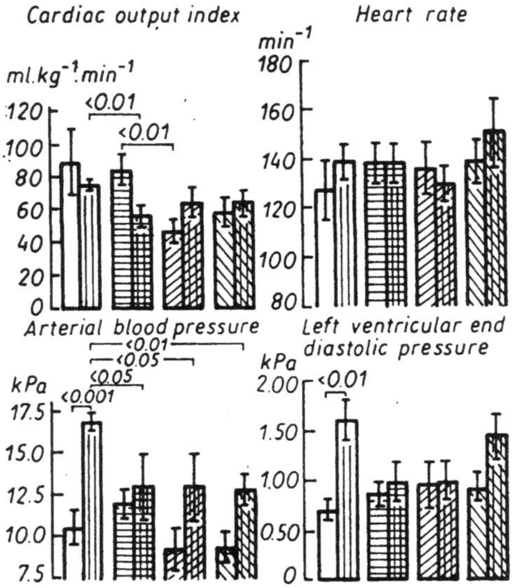

Fig. 7. Haemodynamic variables of the experimental groups.

ventricular diastolic stiffness is originally enhanced, and it decreases when norepinephrine is administered 2 or 48 hours after coronary ligation (Fig. 4, 5). It is well known that diastolic stiffness of ischaemic myocardium decreases at first [10]. Accordingly, the decrease of passive elastic modulus suggest extended infarcted myocardial zone in diabetes. Indeed, the macroscopic findings confirmed this suggestion (Fig. 6). Cardiac output index decreases by norepinephrine administered 2 or 48 hours after coronary ligation only in metabolically healthy animals. In diabetics cardiac output index is originally lower than in healthy ones but it is not influenced by coronary ligation or norepinephrine administration (Fig. 7).

Discussion and conclusion

Vascular reactivity is altered in diabetes in the coronary arteries, too. Altered diabetic coronary reactivity aggrevates necrosis in the infarcted part and it hinders the development of myocardial edema in the non-ischaemic part of myocardium. The observations have clinical importance because the dosage of norepinephrine used is similar to the pathophysiological one released under stress conditions caused by the pain of infarction. In addition the study draws attention to the possibility that not only macroangiopathy, or microangiopathy or cardiovascular manifestations of diabetic neuropathy but altered vascular reactivity may be responsible for the increased incidence and more severe course of ischaemic heart diseases in diabetics.

References

[1] Hyvärinen, A. and E. A. Nikkilä: Clin. Chem. Acta 7 (1962), 140–143
[2] Coulombe, J. J. and L. Favreau: Clin. Chem. 9 (1963), 102–108
[3] Conard, V., J. R. M. Franckson, P. A. Bastenie, J. Kestens and L. Kovács: Arch. Int. Pharmacodyn., **93** (1953), 277–292
[4] Neuweiler, W.: Klin. Wschr. **12** (1933), 869–980
[5] Fegler, G.: Quart. J. Exp. Physiol. **39** (1954), 153–164
[6] Pogátsa, G., E. Dubecz, S. Juhász-Nagy, I. Kolonics and Gy. Gábor: Acta Med. Acad. Sci. Hung. **34** (1977), 71–79
[7] Diamond, G. and J. S. Forrester: Circulation **45** (1972), 11–19
[8] Dubecz, E., S. Juhász-Nagy, G. Pogátsa and Gy. Gábor: J. Res. Comm. Sci. Med. Sci. **3** (1975), 285
[9] Crandall, L. A. jr. and M. X. Anderson: Amer. J. Digest. Dis. Nutr. **1** (1934), 126–131
[10] Nieminen, M. and J. Heikkilä: Brit. Heart. J. **38** (1976), 271–281

Departments of Biochemistry[1] and of Internal Medicine[2], Humboldt-University, Berlin, GDR

Enzyme Pattern in Endomyocardial Biopsies

I. LEHMANN[1], R. A. PARSI[2], B. PAPIES[1], E. LUDWIG[2], M. L. KÖNIG[1], M. NAGI[1] and C. WAGENKNECHT[1]

Introduction

In previous investigations by our group changes in the isoenzyme activities of lactate dehydrogenase (LDH) and aspartate aminotransferase (ASAT) in the blood plasma of patients with chronic ischaemia heart disease (IHD) were found [7, 11]. The purpose of the present investigation was, to test if and to what extent the data obtained in plasma reflect the enzyme activities in the myocardium, to look for alterations in enzyme activities of other main metabolic pathways (glycogenolysis, respiration chain) and to elaborate methods for the homogenization of minute tissue samples, and methods sensitive enough for the measurement of enzyme and isoenzyme activities.

Material and methods

We investigated endomyocardial biopsies from 10 patients with IHD (8 male, 2 female, age 26–55 yr) and 8 patients without pathomorphological alterations (4 male, 4 female, age 25–43 yr). Biopsies were taken from the left ventricle near the apex of the heart using a newly developed technique [8]. The wet weight of the samples was 0.25–1.76 mg (9 samples less than 1 mg). The samples were homogenized in a special Potter homogenizer. The homogenizing media were 200 to 400 μl 0.025 M TRA-buffer/0.07 M NaCl/0.0025 M EDTA (pH 7.6) for LDH, ASAT and succinic cytochrome c reductase and 0.005 M Na-β-glycerophosphate/0.015 M mercaptoethanol/0.001 M EDTA (pH 6.1) for glycogen-phosphorylase. The isoenzymes were differentiated by kinetic methods [3,4], succ.-cyt. c-red. was analyzed according to RAPOPORT [9], glycogen-phosphorylase according to CORI and ILLINGWORTH [2].

Results

The investigated enzyme activities in the endomyocardial biopsies of patients with IHD differed significantly from those of patients without pathomorphological signs of IHD. In the group of patients with IHD the activities of LDH and LDH-H were significantly decreased ($p < 0.05$). The lower ratio of LDH-H/LDH-M in this group indicates an elevated proportion of LDH-M in the total activity (Fig. 1). The total activity of ASAT and the activity of the mitochondrial isoenzyme were significantly decreased ($p < 0.05$) in the group of patients with IHD (Fig. 2). The difference in the activity of succinic cytochrome c reductase between both groups could not be verified statistically (Fig. 3). The activity of glycogen phosphorylase is significantly increased ($p < 0.05$) in the group of patients with IHD (Fig. 3).

Discussion

The decreased activities of LDH and LDH-H, ASAT and mitochondrial ASAT and of succinic cytochrome c reductase may be a result of a rarification of specific myocardial tissue, associated with an increased proportion of fibrous material, of an alteration of membrane permeability or of

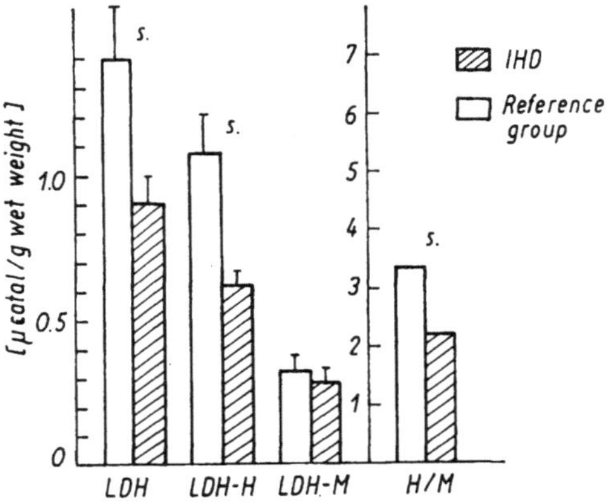

Fig. 1. Activity of LDH isoenzymes.

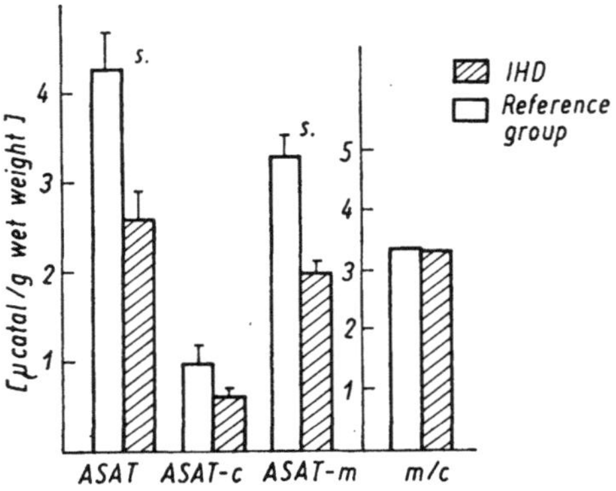

Fig. 2. Activity of ASAT isoenzymes.

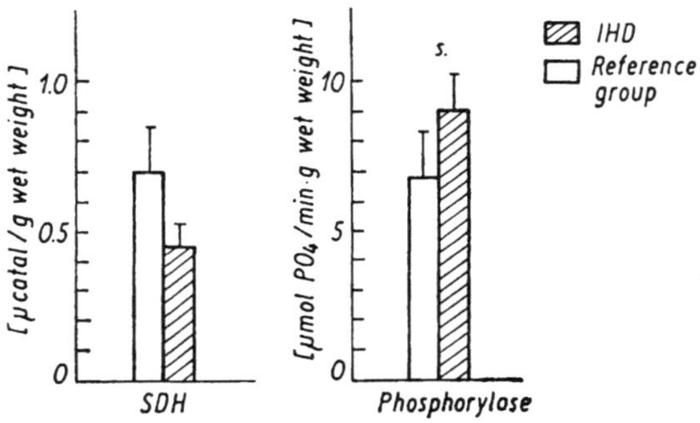

Fig. 3. Activities of succinic-cytochrome reductase and glycogen phosphorylase.

a decreased rate of protein synthesis due to a lack of energy-rich phosphates. The elevated proportion of LDH-M in the total activity suggests an increased synthesis of M-subunits. This is in accordance with results obtained in the myocardium under chronic hypoxic conditions [1] and in myocardial samples of patients with IHD taken during cardiac surgery [5] or by autopsy [10]. The increased activity of glycogen phosphorylase is in agreement with postmortal investigations in which an endoepicardial gradient for glycogen phosphorylase and glycogen in various species was found [6]. The higher activity of glycogen phosphorylase and glycogenconcentration in the endocardium are regarded as an adaption to lower vascularization and hence a larger dependence on anaerobic energy production [6].

References

[1] BALLO, I. M. and I. V. MESSER: Biochem. Biophys. Res. Commun. **33** (1968), 487–491
[2] CORI, G. T. and B. ILLINGWORTH: Biochem. Biophys. Acta **21** (1956), 105–110
[3] GRAUBAUM, H. J., H. FRIEDEMANN, B. NACK, C. WAGENKNECHT, J. ZINSMEYER and E. EGGER: Zbl. Pharm. **111** (1972), 917–931
[4] GRAUBAUM, H. J., K. EHRENBERG and C. WAGENKNECHT: Acta biol. med. germ. **32** (1974), 293–297
[5] HAMMOND, G. L., B. NADAL-GINARD, N. S. TALNER and C. L. MARKERT: Circulation **53** (1976), 637–643
[6] JEDEIKIN, L. A.: Circul. Res. **14** (1964), 202–211
[7] KOTHE, K., P. ROMANIUK, R. NUSSBAUM, I. LEHMANN, M. BÖHM, R. A. PARSI, W. PORSTMANN and C. WAGENKNECHT: Dt. Gesundh.-wesen **34** (1979), 1112–1115
[8] PARSI, R. A., E. LUDWIG and H. J. PECH: Dt. Gesundh.-wesen **36** (1981), 1097–1099
[9] RAPOPORT, S. and Ch. NIERADT: Hoppe-Seyler's Zeitschr. Physiol. Chemie **302** (1955), 156–160
[10] SCHMECHTA, M. and B. KOPETZ: Dt. Gesundh.-wesen **31** (1976), 2075–2078
[11] WAGENKNECHT, C., M. BÖHM, R. A. PARSI, K. KOTHE, I. BLÄTTERLEIN and I. LEHMANN: Dt. Gesundh.-wesen **31** (1976), 2075–2078

Central Institute of Occupational Medicine, Dept. Work Physiology, and Physiol. Institute of the Humboldt University, Dept. Cardiovascular Physiology, 1040 Berlin, GDR

Action of Free Fatty Acids on Contractility and Action Potential of the Heart

G. CAFFIER and R. M. KRÜNES

Introduction

Free fatty acids (FFA) are the preferred substrates for energy production of the myocardium. On the other hand, it has been shown that the force of contraction of isolated heart and skeletal muscle is decreased by FFA [2, 4, 5]. In the present experiments the effect of a selected fatty acid salt, Na-octanoate, on the contractile properties and action potential of isolated rat papillary muscles has been studied to find out some details about the mechanism of action of FFA on the heart.

Methods

Na-octanoate (Ferak) in a concentration of 0.5 mM was added to O_2-bubbled Tyrode solution (140 mM NaCl, 2.7 mM KCl, 1.8 mM $CaCl_2$, 0.5 mM $MgCl_2$, 10 mM Tris-HCl, pH 7.3, 2 g/l glucose, temperature 32 °C) and allowed to act on isolated rat papillary muscles for 1—15 min. The muscles were stimulated electrically by twice threshold square wave pulses of 1 ms duration with a frequency of 0.5 Hz. Extra pulses were interpolated with an interstimulus interval of 400 or 500 ms. Isometric contractions were measured by means of strain gauges. Intracellular glass microelectrodes were used for simultaneous registration of the action potentials. The diastolic tension of the muscles was fixed at 5 mN.

Results

Na-octanoate (0.5 mM) decreased the peak tension, the time to peak tension, and the half relaxation time of the isometric twitch of isolated rat papillary muscles. The effect increased with the time of exposure in octanoate-containing solution. Extra contractions changed in a similar way. When force-velocity curves were constructed from tension and differentiated tension records (c.f. [3]), the curves of octanoate-exposed muscles showed an increase in slope due to the octanoate-induced decrease of contractile tension. V_{max}-values obtained by extrapolating the curves to zero load were not affected.

Postextrasystolic potentiation (PEP) after paired pulse stimulated was more pronounced in fatty acid-exposed muscles. The ability to show restitution of contraction between the beats (R) decreased. The adjustment of a new steady state of contraction lasted longer but there was no significant difference in the time to reach half steady state values of PEP and R.

Action potentials (AP) were shortened by octanoate. The area at 50% repolarization was clearly reduced. The changes were more pronounced in the extrasystolic AP.

Discussion

The depressive effect of Na-octanoate on heart muscle contraction may be due to an alteration of [1] the amount of Ca^{2+} available for contractile activation, [2] the function of the contractile elements, and [3] the supply of sufficient chemical energy from the cellular metabolism.

An alteration of the metabolism cannot be excluded by our experiments. A restriction of metabolic energy, however, should prolong the relaxation time of a twitch. Our experiments do not prove such an assumption. Moreover, the increase in force by paired pulse stimulation requires that a sufficient amount of ATP must be available for contractions.

The functional state of the contractile element can be evaluated by determining its ability to shorten with maximum speed at zero lead, i.e. V_{max} [6]. Since V_{max} is not changed by octanoate, the contractile element should not be altered directly.

It is concluded that Na-octanoate effects the excitation-contraction coupling of the heart muscle cell. The slower restitution and the longer time for adjustment of a new steady state of contraction after paired pulse stimulation suggest a reduced release of Ca^{2+} and/or a smaller replenishment of the stores of activator calcium. The changes of AP may contribute to these effects. The hypothesis is supported by findings on skeletal muscle where the octanoate-induced changes of contraction indicate a reduced release of Ca^{2+} from cellular stores [1].

References

[1] CAFFIER, G., F. KÖSSLER, E. RANSCH and G. KÜCHLER: Acta biol. med. germ. **41** (1982), 205–213

[2] HENDERSON, A. H., R. J. CRAIG, R. GORLIN and E. H. SONNENBLICK: Cardiovasc. Res. **4** (1970), 466–472

[3] KÖHLER, E.: Verh. dt. Ges. Kreislaufforsch. **39** (1973), 144–151

[4] KÖSSLER, F., G. CAFFIER u. G. KÜCHLER: Acta biol. med. germ. **35** (1976), 1327–1334

[5] OPIE, L. H.: Nature (Lond.) **227** (1970), 1055–1056

[6] SONNENBLICK, E. H.: Fed. Proc. Suppl. **21** (1962), 975–990

Julius Bernstein Institute of Physiology, Halle (Saale), GDR

The Influence of Ca^{2+} and Passive Tension on Relaxation Phenomena in the Mammalian Myocardium

M. Wussling and G. Szymanski

Relaxation in the ventricular mammalian myocardium with an effective calcium sequestering system was shown to be load-dependent ([1], load clamp analysis). Load dependent relaxation can be converted into load-insensitive relaxation by retardation of the calcium sequestration, e.g. under the influence of caffeine [2, 3]. — We have proposed a relaxation model in 1980 [4] which is based on two Ca sequestration processes in the myocardial cell. The model was used for the analysis of diastolic oscillations (isometric aftercontractions) observable at low temperature and increased Ca concentration in the bathing solution. The question arises whether or not relaxation is governed by loading conditions at low temperature.

We investigated diastolic oscillations of r.v. rabbit papillary muscles superfused (a) with Krebs-Henseleit-solution (KHS) containing 2.5 mM Ca^{2+} and (b) with KHS containing 5 mM Ca^{2+} and 10^{-5} M noradrenaline (NA), both solutions at 15 °C, in dependence upon the preparation length. Approximations of relaxation time courses by the model [4] allowed to determine relaxation parameters, e.g. the oscillation period T_0 and the damping ratio D.

Contraction as well as relaxation show a very similar hysteresis-like dependence on the preparation length (Fig. 1). It is assumed that the degree of relaxation (e.g. after a rest of 6 sec) is determined by the number of detached cross bridges available within each overlap zone of thick and

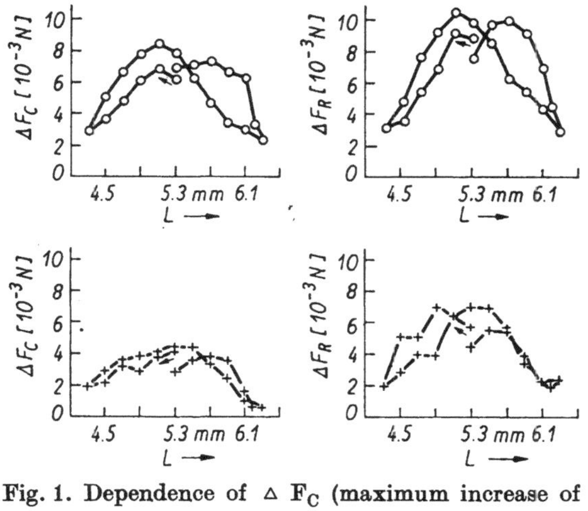

Fig. 1. Dependence of ΔF_C (maximum increase of force during contraction) and ΔF_R (decrease of force during 6 sec relaxation) upon preparation length.
circles: 2.5 mM Ca^{2+}
crosses: 5 mM Ca^{2+}, 10^{-5} M NA

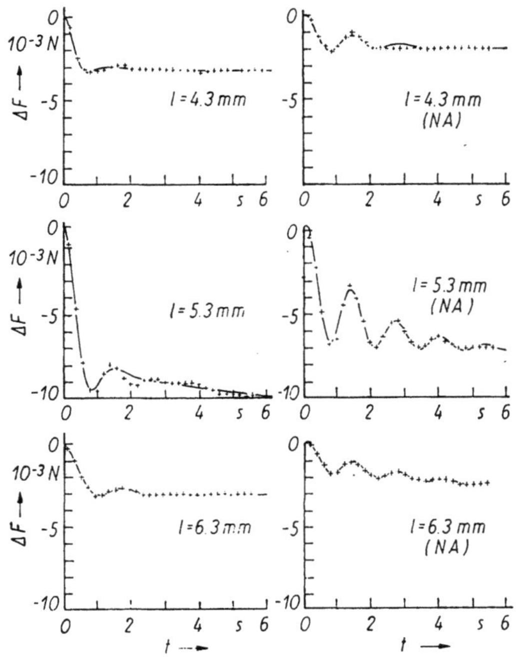

Fig. 2. Influence of preparation length on relaxation.
left: 2.5 mM Ca^{2+}
right: 5 mM Ca^{2+}, 10^{-5} M NA

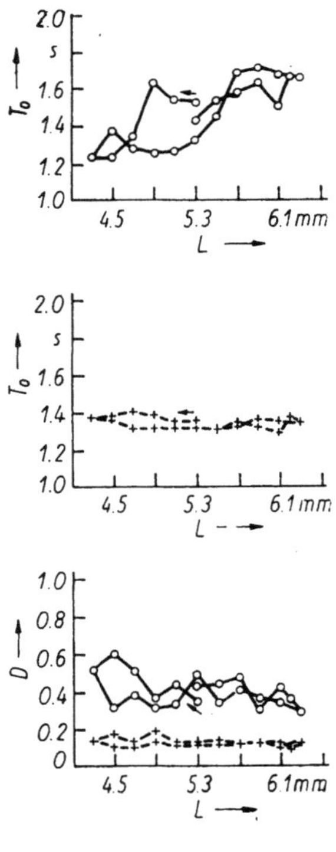

Fig. 3. Dependence of oscillation period T_0 and damping ratio D upon preparation length.
circles: 2.5 mM Ca^{2+}
crosses: 5 mM Ca^{2+}, 10^{-5} M NA

thin filaments. Although load dependence of relaxation was not tested by imposing a sudden change of mechanical conditions in our experiments, we observed a little change of the diastolic oscillation parameters in dependence upon the preparation length thus reflecting load (preload) dependence of relaxation at 15 °C (Fig. 2 and Fig. 3). The influence of NA and increased extracellular calcium concentration leads to a striking change of the relaxation parameters but not to a more evident load dependence (Fig. 3).

It is concluded that inactivation dependence of relaxation is predominant at low temperature compared with load dependence of relaxation.

Acknowledgments

The authors are grateful to Dr. G. Koester for kindly permitting the use of his calculator-programmes which allowed the approximations of oscillation time courses.

References

[1] Brutsaert, D. L., P. R. Housmans and M. A. Goethals: Circulation Res. **47** (1980), 637–652
[2] Hoerter, J., F. Mazet and G. Vassort: J. Mol. Cell. Cardiol. **13** (1981), 725–740
[3] Lecarpentier, Y. C., L. H. S. Chuck, P. R. Housmans, N. M. de Clerck and D. L. Brutsaert: Am. J. Physiol. **237** (1979), H 455–H 460
[4] Wussling, M. and G. Szymanski: Acta biol. med. germ. **39** (1980), 583–590

Institute of Physiology, Humboldt-University of Berlin, Berlin, GDR

Lipid-Diet Induced Changes of the Ca Regulation in the Rabbit Myocardium

J. GÜNTHER, E. STORCH, E. KUTSCHERSKIJ and R. VETTER

A diet containing cholesterol and unsaturated fatty acids can modify electro-mechanical coupling [1, 3, 6, 7, 8, 10, 12]. The development of tension produced by different stimulation patterns shows a time dependence of Ca supply for the activation (Fig. 1). The effectiveness of different stimulation patterns for the development of tension in left ventricular trabeculae of rabbit hearts was investigated with external Ca concentrations (Ca_e) of 1.25 and 2.5 mM. The experiments were carried out on rabbits fed for 12 weeks with a cholesterol-oil diet (ChOD) and on a control group (CG). Similar experiments performed on right ventricular papillary muscles after a rape oil diet (ROD) should show the influence of unsaturated fatty acids only (for methodical details see [4, 5].

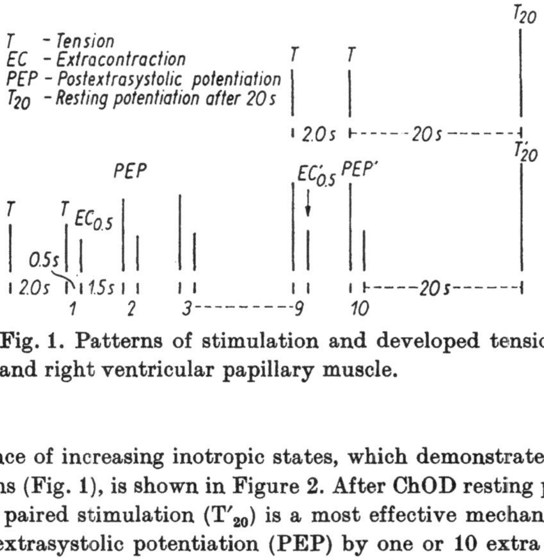

Fig. 1. Patterns of stimulation and developed tension of leftventricular trabeculae and right ventricular papillary muscle.

The sequence of increasing inotropic states, which demonstrate the effectiveness of the stimulation patterns (Fig. 1), is shown in Figure 2. After ChOD resting potentiation following rhythmical (T_{20}) and paired stimulation (T'_{20}) is a most effective mechanism for the enhancement of Ca release. Postextrasystolic potentiation (PEP) by one or 10 extra stimuli (PEP′) is less effective than in CG. Interpolated extra contractions (EC) after one or 10 extra stimuli (EC′) are relatively small exhibiting a delay in the supply of releasable Ca. In contrast to CG the difference of the inotropic states at 1.25 and 2.5 mM Ca_e (columns with slanted lines) after ChOD increasses systematically with the enhancement of Ca release.

In ChOD the mean value of the maximum rate of development and decline of tension ◑ dT/dt_{max} correlates strongly linear with the mean values of tension development in the different inotropic states. In CG these correlations are fitted better by exponential functions.

High values of T_{20} and T'_{20} after ChOD point to a high Ca accumulating ability of the SR as seen for isolated microsomes [7]. Concerning the linear relationship between tension and $\pm dT/$

dt_{max} only one structure, i.e. the SR should determine these parameters. It is assumed that Ca_e after ChOD mainly influences the time dependent Ca supply out of one source, probably the SR too. In CG the influence of Ca_e might be more complex, involving the effects on the time dependence of sarcolemmal Ca entry as well as on the time dependent Ca supply by the SR [13]. After ChOD PEP is small if the Ca loading effect of the Ca entry during the action potential (AP) accompanying the preceding EC contributes less to the PEP [9].

ROD during 12 weeks has a similar effect on PEP as ChOD. Therefore PEP is smaller than in CG (Fig. 3). A maximum PEP is caused by EC with a shorter interval between the rhythmical developed tension T and EC.

The restitution of T is described by increasing EC within the 2-s-interval (Fig. 1). This process is delayed after ROD. The Ca loading effect of the transsarcolemmal Ca influx during the AP accompanying EC is low as after ChOD. This could be connected with a shorter refractory period of AP accompanying T after ROD [5].

Increasing Ca_e between 0.5 and 4.0 mM has a smaller effect on the transsarcolemmal Ca influx during extrasystolic AP measured by the Ca_e dependence of maximum PEP. On the other hand

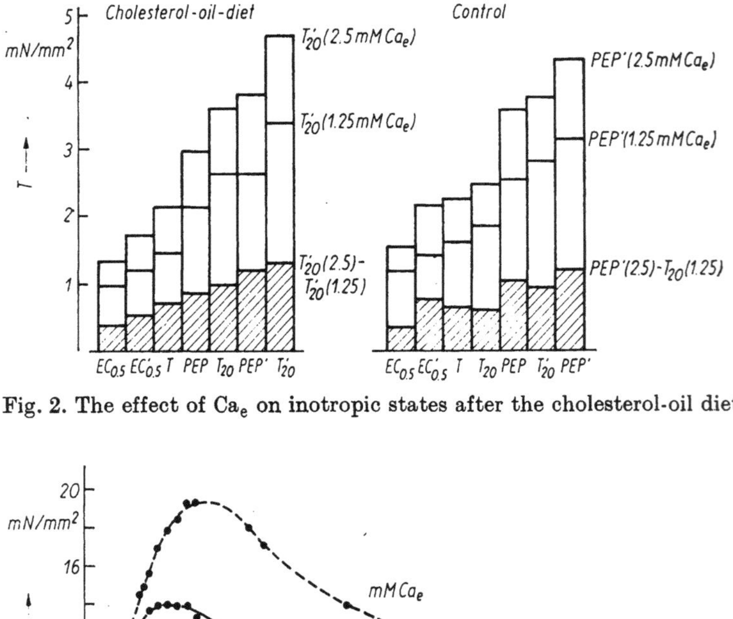

Fig. 2. The effect of Ca_e on inotropic states after the cholesterol-oil diet.

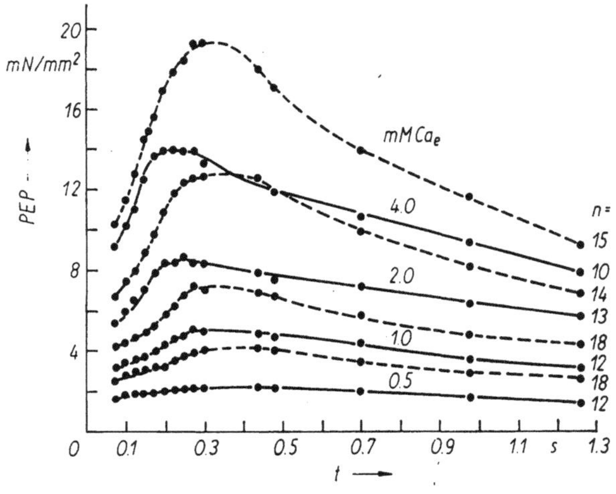

Fig. 3. The effect of Ca_e on the postextrasystolic potentiation PEP after the rape oil diet (———) and in the control group (- - - -) at different time intervals between T and EC.

a higher rate in isometric contraction as well as in relaxation and enhanced resting potentiation point to a more pronounced involvement of SR in Ca regulation [5]. The delay in the restitution of the contractility is similar to its shape in rat myocardium with a more developed SR [2]. The results show that some of the observed alterations of Ca regulation induced by ChOD are attributed to the administration of unsaturated fatty acids as a component of ROD. These alterations in the SR function are in agreement with the high stimulating effect of unsaturated fatty acids on the Ca-ATPase [11].

References

[1] DHALLA, N. S., P. K. DAS and G. P. SHARMA: J. Mol. Cell. Cardiol. **10** (1978), 363–385
[2] GÜNTHER, J., R. KRÜNES, E. KUTSCHERSKIJ, W. SCHOLZ, E. STORCH and R. VETTER: 5. Gemeinschaftstagung der Gesellschaft f. experimentelle Medizin der DDR, Berlin 16. –19. 11. 1981, Kurzreferate Teil 1, V 19
[3] GÜNTHER, J. and E. KUTSCHERSKIJ: Adv. in Myocardiol. **3** (1982), 329–334
[4] GÜNTHER, J., E. KUTSCHERSKIJ, E. STORCH and R. VETTER: Acta biol. med. germ. **41** (1982), 325–331
[5] GÜNTHER, J., E. STORCH and R. VETTER: Acta biol. med. germ. **41** (1982), 333–339
[6] GÜNTHER, J., E. SCHUBERT and E. STORCH: Adv. Myocardiol. **3** (1982), 417–424
[7] GÜNTHER, J. and H. WILL: Acta biol. med. germ. **38** (1979), 1467–1472
[8] INNIS, S. M. and M. T. CLANDININ: Biochem. J. **193** (1981), 155–167
[9] JOHANNSSON, M. and B. WOHLFAHRT: Acta Physiol. Scand. **110** (1980), 241–247
[10] KATZ, A. M. and F. C. MESSINEO: Circulation Res. **48** (1981), 1–16
[11] KORRENBROT, J. I.: Ann. Rev. Physiol. **39** (1977), 19–49
[12] SENGES, I., E. WEIHE, I. BRACHMANN, D. PELZER, H. NIMMRICH and W. KÜBLER: J. Mol. Cell. Cardiol. **13** (1981), 253–264
[13] WOHLFART, B.: Acta Physiol. Scand. **106** (1979), 395–409

Central Institute of Heart and Circulation Research Berlin and Central Institute of Microbiology and Experimental Therapy Jena, Academy of Sciences, GDR

Appearances of Metabolically Influenced Long-term Vasotonus Changes in Coronary Microvessels of Rats

HERRMANN, H.-J., V. MORITZ, T. HECHT, C. NORDEN and P. MÜHLIG

The long term effects of metabolic factors on tonus and structure of coronary microvessels (b.v.) are unknown. Insights into these effects and their susceptibility to vasotonic influences offer a key to a proper understanding of coronary insufficiency and its prevention.

Material and methods

92 1, 2, 3, 4, 6, or 12 month-old male spontaneously hypertensive rats (SHR) and 60 age- and sex-matched normotensive Wistar control rats (NWR) were investigated. Moreover 12 NWR were exercised by tread-mill 3 hours daily for 6 months. After the daily training 6 NWR were stressed by electric foot-shock.

Histomorphometric measurements of changes of wall thickness as morphological correlatives of long-term vasotonus changes in b.v. were made by means of a new morphometric and preparative method using the automatic image analyzing system QUANTIMET (QTM). Changes of wall thickness were detected by significantly changed b.v. number (N) in 3 classes and by changes of wall area (A). Differences in the histochemical development of the reaction product of the LDH- and SDH reaction were detected by measuring areas of heart muscle tissue of a definite gray-level by means of the QTM. Statistical testing by a 2-factorial analysis of variance and Student's t-test. For details s. HERRMANN et al. [1, 2].

Results

Histomorphometric b.v. measurements (Fig. 1) prove morphological appearances of an increased long-term vasotonus of coronary b.v.$_{d<10.5\mu m}$ in the pre-stage of spontaneous hypertension (SH) and their return to signs of long-term vasotonus decrease of b.v.$_{d<21\mu m}$ in the acute phase of SH (2nd-4th month). This phase shows a strong rise of systolic blood pressure (BP) and relative heart weight as well as an increase of heart muscle area with high concentration of LDH-reaction-product in 1-month-old SHR. A further activation of myocardial activity induced by loads of repeated BP measurements from the 1st to the 3rd month, results in a spread of vasotonus decrease in larger b.v. The increase of wall thickness in larger arterioles ($d > 21$ μm) of rats which were not repeatedly measured and in 4-month-old animals demonstrates for the acute phase of SH a concomitant activation of tonic factors in coronary b.v. In b.v. of skeletal muscles the morphologic characteristics of long-term increase of contractile vasotonus of the pre-stage persist (in preparation). After the attenuated rise of myocardial activity (smaller elevation of systolic BP and relative heart weight, insignificant difference of LDH-reaction) beginning with the 4th month the signs of coronary long-term vasotonus increase in the smallest b.v. reappear in 6 month-old rats. They are further strengthened after the 12th month, when the LDH and SDH-activity are extremely decreased. Intense tread-mill exercise results in appearances of long-term decrease of contractile vasotonus (Fig. 2, top). They are opposed by an aversion stress (Fig. 2, bottom), which induces only minor morphological reactions (Fig. 2, middle).

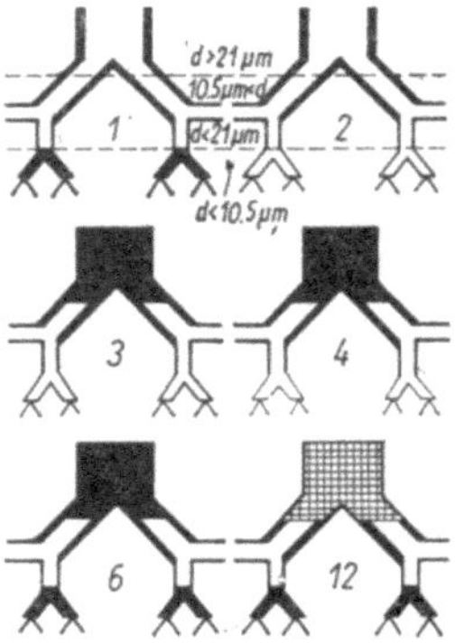

Fig. 1. Schemas of the microvasculature. The schema of 2-month-old SHR [2] also represents the normal state. Solid ramifications: significant increase of wall thickness, beyond that in b.v.$_{d<10.5\mu m}$ an increase of phosphatase activity. Thin-lined ramifications: significant decrease of wall thickness, moreover in b.v.$_{d<10.5\mu m}$ a decrease of phosphatase activity. Hatched and double-lined ramifications represent an insignificant but pronounced increase and decrease, respectively, of the above-mentioned reactions.

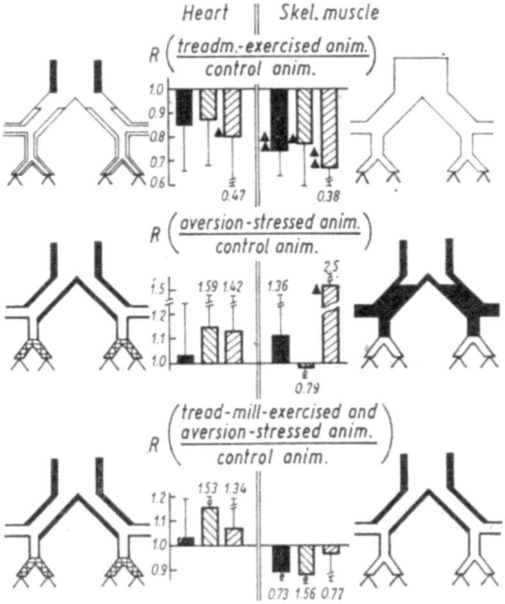

Fig. 2. Mean experimental to control-value ratios (R) of $A^{\Sigma b.v.}$ ( ), $N_{b.v.d<21\mu m}$ ( ), $N_{b.v.d>21\mu m}$ ( ) and their interpretation (Fig. 1) of the heart and skeletal muscle of rats exercised by tread-mill (top), stressed by an electric foot-schock (middle) or exercised and thereafter stressed (bottom) over a period of 6 months.

Conclusions

Long-term rise of myocardial activity causes morphologic changes of b.v. walls to be interpreted as morphological correlative of metabolic long-term vasotonus decrease and a sign of metabolic long-term autoregulation in coronary microvasculature. In the acute phase of SH and in intense physical training the metabolic vasodilatoric mechanisms can predominate on the increased activity of tonic factors. They can be governed by the latter, if the increase of myocardial activity is reduced (e.g. stable phase of SH) and/or the activity of tonic factors is absolutely augmented (e.g. aversion stress in rats exercised by tread-mill). How far an absolute increase of tonic factors has accompanied the decrease of relaxic influences in the chronic SH stage has to be elucidated. The failure of metabolic mechanisms to antagonize the elevated activity of vasotonic factors could result in a vicious circle, possibly contributing to heart insufficiency in SH.

References

[1] HERRMANN, H. J., P. MÜHLIG, Chr. KÜHNE and J. LÄUTER: Exp. Path. **17** (1979), 215–227 and ibid. **18** (1980), 140

[2] HERRMANN, H.-J., Chr. KÜHNE, P. MÜHLIG and J. LÄUTER: Gegenbaurs morph. Jahrb. **126** (1980), 273–276

*Central Institute of Heart and Circulation Research, GDR Academy of Sciences, Berlin-Buch and *Institute of Physiology, Humboldt University Berlin, GDR*

Potentiating Effect of Calmodulin and Cyclic AMP-Dependent Protein Kinase on the Ca^{2+}-Pump of Cardiac Sarcolemma

R. VETTER*, H. HAASE and H. WILL

Introduction

ATP-dependent Ca^{2+}-transport systems located in the sarcolemma (SL) and in the sarcoplasmic reticulum (SR) of cardiac cells participate in the extrusion of Ca^{2+} from the myoplasm during each contraction-relaxation cycle of the myocardium (TSIEN [6], WOLLENBERGER and WILL [9], CARONI and CARAFOLI [1], TRUMBLE et al. [5]). The Ca^{2+}-pump ATPase of SR is stimulated after phosphorylation of membrane protein(s) with cyclic AMP-dependent protein kinase (TADA et al. [5]) and also with Ca^{2+}/calmodulin-dependent protein kinase (KIRCHBERGER and ANTONETZ [3]). These regulations are thought to play important roles in the control of cardiac function by catecholamines and other agents that affect cellular concentrations of Ca^{2+} and cyclic AMP. The present study demonstrates that ATP-dependent Ca^{2+}-transport across SL membranes is also accelerated following preincubation of membranes with MgATP, calmodulin and catalytic subunit of cyclic AMP-dependent protein kinase (C subunit).

Methods

Isolation of SL vesicles, Ca^{2+}-transport measurements, evaluation of membrane sidedness and activity determinations for membrane-bound enzymes were performed as described previously (VETTER et al. [7]).

Results and conclusions

As shown in Table 1 the membrane preparation used is highly enriched in fragments of cardiac SL. This is documented by the activity values of SL marker enzymes Na^+, K^+-ATPase and K^+-pNitrophenylphosphatase (K^+-pNPPase). It is confirmed by the characteristics of the Ca^{2+}-transport systems. As reported earlier by CARONI and CARAFOLI [1] and by TRUMBLE et al. [5] a Na^+/Ca^{2+}-antiporter exists together with an ATP-dependent Ca^{2+}-pump in SL fragments. The ATP-dependent Ca^{2+}-transport in SL vesicles is not stimulated by oxalate and not supported by p-nitrophenylphosphate. Oligomycin, an inhibitor of mitochondrial Ca^{2+}-uptake, does not affect Ca^{2+}-accumulation into SL vesicles, while orthovanadate causes strong inhibition. The data rule out significant contamination of SL membranes with reticular or mitochondrial membranes. They demonstrate that ATP-dependent Ca^{2+}-transport in SL membranes exhibits properties distinct from those of active Ca^{2+}-transport in other membranes.

ATP-dependent Ca^{2+}-transport across SL membranes is increased after preincubation of isolated membranes with MgATP and C subunit (Fig. 1). By contrast ATP-dependent Ca^{2+}-transport does not change significantly following preincubation of SL membranes with MgATP, Ca^{2+} and calmodulin (0.01—0.5 μM). It was found, however, that the calmodulin antagonist trifluoperazine

Table 1
Characterization of sarcolemmal membrane preparations from pig heart

Enzyme activities		ATP-dependent Ca^{2+}-transport		
Enzyme	Activity	Condition	Ca^{2+} uptake (nmoles $Ca^{2+} \cdot$ mg Protein^{-1}) 1 min	10 min
(μmoles $P_i \cdot$ mg Protein$^{-1} \cdot h^{-1}$)				
(Na^+, K^+)-ATPase	87.3 ± 6.6	1 mM ATP	4.6 ± 0.5	18.2 ± 2.1
(Ca^{2+}, Mg^{2+})-ATPase	4.3 ± 0.7	1 mM ATP + 2.5 mM K-oxalate	n.d.	17.3 ± 0.8
K^+-pNPPase	23.0 ± 3.4	3 mM n-ditrophenylphosphate	n.d.	2.4 ± 0.9
Orientation of vesicles	60% right-side-out	35% inside-out		
Na^+/Ca^{2+} exchange	About 90% of Ca^{2+} transported in membrane vesicles is released into the medium by 40 mM NaCl.			
Effect of vanadate	2 μM orthovanadate inhibits Ca^{2+}-transport by about 60%. Complete inhibition occurs at 10 μM orthovanadate.			

Means $\pm$ S.E.M.; n.d. = not determined

inhibits Ca^{2+}-uptake rates by about 30%. The failure to stimulate Ca^{2+}-transport by exogeneous calmodulin might therefore be due to the possible presence of endogeneous calmodulin in the membrane preparation. The most striking effect on ATP-dependent Ca^{2+}-transport into SL vesicles was observed when membranes were preincubated in the presence of 1 mM MgATP, 0.5 μM C subunit, 75 μM $CaCl_2$ and 0.5 μM calmodulin. The initial rate of Ca^{2+}-uptake was increased 1.8-fold following such treatment.

Stimulation of SL Ca^{2+}-transport after prephosphorylation of membranes with C subunit is attributed to phosphorylation of specific SL proteins (WILL et al. [8]). Calmodulin can affect Ca^{2+}-transport systems directly or by stimulation of membrane-bound Ca^{2+}/calmodulin-dependent protein kinases (CARONI and CARAFOLI [2], KIRCHBERGER and ANTONETZ [3]). Irrespective of the mechanisms underlying the potentiating actions of calmodulin and C subunit, the enhancement in active Ca^{2+}-transport across SL membranes should be regarded as a powerful regulatory device for a more effective extrusion of Ca^{2+} from myocardial cells under specific conditions.

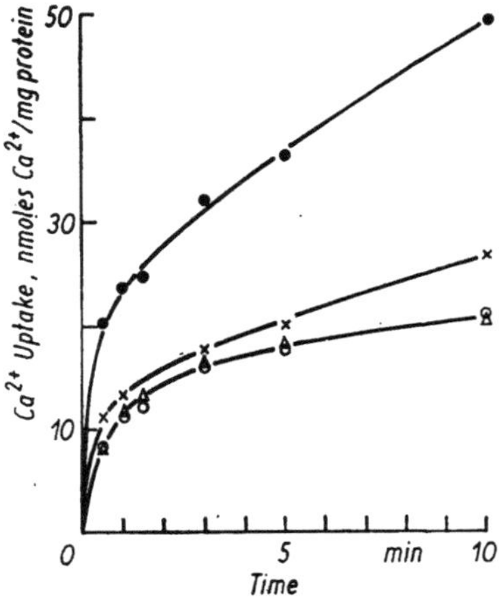

Fig. 1. Stimulation of Ca^{2+}-transport following preincubation of cardiac plasma membranes with MgATP, calmodulin and C subunit.
○ — control, △ — 0.5 μM calmodulin,
× — 0.5 μM subunit, • — 0.5 μM calmodulin and 0.5 μM C subunit

References

[1] CARONI, P. and E. CARAFOLI: Nature **283** (1980), 765–767
[2] CARONI, P. and E. CARAFOLI: J. Biol. Chem. **256** (1981), 3263–3270
[3] KIRCHBERGER, M. A. and T. ANTONETZ: J. Biol. Chem. **257** (1982), 5685–5691
[4] TADA, M., M. A. KIRCHBERGER, D. L. REPKE and A. M. KATZ: J. Biol. Chem. **249** (1974), 6174–6180
[5] TRUMBLE, W. R., I. L. SUTKO and I. P. REEVES: Life Sci. **27** (1980), 207–214
[6] TSIEN, R. W.: Adv. Cyclic Nucl. Res. **8** (1977), 363–420
[7] VETTER, R., H. HAASE and H. WILL: FEBS Let. **148** (1982), 326–330
[8] WILL, H., T. LEVCHENKO and C. KEMSIES: (in this volume)
[9] WOLENBERGER, A. and H. WILL: Life Sci. **22** (1978), 1159–1178

Central Institute of Heart and Circulation Research, Academy of Sciences of the GDR, Berlin-Buch, GDR

Characterization of a Phosphorylated Protein-Lipid Complex of Heart Sarcolemma

M. HOLTZHAUER, H. SYDOW and H. WILL

Introduction

Phosphorylation of membrane components is an important regulatory mechanism in membrane function. Both, proteins and lipids may serve as phosphate acceptors (for review see [1, 4, 5]). With regard to cardiac sarcolemma interest has been focused so far mainly on membrane proteins that are phosphorylated either by cyclic AMP-dependent or calcium and calmodulin-dependent protein kinases [6]. Sarcolemmal fractions contain in addition kinases that act independently of cyclic AMP and calmodulin. The endogenous kinases catalyse ^{32}P-phosphate incorporation into low molecular weight membrane components. The paper gives a first characterization of the respective phosphorylation products.

Methods

Porcine heart sarcolemmal vesicles were prepared by differential and density gradient centrifugations.

Extraction of lipids was performed according to GRIFFIN and HAWTHORNE [3], TLC was done as described by GONZALEZ-SASTRE and FOLCH-PI [2].

For autoradiography dried SDS-PAGE gels and TLC plates were exposed to ORWO X-ray film HS 11 at dry ice. Endogenous phosphorylation was performed at 30 °C for 60 to 90 seconds with 500 to 750 μg membrane protein per ml in the presence of 120 mM KCl, 10 mM $MgCl_2$, 40 mM histidine, pH 6.8, 0.5 mM EGTA, and 0.25 mM [γ-^{32}P]-ATP.

Abbreviations: SDS, sodium dodecyl sulfate; EGTA, ethyleneglycol-bis(2-aminoethylether)-N,N'-tetraacetic acid; PI, phosphatidyl inositol; PI-P, phosphatidyl inositol-4-phosphate; PI-P_2, phosphatidyl inositol-4,5-bisphosphate; PAGE, polyacrylamide gel electrophoresis; TLC, thin-layer chromatography; M_r, relative molecular weight.

Results

Autoradiography of SDS PAGE gels of phosphorylated heart sarcolemma vesicles on polyacrylamide gradients (T 10 to 20%) either in presence or absence of urea shows only one ^{32}P-labeled component with a M_r of about 5000 Dalton. The diffuse band is well stained by Sudan Black and by PAS, and only weak stained by Coomassie Blue.

Digestion of phosphorylated membrane vesicles by different proteases liberates only 30% of the acid precipitable phosphate. About 2/3 of the bound ^{32}P-phosphate may be extracted by acid chloroform-methanol mixtures. TLC of the latter extracts followed by autoradiography reveals two major components, one of which moves identically with phosphatidyl inositol-4-phosphate. There are in addition some minor spots (Fig. 1).

Gel permeation chromatography on Sephacryl S-200 in a denaturating system which ought to break hydrophobic interactions leads to the separation of ^{32}P-phosphate radioactivity into two major parts. The main part appears in the total volume of the column, the minor part elutes at a volume corresponding to a molecule of M_r 10,000 to 12,000. This value is in agreement with the relative molecular weight calculated from the amino acid composition (Table 1) of the electrophoretically purified phosphorylation product.

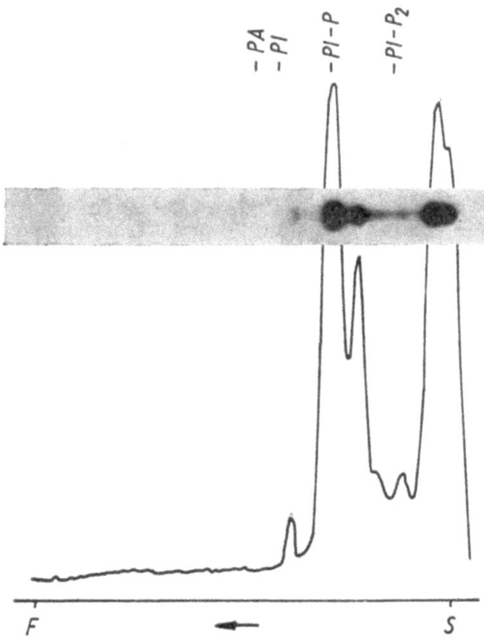

Fig. 1. TLC of an acid chloroform/methanol extract of phosphorylated membranes (autoradiogram and densitogram).

Table 1

Amino acid composition of electrophoretically purified phosphorylated compound of heart sarcolemma (mol-%)

Asp	8.42	Ala	5.64	Tyr	0.91
Thr	5.85	Cys	1.33	Phe	2.54
Ser	10.48	Val	4.85	His	1.63
Glu	12.22	Met	0.87	Lys	5.16
Pro	3.68	Ile	3.42	Arg	3.67
Gly	22.73	Leu	6.75		

Conclusions

Endogenous, calmodulin-independent and cyclic AMP-independent kinases phosphorylate lipids as well as polypeptides of cardiac sarcolemma. It is assumed that lipid phosphorylation and protein phosphorylation are catalysed by different kinases. Phosphorylated lipids and polypeptides appear to be tightly associated. They could not be separated by SDS-PAGE. The type of interactions between phosphorylated lipids and polypeptides and the physiological relevance of the phosphorylation reaction are not known.

References

[1] BÁRÁNY, M. and K. BÁRÁNY: Am. J. Physiol. **241** (1981), H117–H128
[2] GONZALEZ-SASTRE, F. and J. FOLCH-PI: J. Lipid Res. **9** (1968), 532–533
[3] GRIFFIN, H. D. and J. N. HAWTHORNE: Biochem. J. **176** (1978), 541–552
[4] PUTNEY, J. W., jr.: Live Sci. **29** (1981), 1183–1194
[5] TADA, M. and A. M. KATZ: Ann. Rev. Physiol. **44** (1982), 401–423
[6] WILL, H., T. S. LEVCHENKO, D. O. LEVITSKY, V. N. SMIRNOV and A. WOLLENBERGER: Biochim. Biophys. Acta **543** (1978), 175–193

Institute of Physiological Chemistry, Friedrich-Schiller-University Jena, GDR

Activation of (Ca^{2+} + Mg^{2+}) ATPase of Erythrocyte Membranes by Trypsin, Fatty Acids and Ca²/. A Comparisation with Calmodulin Action

R. WETZKER, R. KLINGER, I. FLEISCHER and H. FRUNDER

Introduction

Calmodulin-depleted erythrocyte membranes exhibit a low Ca^{2+}-affinity (Ca^{2+} + Mg^{2+}) ATPase which can be transformed into a high activity and high Ca^{2+}-affinity form by calmodulin. In the absence of calmodulin, this transformation can be brought about by trypsin, phospholipase A_2, fatty acids, acidic phospholipids, and millimolar Ca^{2+} [1—4]. Concomitantly, the increment in ATPase activity caused by calmodulin decreases.

In this communication we present parallel measurements of enzyme activity and calmodulin binding to the membranes in the course of the calmodulin independent activation process. Ca^{2+} concentration dependence on activities of different enzyme forms are compared.

Methods

The techniques for collection of blood, preparation of calmodulin, preparation of calmodulin-depleted ghosts, assay of calmodulin, assay of (Ca^{2+} + Mg^{2+}) ATPase by P_i liberation, assay of calmodulin binding to ghosts, assay of fatty acids, treatment of ghosts with trypsin, Ca^{2+} and fatty acids and calculation of free Ca^{2+} concentration have been described in recent publications [4—6]. Ghosts were preincubated with trypsin (3 μg/ml), Ca^{2+} (2 mM) or oleic acid (1—5 mM). Preincubation was stopped after 1—60 min as indicated in the Figures. Trypsin, Ca^{2+} or oleic acid (not accumulated in ghosts) were removed by washings. Aliquots of the pelleted ghosts were resuspended in assay medium or in calmodulin loading medium and used for determinations of enzyme activity at 2.6 μM free Ca^{2+} and calmodulin binding to ghosts at 50 μM Ca^{2+} and 0.6—6 μM calmodulin.

Results and discussion

The maximum activation of (Ca^{2+} + Mg^{2+})ATPase by trypsin was obtained after 7—10 min preincubation (Fig. 1a). The higher the degree of activation the lower was the increment in enzyme activity caused by calmodulin. In parallel to increasing enzyme activity a progressive decrease of calmodulin binding to ghosts was observed (Fig. 1b). According to recent results of ROUFOGALIS [7] this may be due to proteolytic removal of a splitting product with 22 K containing the calmodulin binding domain of the enzyme. — Figure 2 illustrates the effects of preincubation with 2 mM free Ca^{2+} and 1 mM ATP on enzyme activity and calmodulin binding to ghosts. There are striking similarities between the effects of trypsin (Fig. 1) and Ca^{2+} (Fig. 2). This suggests that high Ca^{2+} concentrations activate a membrane-bound Ca^{2+}-dependent proteinase, which induces similar proteolytic alterations of Ca^{2+}-ATPase as trypsin. This suggestion is supported by the finding (not shown) that the effects of trypsin and Ca^{2+} can be more or less completely abolished by the presence of calmodulin in the preincubation mixture. Furthermore, the effects of Ca^{2+} can be considerably

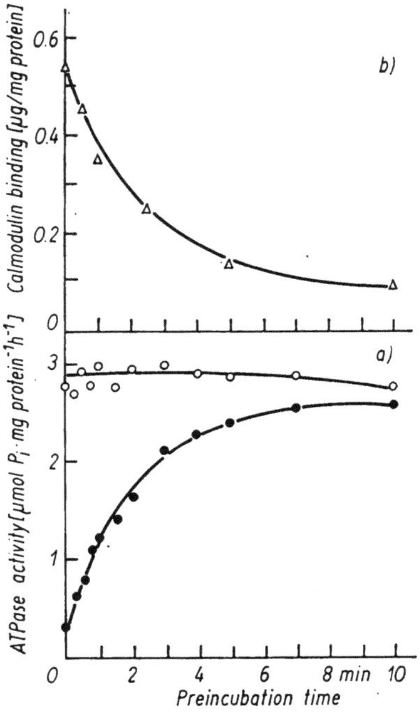

Fig. 1. Time course of the effect of preincubation with trypsin on (Ca^{2+} + Mg^{2+})-ATPase activity (A) and calmodulin binding to ghosts (B).
a: Enzyme activity at 2.6 µM free Ca^{2+} in the absence (•) and in the presence (○) 0.06 µM calmodulin
b: Calmodulin binding to ghosts at 0.6 µM calmodulin and 50 µM free Ca^{2+}

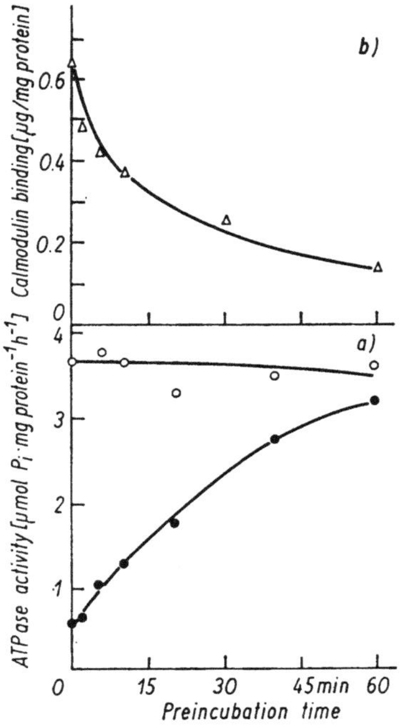

Fig. 2. Time course of the effect of preincubation with 2 mM Ca^{2+} and 1 mM ATP on (Ca^{2+} + Mg^{2+})ATPase activity (a) and calmodulin binding to ghosts (b).
a: Enzyme activity at 2.6 µM free Ca^{2+} in the absence (•) and in the presence (○) of 0.06 µM calmodulin
b: Calmodulin binding to ghosts at 0.6 µM calmodulin and 50 µM free Ca^{2+}

diminished by the addition of leupeptin. These results point to a possible involvement of calpain in enzyme activation and decrease of calmodulin binding during preincubation of ghosts in the presence of high Ca^{2+} concentrations. Calpain has been found in all cells so far examined and was characterized recently by MURAKAMI et al. [8].

In the absence of calmodulin, maximum stimulation by oleic acid of $(Ca^{2+} + Mg^{2+})$ATPase activity was obtained at 0.75 μmol oleic acid/mg protein (Fig. 3A). Higher concentrations of oleic acid progressively inhibited enzyme activity. In the presence of calmodulin, small concentrations

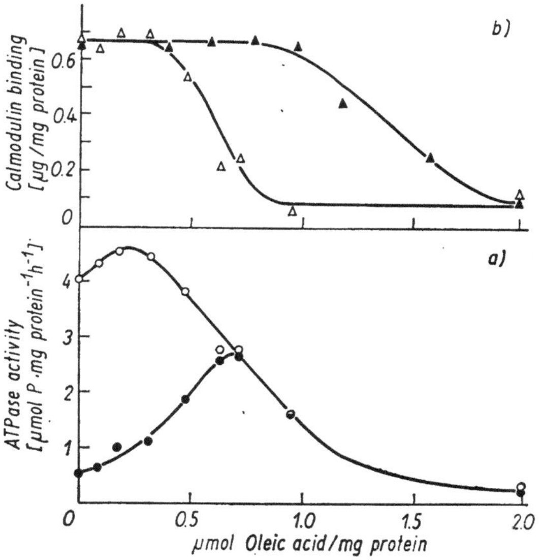

Fig. 3. Concentration dependence of the effect of oleic acid on $(Ca^{2+} + Mg^{2+})$ATPase activity at 2.6 μM free Ca^{2+} (A) and on calmodulin binding to ghosts at 50 μM free Ca^{2+} (b).

a: Enzyme activity in the absence (•) and in the presence (○) of 0.18 μM calmolin

b: Calmodulin binding to ghosts in the presence of 0.6 (△) and 6 (▲) μM calmodulin

of oleic acid induced an additional stimulation of enzyme activity, which proceeded to a progressive inhibition at further increasing concentrations. Calmodulin binding to ghosts decreased progressively at increasing oleic acid concentrations (Fig. 3b). This can be almost completely abolished by increasing calmodulin concentrations, indicating, that there is a competitive interaction of fatty acids and calmodulin with the regulatory domain of the membrane-bound Ca^{2+}-ATPase. In contrast to it, after preincubation of the membranes with trypsin or Ca^{2+} the decreased calmodulin binding to ghosts can only be partly restored by high calmodulin concentration (not shown).

Table 1 summarizes our experimental data on Ca^{2+} concentration dependence of native and transformed Ca^{2+}-ATPase as calculated parameters of the Hill equation. In the absence of calmodulin, the native enzyme of calmodulin-depleted ghosts exhibited low V_{max} and low Ca^{2+}-affinity, which were increased severalfold after transformation by trypsin, millimolar Ca^{2+} and oleic acid. The Hill coefficient under these conditions is about 1. The activation by Ca^{2+} of the native enzyme in the presence of calmodulin seemed to be highly cooperative. In a recent publication the question was examined, whether this behavior may be due to cooperative formation of an activating calmodulin-Ca_n^{2+} species (see [6]). The results have shown that calmodulin-Ca_3^{2+} is the activating species, which is produced in a cooperative manner in dependence on Ca^{2+} concentration. The dependence of the enzyme activity on the calmodulin-Ca_3^{2+}-complex follows a hyperbolic kinetics.

$K_{0.5Ca}$, which considerably decreased by enzyme transformation, can be taken as a measure for the affinity of the Ca^{2+} binding site of the enzyme in the absence of calmodulin. In the presence of calmodulin, however, $K_{0.5Ca}$ is a measure of the concentration of the activating calmodulin-Ca_3^{2+} species. A possible role of an additional Ca^{2+} binding site of the calmodulin-activated enzyme for enzyme activity remains to be established.

Table 1

Kinetic parameters of Ca^{2+}-activation of the native and transformed (Ca^{2+} + Mg^{2+})-ATPase

Enzyme form	V_{max} (µmol P_i · mg^{-1} xh^{-1})	$K_{0.5Ca}$ (µM)	dn_H
A: Without calmodulin native	~ 1	~ 3	~ 1
after transformation by trypsin	4.5	0.5	1.2
mM Ca^{2+}	4.4	0.4	1.1
oleic acid	3.4	0.6	1.2
B: with 6 µM calmodulin native	4.4	0.3	2.9

References

[1] TAVERNA, R. D. and D. J. HANAHAN: Biochem. Biophys. Res. Commun. **94** (1980), 652–659
[2] NIGGLI, V., E. S. ADUNYAH and E. CARAFOLI: J. Biol. Chem. **256** (1981), 8588–8592
[3] NIGGLI, V., E. S. ADUNYAH, J. T. PENNISTON and E. CARAFOLI: J. Biol. Chem. **256** (1981), 395–401
[4] KLINGER, R., R. WETZKER, I. FLEISCHER and H. FRUNDER: Cell Calcium **2** (1981), 553–560
[5] KLINGER, R., R. WETZKER, I. FLEISCHER and H. FRUNDER: Cell Calcium **1** (1980), 229–240
[6] WETZKER, R., R. KLINGER, G. CUMME, H. HOPPE and H. FRUNDER: Biochem. Intern. **4** (1982), 385–390
[7] ROUFOGALIS, B. D.: personal communication
[8] MURAKAMI, T., M. HATANAKA and T. MURACHI: J. Biochem. **90** (1981), 1809–1816

Institute of Physiological Chemistry, Medical Academy, Magdeburg, G.D.R.

Simultaneous Oxidation of Pyruvate and Fatty Acids by Rat-Heart Mitochondria at Limiting Substrate Supply

P. Schönfeld, D. Petzold and W. Kunz

Statement of problem

The energy demand of the cardiac muscle is supported by mitochondrial oxidative phosphorylation, predominantly.

Pyruvate and fatty acids are the most important fuels of mitochondrial energy transformation. In the presence of saturating fatty acid concentrations pyruvate oxidation is inhibited as shown in experiments with isolated mitochondria as well perfused organs (e.g. [1] for review). However, a lack of informations exists concerning simultaneous oxidation of pyruvate and fatty acids under conditions of a limited substrate supply. In this study it was investigated experimentally if the supply of fatty acids influences the oxidation of pyruvate and vice versa.

Methods and materials

Rat-heart mitochondria (RHM) were isolated according to Schaller et al. [2]. Limiting concentrations of pyruvate, octanoate and palmitoylcarnitine were supplied to RHM by means of a perifusion procedure as recently described by Schönfeld et al. [3]. The incubation medium contained (in mM): 110 sucrose, 60 Tris, 60 KCl, 10 KH_2PO_4, 5 $MgCl_2$, 0.5 EDTA. The pH was adjusted to 7.4 with HCl. All experiments were performed at 25 °C.

Results and discussion

Incubation of isolated mitochondria in closed polarographic vessels results in a continuous disappearance of substrates by its oxidation. Therefore investigations in presence of limiting fatty acid concentrations canot performed in this manner. A permanent supply of substrates realized with the mentioned perifusion procedure (Fig. 1) offers the possibility to study simultaneous steady state oxidation of fatty acids and pyruvate down to very low concentrations.

In Figure 2 the influence of increasing concentrations of octanoate or palmitoylcarnitine on pyruvate oxidation in the active state is shown. As seen pyruvate oxidation is already suppressed by very low fatty acid concentration. Furthermore higher concentrations of fatty acids diminish pyruvate oxidation only to about 60 or 85 percent, respectively. Both fatty acids differ in their maximal inhibitory action. The increased respiration observed at presence of fatty acids points to a simultaneous oxidation of both substrates. In Figure 3 mitochondria were supplied with an octanoate concentration near to its apparent K_M value (6—8 μM). The apparent K_M for octanoate oxidation in the active state was determined in separate perifusion experiments (not shown). As seen the rate of respiration is doubled by addition of pyruvate.

Further increase of pyruvate concentration in the medium is paralled by an increase of the rate of pyruvate oxidation whereas the respiration rate is not enhanced. However an increase of pyruvate oxidation at constant rate of respiration is only compatible with a suppressed octanoate oxidation.

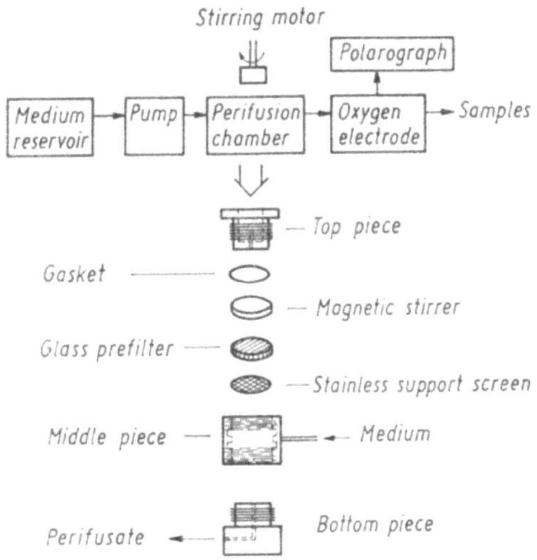

Fig. 1. Scheme of perifusion procedure.
Isolated rat heart mitochondria (RHM) were immobilized adsorptively on a glass prefilter (Type: AP 25, Fa. Millipore/USA) by injection of a portion of RHM suspension to the flow of air-saturated incubation medium. The amount of mitochondria immobilized on the glass prefilter was determined by a biuret method. Rates of respiration (V_{Resp}) and pyruvate oxidation (△ Pyr.) were calculated from the concentrations of oxygen and pyruvate in the efflux medium, the amount of immobilized mitochondria on the filter and the flow rate of the medium. Oxygen and pyruvate concentrations were determined polarographically and enzymatically, respectively.

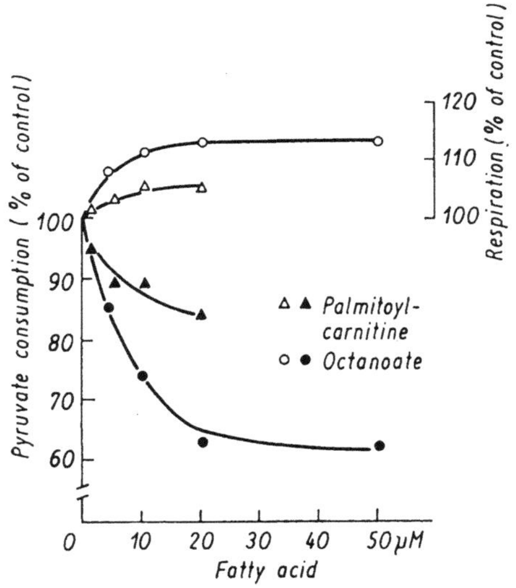

Fig. 2. Influence of fatty acids on pyruvate oxidation and respiration.
Immobilized mitochondria (2.5 mg protein) were perifused with incubation medium (flow rate 1.5 ml/min) containing pyruvate (100 μM), malate (100 μM) and ADP (0.5 mM). Increasing amounts of octanoate or palmitoylcarnitine were added, respectively. 100% of pyruvate consumption (▲, •) and respiration (△, ○) amounts to 23.3 ± 1.3 nmol/mg · min and 49.4 ± 1.6 nmol O_2/mg · min (means ± SEM).

The rate of octanoate oxidation in dependence of pyruvate concentration was calculated from the rates of pyruvate oxidation, rate of respiration and the ratios of oxygen consumption and amount of substrate oxidized. According to this an increase of pyruvate concentration to 200 μM suppresses octanoate oxidation to one half.

From this study it is concluded that pyruvate and fatty acids compete at conditions of a limited availability for supply of reducing equivalents to the system of mitochondrial energy transformation.

Experimental results by TAEGTMEYER et al. with perfused working rat-hearts are in line with this [4].

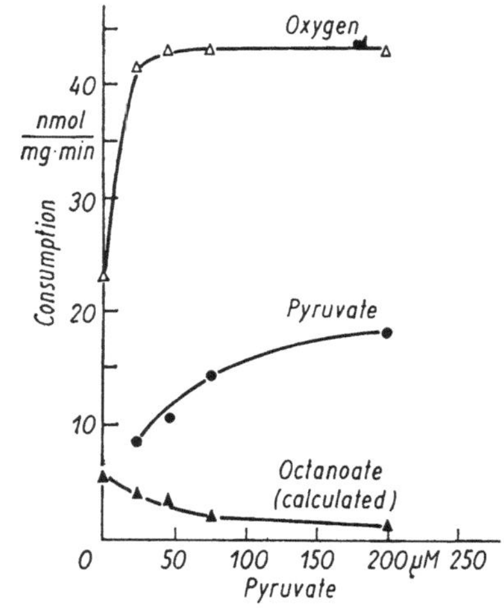

Fig. 3. Respiration, pyruvate and octanoate oxidation in dependence on pyruvate concentration.
Immobilized mitochondria (2.9 mg protein) were perifused with incubation medium (flow rate 1.6 ml/min) containing malate (100 μM), octanoate (5 μM) and ADP (0.5 mM). Increasing amounts of pyruvate were added to the medium. The rate of octanoate oxidation (Δ Oct.) was estimated according to:

$$\Delta \text{ Oct} = (2 \cdot V_{Resp} - F_{Pyr} \cdot \Delta \text{ Pyr})/F_{Oct}$$

with $F_{Pyr} = 4.5$ and $F_{Oct} = 11$ and rate of respiration expressed in nmol O_2/mg · min. F_{Pyr} and F_{Oct} are defined as the ratios of oxygen consumption and the amount of substrate oxidized. This ratios were determined in separated experiments by addition of exact know amounts of substrates to RHM incubated in a closed polarographic vessel (not shown).

References

[1] NEELY, J. R. and H. E. MORGAN: Ann. Rev. Physiol. **36** (1974), 413–453
[2] SCHALLER, H., G. LETKO and W. KUNZ: Acta biol. med. germ. **37** (1978), 31–38
[3] SCHÖNFELD, P. and U. KÜSTER: Acta biol. med. germ. **38** (1979), 1307–1314
[4] TAEGTMEYER, H., R. HEMS and H. A. KREBS: Biochem. J. **186** (1980), 701–711

Department of Pharmacology, University Medical School, Szeged, Hungary

Protecting Effect of Adrenergic β-Blocking Agents on the Energy Metabolism of Ischaemic Myocardium

I. Takáts and L. Szekeres

Before introducing a new cardioactive drug into clinical practice generally the haemodynamic, electrophysiological and other pharmacological effects of the new compound are studied. Only a limited number of observations consider also their effect on the metabolic changes produced by pathological processes.

As it is well known the breakdown of ATP is the primary source of the contraction energy. Anoxia or ischaemia leads to a rapid change in the high-energy phosphates: creatine phosphate (CP) and ATP decrease, while ADP, AMP, inorganic phosphate (IP) and lactate levels increase. The extent of these changes is related to the degree of ischaemic lesion.

Our present study was devoted to the question whether the different β-blocking agents may affect the metabolism of ischaemic changes mentioned above.

The experiments were performed in anaesthetized (nembutal 45 mg/kg i.p.), thoracotomized and artificially respirated male rats. With the aid of a Wollenberger clamp cooled in liquid nitrogen samples were taken from the left ventricle. The frozen tissue samples were pulverized and extracted with 0.5 N perchloric acid. After centrifugation and neutralization aliquots were taken for the estimation of the above-mentioned components. IP and CP were determined by the method of Wahler and Wollenberger [6]. ATP was determined according to Dennemann [1], ADP and AMP according to Jaworek et al. [4] with the aid of Boehringer Test-combination. Lactate content was determined also enzymatically with LDH according to Hohorst [3].

The biochemical protecting effects of β-blocking agents: propranolol (0.5 mg/kg), pindolol (0.025 mg/kg), practolol (2 mg/kg) and atenolol (1 mg/kg) were studied. The drugs were administered i.v. 10 min before the experiments.

None of the drugs studied and given in the above doses had significant influence on the energy metabolism of the normal myocardium. The protective effect of the drugs was examined on the "isolated ischaemic heart model" elaborated by Takáts et al. [5]. Ten minutes after the administration of the drug (or physiological saline solution in control experiments) we cut out the left ventricle of the heart, incubated the tissue in mammalian Ringer solution of 37 °C exactly for one minute, then freezed it by means of a pair of cooled Wollenberger tongue.

The protective effect of the above-mentioned drugs on the IP, CP, ATP, ADP, AMP and lactate content of the ischaemic myocardium is summarized in Table. 1.

CP concentration, which is a highly sensitive indicator of the ischaemic state, was increased by all applied drugs; atenolol was the most effective, the other drugs exerted also significant protective action.

In contrast to CP, ATP concentration showed less change in this type of hypoxia. In our experiments propranolol pretreatment proved to exert a significant protective effect against ischaemic diminution.

The increased ADP and AMP level in the ischaemic state points to the extent of ATP degradation, on the other hand, it hints to the possible sources of the resynthesis of ATP. We measured the lowest ADP level after the administration of propranolol and pindolol.

Table 1

The effect of different β-blockers on the CP, ATP, ADP, IP and lactate content and on the Bioenergetic Index of ischaemic myocardium

Experimental groups	CP	ATP	ADP	AMP	IP	L	B.I.
Controls in situ	5.82 ± 0.29 (7)	4.24 ± 0.14 (8)	1.41 ± 0.15 (8)	0.76 ± 0.07 (7)	3.78 ± 0.29 (9)	3.32 ± 0.26 (7)	122.65 ± 20.05 (5)
Ischaemia	1.80 ± 0.21 (7]	3.57 ± 0.13 (6)	1.72 ± 0.14 (8)	1.13 ± 0.14 (8)	8.29 ± 0.39 (8)	5.50 ± 0.41 (6)	21.83 ± 5.43 (6)
Propranolol 0.5 mg/kg	b 3.20 ± 0.35 (10)	a 3.93 ± 0.08 (12)	a 1.43 ± 0.05 (12)	a 0.79 ± 0.04 (12)	c 6.35 ± 0.29 (10)	N.S. 6.07 ± 0.34 (11)	a 35.24 ± 3.70 (6)
Pindolol 0.025 mg/kg	c 3.59 ± 0.25 (14)	N.S. 3.70 ± 0.25 (14)	c 1.15 ± 0.06 (14)	N.S. 0.97 ± 0.08 (15)	c 5.81 ± 0.19 (14)	a 6.78 ± 0.38 (13)	c 47.89 ± 4.21 (15)
Practolol 2 mg/kg	c 3.89 ± 0.11 (6)	N.S. 4.28 ± 0.39 (6)	N.S. 1.84 ± 0.09 (5)	N.S. 1.06 ± 0.08 (5)	N.S. 7.50 ± 0.22 (6)	a 3.90 ± 0.36 (5)	a 45.46 ± 2.98 (5)
Atenolol 1 mg/kg	c 6.78 ± 0.16 (6)	N.S. 3.89 ± 0.25 (7)	N.S. 1.62 ± 0.15 (6)	N.S. 0.87 ± 0.12 (7)	c 4.33 ± 0.21 (6)	a 3.71 ± 0.48 (6)	c 115.26 ± 5.89 (6)

Results are given in μmoles/g w · wt and represent means ± S.E.M.
d = ( ) — the number of single measurements
Differences against the ischaemic group are significant
with a = $p < 0.05$ b = $p < 0.001$ c = $p < 0.005$
B.I. = Bioenergetic Index; L = lactate

Propranolol also decreased significantly the AMP content. The applied drugs influenced the increased myocardial IP concentration after the degradation of high-energy phosphate compounds. Significant decrease was observed after pretreatment by propranolol, pindolol and atenolol.

The cardioselective β-blockers: practolol and atenolol afforded significant protection against the increase in lactate content which is an important indicator of ischaemia. Pindolol and propranolol were not effective in this respect.

When to compare the influence of drugs with different mode of action, the evaluation of the specific effect of these drugs is based upon the parameters as mentioned before. Several attempts have been made until now to work out uniform and objective criteria which would involve and integrate the different metabolic indicators. In our present work we used the so called "Bioenergetic Index" elaborated by FEDELEŠOVÁ and ZIEGELHÖFFER [2]. The indexes were calculated from the data demonstrated before. Accordingly atenolol exerted the best protective effect against the rapid decrease of the bioenergetic index in anoxia. Pindolol, propranolol and practolol had a smaller effect.

The protective metabolic effect of some β-blockers were examined on "isolated ischaemic heart model". All of the studied drugs had remarkable protective effect against the alterations of energy metabolism in ischaemic myocardium but only practolol and atenolol improved simultaneously the energetic state and reduced the increased lactate level in ischaemic heart tissue.

Importance of these results lies in the demonstration of the fact that numerous drugs are able to give a more or less expressed protection against the metabolic alterations occuring in the ischaemic myocardium. We assume that this positive metabolic action may also play an important role in the anti-ischaemic effect of the drugs in question.

References

[1] DENNEMANN, H.: Zeitsch. ges. Exp. Med. **134** (1961), 335–340

[2] FEDELEŠOVÁ, M., and A. ZIEGELHÖFFER: Bratisl. Lek. Listy **65** (1976), 312–319.

[3] HOHORST, H.-J.: In: BERGMEYER, H. U.: Methods of enzymatic analysis. Academic Press, New York and London, (1965), p. 266–270

[4] JAWOREK, D., W. GRUBER and H. U. BERGMEYER: In: BERGMEYER, H. U.: Methods of enzymatic analysis. 2nd. ed. Academic Press, New York and London, (1974), p. 2127–2130

[5] TAKÁTS, I., P. VÁGHY and L. SZEKERES: Acta physiol. Acad. Sci. Hung. **44** (1973), 410

[6] WAHLER, B. E. and A. WOLLENBERGER: Biochem. Zeitsch. **329** (1958), 508–520

Department of Pharmacology, University Medical School of Szeged, Szeged, Hungary+ and Department of Pharmacology and Cell Biophysics, University of Cincinnati, Cincinnati, Ohio, USA

Diltiazem is a Selective Inhibitor of the Na^+-Ca^{2+} Antiporter in Heart Mitochondria*

P. L. Vághy*, M. A. Matlib and A. Schwartz

Introduction

We recently reported that Ca^{2+} antagonist drugs inhibit Na^+-induced Ca^{2+} release from isolated heart mitochondria, Vághy et al. [14]. Among the drugs studied only diltiazem was able to inhibit the Na^+-induced Ca^{2+} release without also affecting the Ca^{2+} uptake. The effects of other Ca^{2+} antagonists, which included fendiline, prenylamine, nifedipine and verapamil, were less selective since, at concentrations that produced more than a 60% inhibition of the Na^+-induced Ca^{2+} release, they also inhibited mitochondrial Ca^{2+} uptake. Apart from Na^+, the Ca^{2+} ionophore, A23187, uncoupling agents, inorganic phosphate and a shift in the mitochondrial NAD(P)H NAD(P) ratio are all known to produce a release of Ca^{2+} from mitochondria, Carafoli [3]. Moreover, we have demonstrated that diltiazem does not inhibit either the A23187 or the uncoupler-induced Ca^{2+} release processes, Vághy et al. [14]. In this paper we present evidence which indicates that diltiazem, at a concentration that results in more than a 90% inhibition of Na^+-induced Ca^{2+} release, does not affect the Ca^{2+} release from heart mitochondria induced either by inorganic phosphate or by the oxidation of mitochondrial pyridine nucleotides.

Local anesthetics such as dibucaine, have been shown to inhibit Ca^{2+} release from mitochondria, Dawson et al. [9], Palmer and Pfeiffer [12], Cockrell [4]. Therefore, the effects of dibucaine on mitochondrial Ca^{2+} transport processes were also investigated.

Materials and methods

d-cis-/+/-diltiazem was supplied by Marion Research Laboratories, Inc., Kansas City, MO.

The isolation of rabbit heart mitochondria, measurement of mitochondrial Ca^{2+} transport using the Ca^{2+} indicator dye, arsenazo III, and the atomic absorption spectroscopic determination of Ca^{2+} were carried out as described previously, Vághy et al. [14]. Protein was determined according to Lowry et al. [11]. The redox state of mitochondrial pyridine nucleotides was determined by measurements of the differential light absorbance changes at the wavelength pair 340 and 370 nm using an Aminco DW 2a dual wavelength spectrophotometer as described by Lehninger et al. [10]. The assay medium for Ca^{2+} transport studies contained 120 mM KCl, 10 mM 4-morpholine-propanesulfinic acid (MOPS)-potassium hydroxide buffer, pH 7.0, 5 mM potassium glutamate and 5 mM potassium malate. Where indicated, glutamate and malate were omitted from the mixture. All experiments were carried out at 37 °C and pH 7.0.

Results

Figure 1 demonstrates the effects of ruthenium red alone and diltiazem alone on the steady state extramitochondrial Ca^{2+} concentration maintained by isolated heart mitochondria. In the presence of the oxidizable substrates, (glutamate and malate) mitochondria took up Ca^{2+} from the

* This study has been carried out in the Department of Pharmacology and Cell Biophysics, University of Cincinnati, Cincinnati, Ohio 45267, USA

test medium, as it was indicated by a small decrease in the differential light absorbance, even. if only a contaminating amount of Ca^{2+} was present (4.03 ± 0.48 μM Ca^{2+}). When the extramitochondrial Ca^{2+} concentration reached a constant level, Ca^{2+} was added to the medium. The mitochondria then accumulated all the added Ca^{2+} as indicated by a decrease in the extramitochondrial Ca^{2+} concentration to the level measured before the addition of Ca^{2+}. A subsequent addition of Na^+ induced a partial release of Ca^{2+}. from the mitochondria. The extramitochondrial Ca^{2+} concentration then remained at a constant but higher level (Fig. 1 solid line). The constant extramitochondrial Ca^{2+} concentration observed subsequent to the Na^+- induced partial release

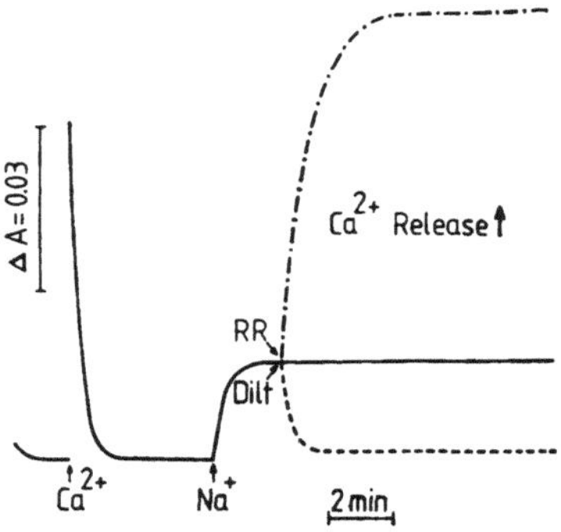

Fig. 1. Effects of ruthenium red and diltiazem on the steady state extramitochondrial Ca^{2+} concentration. Fifty μM arsenaso III was added to 3 ml test medium containing glutamate and malate. The experiments were started by the addition of 2 mg mitochondrial protein. The results of 3 different experiments are superimposed in this Fig. Where indicated by arrows, 40 nmol $CaCl_2$ (Ca^{2+}), 10 mM NaCl (Na^+), 1 μM ruthenium red (RR) or 200 μM diltiazem (Dilt) were added. Downward and upward deflections correspond to the decrease and increase in the extramitochondrial Ca^{2+} concentration, respectively.

of Ca^{2+} may indicate either the absence of both Ca^{2+} uptake and Ca^{2+} release processes or a continuous uptake and release of Ca^{2+} across the mitochondrial inner membrane where the two oppositely directed processes are balancing each other. To test this latter possibility, after the steady state extramitochondrial Ca^{2+} concentration had been established, ruthenium red was added to selectively inhibit the Ca^{2+} uptake process. As it is shown on Figure 1 (dashed-dotted line), the addition of ruthenium red resulted in a net release of Ca^{2+} from mitochondria. Since ruthenium red has no effect on Na^+-induced Ca^{2+} release, the net Ca^{2+} release measured upon the addition of the ruthenium red indicates that both Ca^{2+} uptake and Ca^{2+} release processes were indeed operating at the same time, even though the extramitochondrial Ca^{2+} concentration was maintained at a constant level. If, however, we accept that the constant extramitochondrial Ca^{2+} concentration measured in the presence of Na^+ represents a dynamic steady state where the Ca^{2+} is cycling across the mitochondrial inner membrane, then it would be expected that a selective inhibition of the Na^+-induced Ca^{2+} release process will have an opposite effect to that induced by ruthenium red. The results shown in Figure 1 (broken line) show that diltiazem treatment resulted in a net uptake of Ca^{2+} by the mitochondria provided that the drug was added after the steady state extramitochondrial Ca^{2+} concentration had been established in Na^+-treated mitochondria. This result suggests that diltiazem is a selective inhibitor of the Na^+-induced Ca^{2+} release process in heart mitochondria.

It has been known, however, that Ca^{2+} can be released from mitochondria by several agents and conditions as recently reviewed by CARAFOLI [3]. Therefore, the next questions to study was, whether or not diltiazem inhibits the Ca^{2+} release from mitochondria induced by Ca^{2+} releasing agents other than Na^+. Figure 2 shows the effect of diltiazem on inorganic phosphate induced Ca^{2+} release. In these experiments heart mitochondria were treated with ruthenium red after the accumulation of externally added Ca^{2+} was completed in order to prevent the interaction of Ca^{2+} uptake with the inorganic phosphate induced Ca^{2+} release process. The results indicate that diltiazem had little effect on the Ca^{2+} release process induced by inorganic phosphate. On the other hand, dibucaine, a local anesthetic drug, significantly inhibited the inorganic phosphate induced Ca^{2+} release process. These data suggest that diltiazem and dibucaine may act in different ways. Next, we studied the effects of these drugs on the Ca^{2+} release induced by the oxidation of mitochondrial pyridine nucleotides. The results demonstrated in Figure 2 show that rabbit heart mitochondria incubated in the absence of exogenous substrates were still able to accumulate Ca^{2+}, but that this process was followed shortly by a spontaneous release of Ca^{2+} from the mitochondria. A parallel recording of the NAD(P)H/NAD(P) ratio suggested that, at the beginning of these experiments the mitochondria had some endogenous substrates, since the presence of reduced pyridine nucleotides was apparent. As soon as the mitochondrial pyridine nucleotides became oxidized, however, the mitochondria began to lose Ca^{2+}. It should be emphasized that this type of Ca^{2+} release could not be measured when external substrates were included in the test medium (Fig. 2), which suggests that an exhaustion of the endogenous substrates was responsible for the oxidation of mitochondrial pyridine nucleotides, State 2 respiration had thus developed. These data indicate that an oxidation of mitochondrial pyridine nucleotides is accompanied by a release of Ca^{2+} from mitochondria as it has been suggested by LEHNINGER et al. [6]. Diltiazem had no effect on this type of Ca^{2+} release (Fig. 3). On the other hand, dibucaine was not only unable to prevent the Ca^{2+} release, but it accelerated both the oxidation of mitochondrial pyridine nucleotides and the release of Ca^{2+} from mitochondria. These experiments again indicate that the effects of diltiazem and dibucaine are different.

The effect of diltiazem on the kinetics of Na^+-induced Ca^{2+} release was determined in the presence of 2.5 mM $MgCl_2$. Double reciprocal plots are shown in Figure 4. The maximum velocity of the Na^+-induced Ca^{2+} release was found to be 26 nmol $Ca^{2+} \times min^{-1} \times$ mg protein^{-1} and the Km for Na^+ was 100 mM^2 i.e. a half maximal activation of Ca^{2+} release could be measured at 10 mM Na^+ concentration. Diltiazem did not change the km, but lowered the maximum velocity of the Na^+-induced Ca^{2+} release suggesting that the drug is a noncompetitive inhibitor of Na^+ in this process. From the data presented an apparent K_i of 19 μM was calculated.

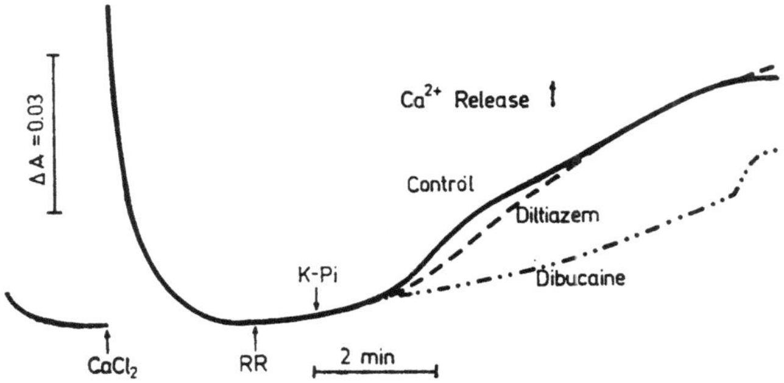

Fig. 2. Effects of diltiazem and dibucaine on the inorganic phosphate induced Ca^{2+} release process. The experimental conditions were the same as described in Fig. 1. The results of 3 different experiments are superimposed in this Fig. Where indicated by arrows, 40 nmol $CaCl_2$ (Ca^{2+}), 1 μM ruthenium red (RR) and 15 mM potassium phosphate buffer pH 7 were added. When the effects of a drug was studied, it was added 1 min before the addition of mitochondria.

———, control experiment, no drug was added. – – –, the effect of 200 μM diltiazem. — · · —, the effect of 200 μM dibucaine

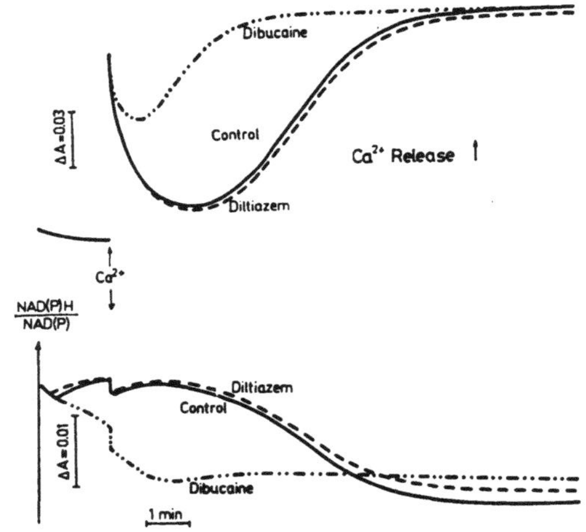

Fig. 3. Effects of diltiazem and dibucaine on the Ca^{2+} release which is related to the oxidation of mitochondrial pyridine nucleotides. The assay medium did not contain glutamate and malate. Upper part, uptake and release of Ca^{2+} as measured by arsenazo III. Lower part, changes in the mitochondrial NAD(P)H/NAD(P) ratio that was measured under identical conditions as the Ca^{2+} transport. Downward deflection corresponds to the oxidation of mitochondrial pyridine nucleotides. Where indicated by arrow 40 nmol $CaCl_2$ (Ca^{2+}) was added. The results of 3 different experiments are superimposed in this Fig.
———, control experiment, no drug was added. – – –, the effect of 200 μM diltiazem. — · · —, the effect of 200 μM dibucaine

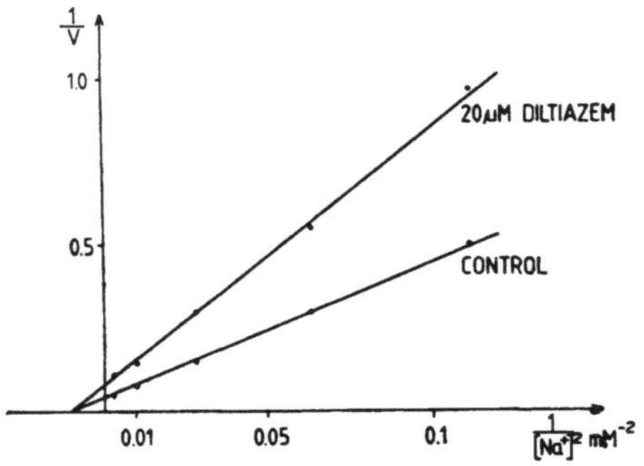

Fig. 4. Effect of diltiazem on the initial rates of Ca^{2+} release induced by different extramitochondrial Na^+ concentrations. Mitochondria were incubated in an assay medium containing 5 mM glutamate plus 5 mM malate, 2.5 $MgCl_2$ and 1 μM ruthenium red. Ca^{2+} release was induced by the addition of different Na^+ concentrations; v is the initial velocity of Ca^{2+} release (nmol $Ca^{2+} \times min^{-1} \times$ mg $protein^{-1}$) at 37 °C

Discussion

It was first demonstrated by CARAFOLI et al. [2] that Na^+ can cause the release of Ca^{2+} from isolated heart mitochondria. Subsequent studies by CROMPTON et al. [5—8] have provided experimental evidence indicating the existence of a Na^+/Ca^{2+} antiporter distinct from the Ca^{2+} uniporter in the mitochondrial inner membrane of excitable tissues. The Ca^{2+} uniporter, which is responsible for Ca^{2+} uptake by mitochondria, can be selectively inhibited by ruthenium red. Several agents have been found recently which inhibit the Na^+-induced Ca^{2+} release from mitochondria without affecting the Ca^{2+} uptake process. It has been demonstrated by DAWSON et al. [9] that local anesthetics like dibucaine and tetracaine are inhibitors of the Ca^{2+} release processes in both rat brain and liver mitochondria. These local anesthetics were, however, unable to produce more than a 70% inhibition of the Ca^{2+} release without inhibiting the Ca^{2+} uptake process. The data presented in this paper show that dibucaine inhibits the inorganic phosphate induced Ca^{2+} release from heart mitochondria which indicates that the effect of this drug is not selective for a particular Ca^{2+} release process. It has been suggested by BEATRICE et al. [1] and PALMER and PFEIFFER [12] that dibucaine, an inhibitor of phospholipase A_2 activity, preserves the integrity of the mitochondrial inner membrane thereby preventing the loss of Ca^{2+} from mitochondria. It is also apparent from this study that dibucaine actually enhances the release of Ca^{2+} from heart mitochondria that is coupled to the oxidation of mitochondrial pyridine nucleotides, provided that the mitochondria are incubated in the absence of oxidizable substrates.

We have recently demonstrated that some Ca^{2+} antagonists like fendiline, prenylamine, nifedipine and verapamil are able to produce a 60% inhibition of the Na^+-induced Ca^{2+} release from heart mitochondria without affecting the Ca^{2+} uptake process, VÁGHY et al. [14]. These Ca^{2+} antagonists appear to act somewhat similarly to local anesthethics. Notwithstanding that, further studies are needed to prove or refuse this possibility.

One Ca^{2+} antagonist drug, diltiazem is different from these compounds with respect to its effectiveness and its selectivity of action on the Na^+-induced Ca^{2+} release process. In the absence of Mg^{2+}, 7 μM diltiazem produces a 50% inhibition of the ruthenium red-insensitive, Na^+-induced Ca^{2+} release process as it has recently been demonstrated by VÁGHY et al. [14]. The kinetic studies presented in this paper indicate that diltiazem is a noncompetitive inhibitor of the Na^+/Ca^{2+} exchange reaction with respect to Na^+. It has previously been demonstrated by VÁGHY et al. [13] that diltiazem concentrations lower than 200 μM have no effect on oxidative phosphorylation of isolated heart mitochondria. This drug does not influence either the respiration dependent Ca^{2+} uptake process or the Ca^{2+} release processes induced by the Ca^{2+} ionophore, A23187, or by the uncoupler, FCCP, VÁGHY et al. [14]. The results presented here demonstrate that diltiazem has no effect on the Ca^{2+} release from heart mitochondria induced either by inorganic phosphate or by the oxidation of mitochondrial pyridine nucleotides. Our data do suggest, however, that diltiazem is a selective inhibitor of the Na^+/Ca^{2+} antiporter in heart mitochondria.

Summary

The effects of diltiazem and dibucaine on the uptake and release of Ca^{2+} by isolated rabbit heart mitochondria were investigated. Neither of these drugs inhibited the Ca^{2+} uptake process at concentrations lower than 200 μM. Inorganic phosphate induced Ca^{2+} release was indibited by dibucaine but not by diltiazem. Ca^{2+} release induced by the oxidation of mitochondrial pyridine nucleotides was stimulated by dibucaine, but was not affected by diltiazem. Since dibucaine is known to inhibit Ca^{2+} release from mitochondria induced by several Ca^{2+} releasing agents including Na^+, it is suggested that this drug does not selectively affect any particular Ca^{2+} release process. On the other hand, diltiazem inhibited only Na^+-induced Ca^{2+} release. Our results indicate that this drug is a selective inhibitor of the Na^+/Ca^{2+} antiporter in heart mitochondria. Our kinetic studies suggest that diltiazem is a noncompetitive inhibitor of Na^+ in the mitochondrial Na^+/Ca^{2+} exchange reaction.

References

[1] Beatrice, M. C., J. W. Palmer and D. R. Pfeiffer: J. Biol. Chem. **255** (1980), 8663–8671
[2] Carafoli, E., R. Tiozzo, G. Lugli, F. Crovetti and C. Kratzing: J. Mol. Cell. Cardiol. **6** (1974), 361–371
[3] Carafoli, E.: In: Membrane Transport of Calcium. (Edited by Carafoli, E.) Academic Press, London (1982), 109–138
[4] Cockrell, R. S.: FEBS Lett. **144** (1982), 279–282
[5] Crompton, M., M. Capano and E. Carafoli: Eur. J. Biochem. **69** (1976), 453–462
[6] Crompton, M., M. Künzi and E. Carafoli: Eur. J. Biochem. **79** (1977), 549–558
[7] Crompton, M., R. Moser, H. Lüdi and E. Carafoli: Eur. J. Biochem. **82** (1978), 25–31
[8] Crompton, M. and I. Heid: Eur. J. Biochem. **91** (1978), 599–608
[9] Dawson, A. P., M. J. Selwyn and D. V. Fulton: Nature **277** (1979), 484–486
[10] Lehninger, A. L., A. Vercesi and E. A. Bababunmi: Proc. Natl. Acad. Sci. U.S.A. **75** (1978), 1690–1694
[11] Lowry, O. H., N. J. Rosebrough, A. L. Farr and R. J. Randall: J. Biol. Chem. **193** (1951), 265–275
[12] Palmer, J. W. and D. R. Pfeiffer: J. Biol. Chem. **256** (1981), 6742–6750
[13] Vághy, P. L., M. A. Matlib, L. Szekeres and A. Schwartz: Biochem. Pharmacol. **30** (1981), 2603–2610
[14] Vághy, P. L., J. D. Johnson, M. A. Matlib, T. Wang and A. Schwartz: J. Biol. Chem. **257** (1982), 6000–6002

Institute of Physiology, Wilhelm-Pieck-University, Rostock, GDR

Rest Versus Frequency Loaded Contractions in the Myocardium of Rats

C. Pfeiffer and Ch. Huckstorf

All changes in the contractile force of myocardial preparations produced by rate and rhythm of the stimulation are due to the excitation-contraction coupling mechanism. Up to now it is not definitely clear what special steps of active or passive movements of the coupling calcium are involved [4]. Recent experimental results, however, show that not only regular short time effects exist of certain changes of the stimulation pattern on the amplitude of the contraction (postextrasystolic potentiation, interval-force relationship e.g.) but there are also evident species differences of these relations. Because of the relativity of all stimulation effects the so called rested-state contraction usually serves as a standard value [2]. The present investigation, therefore, examined the rest contractions in myocardial preparations gained from normal Wistar (NWR) and spontaneously hypertensive rats (SHR).

Methods

Isometric working papillary muscles from the left ventricle of rats were used. The preparations worked for 1 hour in oxygenated Ringer-solution with 1.5 g glucose per liter and Tris-puffer at a stimulation frequency of 30 beats per minute before the contraction rate had been changed. The rectangular stimulation impulses alternating in polarization were applicated by platinum field electrodes. The temperature of the bathing solution was kept at 32°C. With a view to a longer restitution interval after 30 rhythmical beats of 0.5 Hz the stimulation was interrupted during different time periods (0.25 to 200 sec.). The amplitude of the first contraction after the stimulation pause could then be expressed in percent of the previous 0.5 Hz-contractions. The relative contraction values thus obtained were recombined subsequently to a restitution curve [3] extended beyond the duration of the previous contraction interval. Those curves were measured also under 1, 2 and 3 Hz prestimulation rates. For this purpose a short interval of rhythmical high frequency contractions (15—30 beats resp.) was interpolated between the basic 0.5 Hz-phase and the corresponding period of rest.

Results

Measuring phases consisted of 1 minute equilibration at 0.5 Hz stimulation frequency and a period of rest without or with previous high frequency adaptation. The contraction amplitude showed signs of fatigue if the prestimulation frequency exceeded 1 Hz (Fig. 1). At the end of the whole measuring cycle the contraction amplitude amounted to 60% of the starting value. Therefore it seems to be useful to relate all restitution values to the actual previous contraction amplitude at 0.5 Hz.

Under these circumstances extended restitution curves came about having a maximum of 200 to 400% at a resting interval of about 20 sec. (Fig. 2). The amplitudes at the frequency related intervals (0.33 sec. at 3 Hz, 0.5 sec. at 2 Hz, and so on) form part of the interval-force relationship.

If one puts together all maximum values of the restitution curves the arising synopsis of mean values showed that the race of the rats, their age, and the stimulation rate can influence the contraction amplitudes after a rest of 20 sec. (Fig. 3). The statistical significance of this statement is shown in Tables 1 and 2.

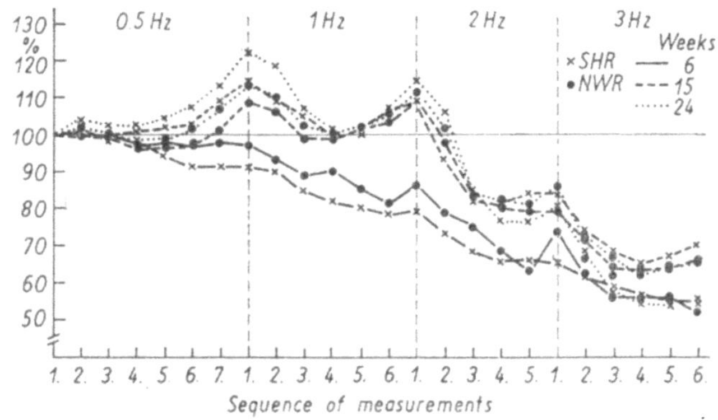

Fig. 1. Fatigue during the application of resting periods of different delay under an increasing basic contraction rate. Spontaneously hypertensive rats (SHR) and normotensive Wistar rats (NWR) of 6—15—24 weeks of age.
n = 11—15

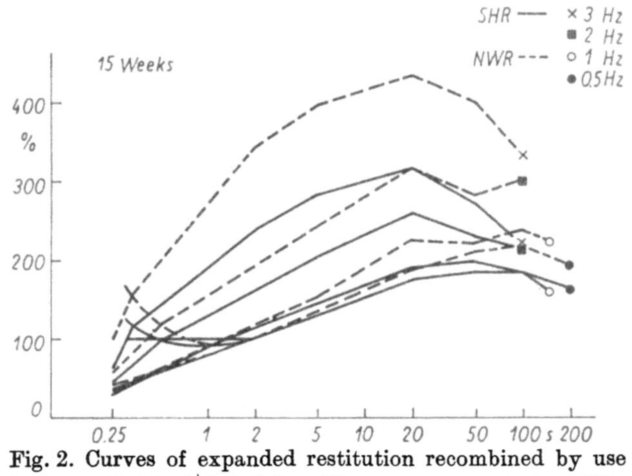

Fig. 2. Curves of expanded restitution recombined by use of rest contractions of different (0.25—200 s) delay. The measurements in SHR and normal Wistar rats started at 4 different stimulation rates (0.5—1—2—3 Hz).
n = 11—15

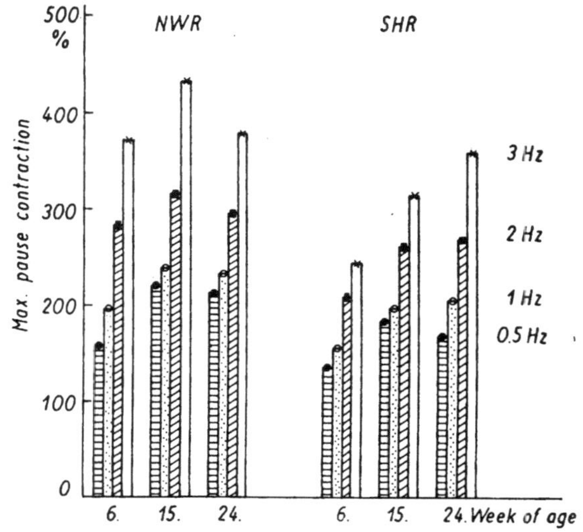

Fig. 3. Maxima of the curves of expanded restitution in NWR and SHR at 4 different basic frequencies and at 3 different ages.

Table 1

Distinctions among the groups of different ages at the 4 used frequencies (Wilcoxon-test for 2 independent assays; $2\alpha = 5\%$)

Weeks of lifetime

Stimulation rate (Hz)	6 vrs. 15	6 vrs. 24	15 vrs. 24	6 vrs. 15	6 vrs. 24	15 vrs. 24
0.5	5	5	—	5	5	—
1	—	—	—	5	5	—
2	—	—	—	—	5	—
3	—	—	—	—	5	—
		NWR			SHR	

Table 2

Distinctions among the groups of different frequencies at the 3 used age-groups (Wilcoxon-test for 2 independent assays; $2\alpha = 5\%$)

Stimulation rate (Hz)

Weeks of lifetime	0.5 vrs. 1	0.5 vrs. 2	0.5 vrs. 3	1 vrs. 2	1 vrs. 3	2 vrs. 3	
6	—	5	5	—	5	—	
15	—	5	5	5	5	5	NWR
24	—	5	5	—	5	—	
6	—	5	5	5	—	—	
15	—	5	5	—	5	—	SHR
24	—	5	5	5	5	5	

Discussion

Frequency tests need a reference value. The rested-state contraction recommended by BLINKS and KOCH-WESER [2], however, can not be used without problems. The rested-state contraction is meant to provide a contraction value that is uninfluenced by the previous contraction rate. But such a value cannot be found in the rat myocardium by using intervals smaller than 200 sec. During these 200 sec. the curve of expanded restitution, recombined by pause-contractions of different intervals, shows a maximum. This maximum is not constant but depends on the previous stimulation rate, the race, and the age of the rats. The existence of a maximum in the restitution curve of the rat ventricle myocardium means that in this case it is not possible to speak of rested state contraction in the proper sense of this term without taking into consideration an interval of at least 200 sec. It is likely that all curves in Figure 2 converge to a contraction amplitude which then could be defined as rested-state contraction. Such a long interval, however, proves to be very inconvenient as a standard. For that reason it seems more practical to use as a reference value (like in our case) a slow rhythmical contraction rate of 0.5 Hz. On the other side the maximum of the restitution of contraction depends significantly on the previous stimulation rate. This correlates with the well known dependence of the velocity of restitution on stimulation frequency [1]. In our opinion the dependence of the above mentioned maximum on the race of the used rats and on their age is a new fact. It shows that the mechanisms of the excitation-contraction coupling are involved in the transformations taking place within the myocardium during the development of hypertension or in the course of aging.

References

[1] BLINKS, J. R. and J. KOCH-WESER: J. Pharmacol. **134** (1961), 373–389
[2] KOCH-WESER, J. and J. R. BLINKS: Pharm. Rev. **15** (1963), 601–652
[3] KRUTA, V. and P. BRAVENY: Arch. int. Physiol. **69** (1961), 645–667
[4] WOHLFART, B.: Acta Physiol. Scand. **106** (1979), 395–409

Julius Bernstein Institute of Physiology, Martin-Luther University Halle-Wittenberg, Halle (Saale), GDR

Influence of Noradrenaline and Caffeine on Potentiation and Staircase Phenomena

WUSSLING, M. and G. SZYMANSKI

Potentiation and staircase phenomena observed on heart muscle preparations of mammalia can be interpreted by transsarcolemmal and intracellular Ca movements [1, 2, 3, 4, 5, 6]. The aim of this study is to elucidate the effects of noradrenaline (NA) and caffeine on these Ca movements.

Figure 1 (panels A, B, C) demonstrates a part of a double rest programme which was shown to be appropriate for testing the "two Ca store hypotheses" [7]. In Figure 1 A is shown evident postextrasystolic potentiation of a r.v. rabbit papillary muscle superfused with Krebs-Henseleit-

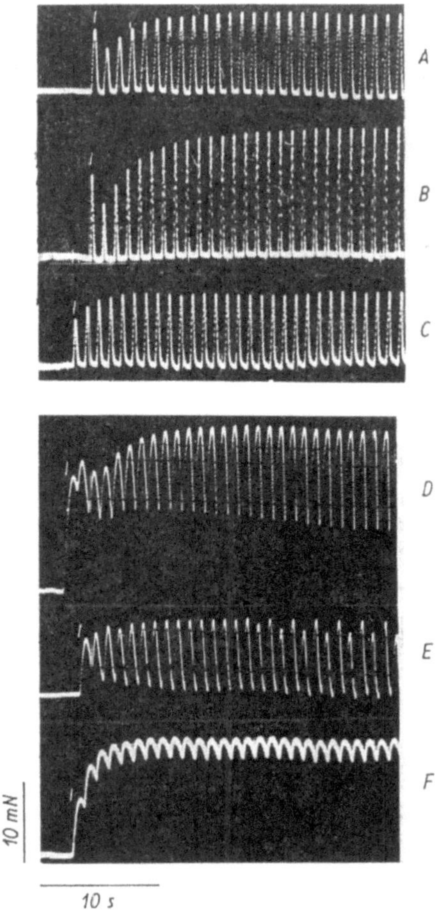

Fig. 1. Isometric contractions of r.v. rabbit papillary muscle, temperature 30 °C, stimulation interval 1 sec.
A (KHS), B (KHS + NA), C (KHS + NA + caffeine); note the effects of extrasystoles and rests
D (KHS), E (KHS + NA + caffeine); note the effects of an extrasystole

solution (KHS) of 30 °C. Figure 1B shows that the positive inotropic effect of NA (3 mg/l) in KHS is accompanied by a decreased potentiation related to the contraction values before rest. The situation is completely changed after the addition of caffeine (1 g/l) to the solution (see Fig. 1C). The absence of every potentiation in this solution can be demonstrated already by a single extrasystole without pause (see Fig. 1E in comparison to Fig. 1D showing potentiation and negative treppe of the preparation in KHS).

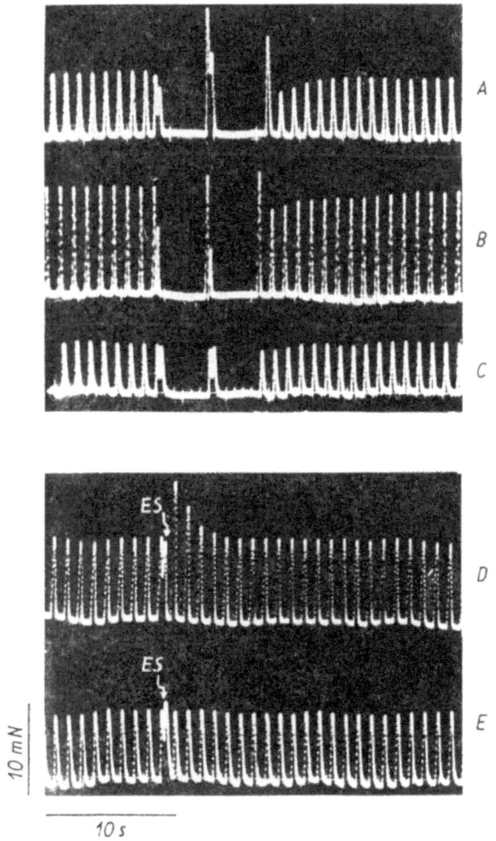

Fig. 2. Staircases of the r.v. rabbit papillary muscle after a rest of 1 minute.
A (KHS), B (KHS + NA), C (KHS + NA + caffeine): 30 °C
D (KHS), E (KHS + NA), F (KHS + NA + caffeine): 18 °C

Examples of staircases after a rest of 1 minute are given in Figure 2. The first beat is called "I" in all registrations. A (KHS), B (KHS + NA), and C (KHS + NA + caffeine) result from papillary muscles at a temperature of 30 °C. It is striking that the staircase in panel C is monotonously. Registrations D, E, F result form A, B, and C, respectively, after lowering the temperature to 18 °C. During the relaxation one can observe diastolic oscillations (aftercontractions) in many cases (not shown in Fig. 2) which disappear in the presence of caffeine. Unpublished laser diffraction studies have demonstrated that the sarcomere length in resting r.a. trabeculae of rabbits is changed by caffeine insignificantly.

The results shall be summarized and interpreted using a three compartment model which can be verified by the hardware analog on the bottom of Figure 3.

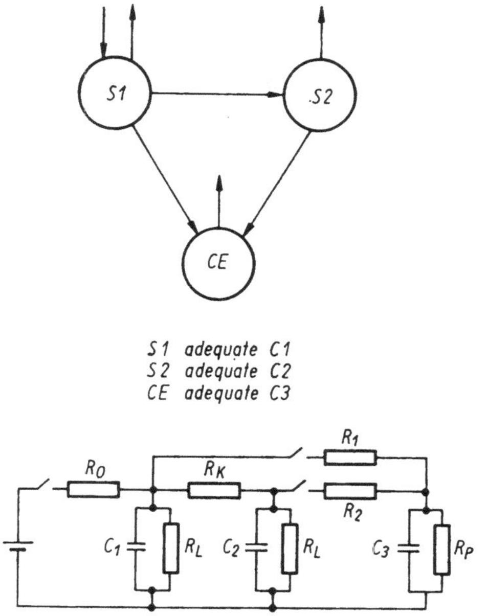

Fig. 3. Scheme indicating supposed Ca movements on the cellular level of the mammalian heart muscle (S_1, S_2 = Ca stores and CE = contractile system) verified by an electrical hardware analog.

1. Potentiation and staircase phenomena are due to the cooperation of Ca stores and the contractile system (S_1, S_2, CE). In the presence of NA potentiation after rest is decreased (hypothesis: influence of S_1 to CE greater than that of S_2). Addition of caffeine leads to total disappearance of potentiation (hypothesis: function of S_2 restricted).
2. At deep temperature staircase phenomena are determined by incomplete relaxation (especially in the presence of caffeine caused by the diminution of the fast Ca sequestration velocity). Caffeine (1 g/l) seems not to prevent the complete relaxation after a long time (caused by the slow Ca sequestration, see [8]).

References

[1] ALLEN, D. G., B. R. JEWELL and E. H. WOOD: J. Physiol. (Lond.) **254** (1976), 1–17
[2] KOESTER, G.: Wiss. Beiträge der Martin-Luther-Universität Halle–Wittenberg **18** (R 61) (1980), 106–116
[3] NAYLER, W. G. and P. GRINWALD: Federation Proc. **40** (1981), 2855–2861
[4] SZYMANSKI, G. and M. WUSSLING: Zool. Jb. Physiol. **82** (1978), 515–529
[5] WOHLFAHRT, B.: Acta Physiol. Scand. **106** (1979), 395–409
[6] WUSSLING, M. and G. SZYMANSKI: studia biophysica (Berlin) **34** (1972), 121–130
[7] WUSSLING, M. and G. SZYMANSKI: Nova Acta Leopoldina, Neue Folge, **211** (1973), 141–173
[8] WUSSLING, M. and G. SZYMANSKI: Acta biol. med. germ. **39** (1980), 583–590

Institute of Pharmacology and Toxicology, Ernst-Moritz-Arndt-University, Greifswald, GDR

Dissociation of Isoproterenol-Induced cAMP-Increase and Vascular Relaxation in Isolated Coronary Arteries under the Influence of DFP

K.-U. Möritz, R. Fermum and U. Tofelde

The biologic roles of cyclic nucleotides in smooth muscle function presently represent a controversial issue. Cyclic AMP is thought to be the second messenger in β-adrenergic relaxation of vascular smooth muscle [2]. On isolated coronary arteries from cattle isoproterenol increased cyclic AMP formation and decreased muscle tension [4, 6]. We tested the hypothesis according that cyclic AMP mediates vasodilation induced by β-adrenergic agents. For this purpose we used diisopropylfluorophosphate (DFP) as a tool, because this substance has been shown to be a potent inhibitor of adenylate cyclase [1].

Experimental procedures

Relaxations studies: Left coronary arterial segments from cattle (Ramus interventricularis anterior) were used for isometric measurement of muscle tension [4].
Adenylate cyclase assay: Adenylate cyclase activity in the particulate fraction ($1000 \times g$) of bovine coronary arteries was determined by measuring the formation of [^{3}H] cyclic AMP from [^{3}H]-ATP [3].
Cyclic AMP formation in vessel segments: The formation of cyclic AMP in incubated vessel segments was measured by pulse-labelling of ATP in the vessel with [8-^{14}C] adenine [7].
Cyclic AMP content: The concentrations of cyclic AMP in coronary artery segments were assayed by the cyclic AMP-binding protein method [5].

Results and discussion

Under the influence of DFP a dissociation between biochemical and relaxing effects of isoproterenol could be observed. The relaxing action of isoproterenol was entirely uneffected by DFP (Fig. 1). In contrast to this finding the stimulatory effects of isoproterenol on adenylate cyclase, cyclic AMP content (not shown) and formation of ^{14}C-cyclic AMP in the intact tissue (not shown) were completly abolished by DFP (Fig. 2).

The results disagree with the opinion according that β-adrenergic relaxation is mediated by cyclic AMP but suggest that isoproterenol induced effects on cAMP system and muscle tension are not connected in series.

Summary

In coronary arteries from cattle isoproterenol stimulates the adenylate cyclase both in the cell free system and in the intact vessel. It increases the cyclic AMP content and decreases muscle tension. Under the influence of DFP, a dissociation between biochemical and relaxing effects can be observed. The biochemical effects are completly prevented and the relaxing properties remain entirely uneffected.

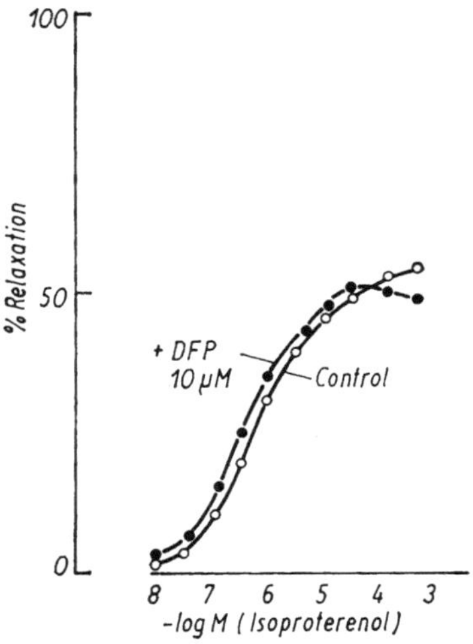

Fig. 1. Change in smooth muscle tension of isolated coronary vessels under the influence of isoproterenol in the presence or absence of DFP (cumulative dose-response curves).

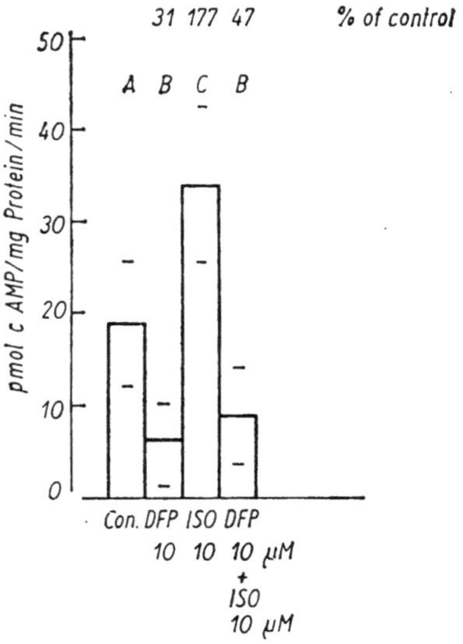

Fig. 2. Influence of DFP on basal and isoproterenol-stimulated activity of adenylate cyclase in the cell-free system. Different letters above columns indicate significant differences.

References

[1] BLEYER, H., K.-U. MÖRITZ and A. GRISK: Acta biol. med. germ. **35** (1976), 87—92
[2] DIAMOND, J. and K. S. BLISARD: Mol. Pharmacol. **12** (1976), 688—692
[3] DRUMMOND, G. I. and L. DUNCAN: J. biol. Chem. **245** (1970), 976—983
[4] FERMUM, R. and K.-U. MÖRITZ: Acta biol. med. germ. **38** (1979), 1211—1223
[5] GILMAN, A. G.: Proc. natl. Acad. Sci. USA **67** (1970), 305—312
[6] GRISK, A., R. FERMUM and K.-U. MÖRITZ: 7. Int. Congr. Pharmacology, Paris 1978
[7] SHIMIZU, H., J. W. DALY and C. R. CREVELING: J. Neurochem. **16** (1969), 1609—1619

Department of Pharmacology and Toxicology, Martin Luther University Halle—Wittenberg, Halle, GDR

Influence of Dietary Linoleate on the Adrenergic Response of Isolated Rat Hearts

P. Hoffmann, P. Mentz and W. Förster

There is good evidence that dietary polyunsaturated fatty acids possess a preventive effect on the development of ischaemic heart disease and hypertension [1, 2]. But little is known about the effectiveness of cardiovascular drugs in conjunction with changes in dietary polyunsaturated fatty acids. Therefore, experiments were carried out in order to gain information on whether the effect of the sympathomimetic isoprenaline on isolated perfused rat hearts can be influenced by diets containing differing amounts of linoleic acids (LA). We chose isoprenaline because recent papers have concerned themselves the links between dietary LA and the activity of the sympathetic nervous system [4]. Furthermore isoprenaline affects *in vitro* prostaglandin (PG) biosynthesis [3].

Methods

Male Wistar rats (100 g) were fed a diet rich in LA (13.3 J% LA; 14 g sunflower oil/100 g dry weight) and a diet deficient in LA (0.5% LA; 14 g hydrogenated palm kernel fat/100 dry weight), respectively, for 10 weeks ad libitum. Diets were complemented by casein (20 g), starch (58 g), and cellulose (5 g). Minerals and vitamins were added in sufficient amounts. Control animals were fed a standard lab chow (3.6% fat, 39,8% of all fatty acids LA). The hearts were quickly excised and perfused according to the Langendorff method at a pressure of 8 k Pa (= 60 Torr) with 310 K (= 37 °C) oxygenated Tyrode solution. Coronary flow rate was measured by photoelectrical drop counting and force of contraction was recorded quasi-isometrically by a stiff displacement transducer.

The concentration of prostaglandin like substances (PLS) in the perfusate was estimated biologically after extraction by means of two rat stomach strips and a rat colon as originally proposed by [5]. The maximum effects of 100 ng isoprenaline (VEB Berlin Chemie) were registered.

Results

The hearts of the rats fed on a diet rich in LA showed compared with LA deficient and pellet fed rats an increase in coronary flow rate and a reduced spontaneous beating frequency (Fig. 1). Force of contraction was insignificantly increased with growing amounts of LA in the diet. From the hearts of the LA rich fed animals distinctly higher amounts of PLS (7.95 ± 1.56 ng/min) were released compared with LA deficient (3.4 ± 0.5 ng/min, $p < 0.05$) and pellet fed rats (3.3 ± 0.8 ng/min, $p < 0.05$).

Compared to the initial values shown in Figure 1 100 ng isoprenaline increased contractile force, heart rate and coronary flow rate in the three dietary groups ($p < 0.01$, Fig. 2). But in the LA rich rats the increase in contractile force and in tendency the increase in heart rate were dimin-

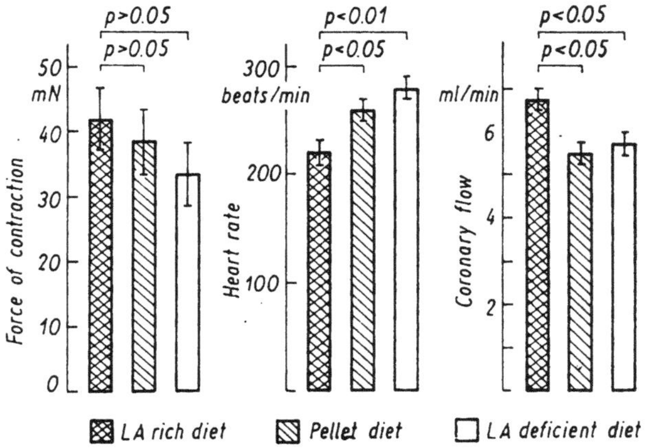

Fig. 1. Influence of dietary linoleic acid (LA) on cardiac function after a ten-week feeding period (n = 10—13).

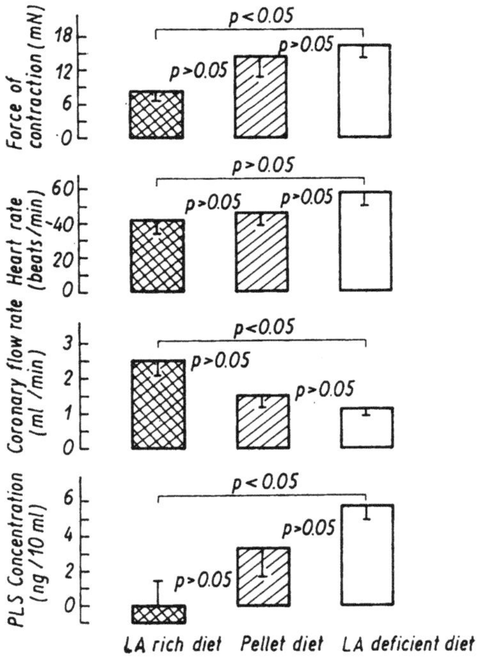

Fig. 2. Increase by 100 ng isoprenaline of the force of contraction, heart rate, and coronary flow rate as well as the effect of isoprenaline on the concentration of prostaglandin like substances (PLS) in the perfusate of isolated rat hearts after ten weeks feeding of diets with different linoleic acid (LA) content (n = 9—14).

ished, whereas the increase in coronary flow was doubled compared with LA deficient rats. Isoprenaline injection caused a marked increase in PLS in the perfusate of LA deficient fed rats ($p < 0.025$, Fig. 2). This effect was weakened in pellet fed rats ($p > 0.05$) and abolished in the LA rich animals.

Discussion

Our results show that different amounts of dietary LA modify not only cardiac functions as described earlier [6, 7], but also the effect of isoprenaline on isolated perfused rat hearts. The mechanism(s) by which dietary LA has these influences is still unknown. Effects on cardiac β-adrenoceptors, alterations of biological membranes, modifications of intracellular transmission systems (e.g. adenylate cyclase, PG system), influences on isoprenaline inactivation as well as interactions with intramural catecholamines could play a role.

References

[1] LEREN, P.: Acta Med. Scand. **466** (Suppl.) (1966), 1–6
[2] HOFFMANN, P. and W. FÖRSTER: Adv. Lipid Res. **18** (1981), 203–227
[3] FÖRSTER, W.: Beiträge zur Wirkstofforschung 6, Akademie-Industrie-Komplex Arzneimittelforschung, Berlin (1979), 61
[4] HOFFMANN, P., Ch. TAUBE, K. PÖNICKE, W. FÖRSTER, L. SOMOVA, V. ORBETZOVA and D. KIPROV: Naunyn-Schmiedebergs Arch. Pharmacol. (1981), 317, 78–80
[5] VANE, J. R.: Br. J. Pharmacol. 23 (1964), 360–373
[6] DE DECKERE, E. A. M. and F. TEN HOOR: Nutr. metabol. 24 (1980), 396–408
[7] HOFFMANN, P., P. MENTZ and W. FÖRSTER: J. Molec. Cell. Cardiol. **9** (Suppl.) (1977), 36

Institute of Physiological Chemistry, Medical Academy, Magdeburg, GDR

Importance of Mitochondrial Creatine Kinase Localization for Securing the Stimulation of Mitochondrial ATP-Production

F. N. GELLERICH and M. SCHLAME

Introduction

Recently it was shown by GELLERICH, BOHNENSACK and KUNZ [2] that the amount of control exerting the adenine nucleotide translocator on the respiration rate [1, 5] depends on the complexity of the metabolic system. Investigations on the importance of mitochondrial creatine kinase for mitochondrial respiration should therefore include a second ATP-producing reaction simulating the glycolytic ATP formation. GOSALVEZ et al. [4] and GELLERICH et al. [2] have shown for rat liver mitochondria that muscle pyruvate kinase/phosphoenolpyruvate is suitable to adjust stationary states of respiration in the presence of hexokinase. In this communication evidences are presented showing the usefulness of this alternative ATP-regenerating system for adjusting stationary states of creatine kinase or hexokinase stimulated respiration of heart mitochondria. The recently published effect that mitochondrial creatine kinase is able to stimulate the mitochondrial respiration even in the presence of a high exess of pyruvate kinase [3] is confirmed here with a more exact measurement of mitochondrial respiration by means of rate meter and metabolite determinations.

Materials and methods

Rat heart mitochondria were isolated as described earlier by SAKS et al. [3]. The rates of respiration were measured using a closed Clark-type electrode and a rate meter.

Incubation medium: 0.25 M sucrose, 10 mM HEPES, pH 7.4, 3 mM Mg-acetate, 0.37 mM dithiothreitol, 4 mM potassium phosphate, 0.3 mM EGTA, 5 mM PEP, 0.1 or 10% bovine serum albumin, 4 mM glutamate, 2 mM malate and either 25 mM creatine or 10 mM glucose.

Results and discussion

Experiments shown in Figure 1 and 2 demonstrate the possibility to adjust all stationary states of respiration between state 3 and state 4 by variation of the relative activities of pyruvate kinase and creatine kinase or hexokinase. Without creatine (Fig. 1) it is even possible to adjust rates of respiration which are comparable to that obtained after inhibition of the adenine nucleotide translocator with carboxyatractyloside. The reason is the virtual high state 4 respiration which is caused by extramitochondrial ATPase present in most preparations of heart mitochondria. Additions of exceeding amounts of pyruvate kinase completely suppress both ATPase and hexokinase stimulated respiration. Pyruvate kinase however is not able to suppress the mitochondrial creatine kinase stimulated respiration completely (Fig. 2 and Table 1). Whereas yeast hexokinase is localized in the bulk phase together with pyruvate kinase, the mitochondrial creatine kinase is bound at the outer side of mitochondrial inner membrane and seems to generate a compartmentation of ADP between the space near the adenine nucleotide translocator and the bulk phase, resulting in a privileged

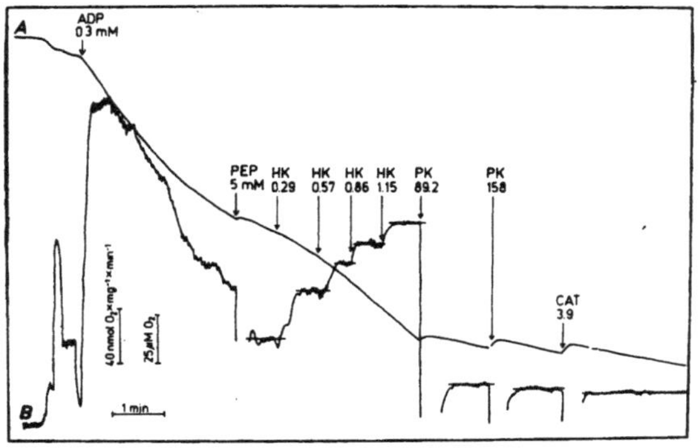

Fig. 1. Stimulation of mitochondrial respiration by yeast hexokinase and its complete repression by pyruvate kinase.
Incubation of rat heart mitochondria (0.3 mg protein/ml) in standard medium without creatine. Stationary states of respiration were adjusted by additions of yeast hexokinase [HK (I.U./mg protein)]. Addition of pyruvate kinase [PK (I.U./mg protein)] decreases respiration velocity at 34 nmol O_2/mg protein · min and the following inhibition by carboxyatractyloside [CAT (nmol/mg protein)] does not change the respiration rate significantly.

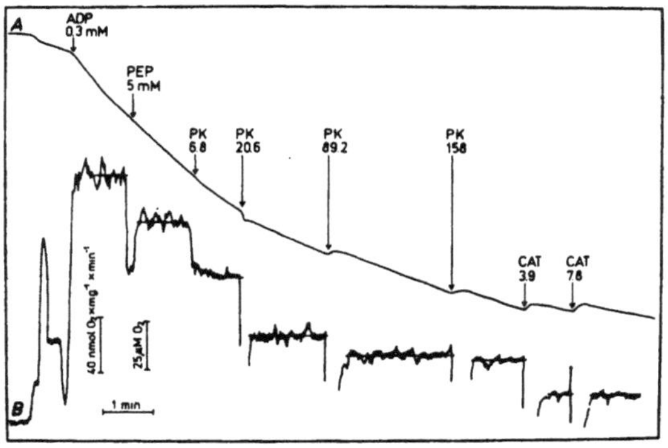

Fig. 2. Limited ability of pyruvate kinase to repress creatine kinase stimulated mitochondrial respiration.
In a parallel experiment to that shown in Fig. 1 mitochondria were incubated in the presence of 25 mM creatine. The creatine kinase stimulated respiration (157 nmol O_2/mg protein · min) comparable to that adjusted with hexokinase in Fig. 1, is decreased at 55.5 nmol O_2/mg protein · min by the same activity of pyruvate kinase as in Fig. 1. Consequently the addition of carboxyatractyloside leads to a further inhibition of respiratory rate at 31 nmol O_2/mg protein · min.

supply of oxidative phosphorylation with ADP. This conclusion is further supported by the results shown in Table 1. Hexokinase stimulates the mitochondrial respiration in the presence of pyruvate kinase at 28.5 nmol O_2/mg · min, whereas creatine kinase with the half of this activity is sufficient for stimulating the respiration at 75.5 nmol O_2/mg · min. Hexokinase in the same compartment as pyruvate kinase mostly use ATP generated by the pyruvate kinase reaction and not by the oxidative phosphorylation as it is indicated by a respiratory rate near to that after inhibition with carboxyatractyloside. Mitochondrial localization of creatine kinase ensures the use of mitochondrial ATP by creatine kinase also at extrem conditions in the presence of high activities of extramitochondrial ATP generating capacity. These results are in line with the hypothesis of energy channeling from heart mitochondria into cytoplasm via creatine kinase [6]. The mechanism of this compartmentation, however, has to be analysed in further investigations.

Table 1

Stationary rates of mitochondrial respiration and fluxes of ATP consuming reactions in the presence of exceeding activities of pyruvate kinase (109 I.U./mg protein) of one representative experiment

Incubation of rat heart mitochondria (0.5 mg protein/ml) in standard medium containing 10% bovine serum albumin. 5 minutes after starting the reactions with 0.3 mM adenine nucleotides two samples were withdrawn for determinations of metabolites. The state 3 and the carboxyatractyloside inhibited respiratory rates were 122 and 26 nmol O_2/mg protein · min respectively. Values in nmol O_2, G-6-P or CP/mg protein · min

Respiration stimulated by:	Respiratory rate	Formation of G-6-P	Formation of CP
Yeast hexokinase	28.5	584 ± 24	–
Mitochondrial creatine kinase	75.5	–	279 ± 21
Yeast hexokinase plus mitochondrial creatine kinase	80.0	633 ± 21	321 ± 23

References

[1] Davis, E. J. and L. Lumeng: J. Biol. Chem. **250** (1975), 2275–2282

[2] Gellerich, F. N., R. Bohnensack and W. Kunz: Biochim. Biophys. Acta submitted (1982)

[3] Gellerich, F. N. and V. A. Saks: Biochem. Biophys. Res. Commun. **105** (1982), 1473–1481

[4] Gosalvez, M., J. Perez-Garcia and S. Weinhouse: Eur. J. Biochem. **46** (1974), 133–140

[5] Kunz, W., R. Bohnensack, G. Böhme, U. Küster, G. Letko and P. Schönfeld: Arch. Biochim. Biophys. **209** (1981), 219–229

[6] Saks, V. A., V. V. Kuprianov, V. G. V. Elizarova and W. E. Jacobus: J. Biol. Chem. **255** (1980), 755–763

Institute of Physiological and Biological Chemistry,[1] and Clinic of Surgery, Cardiovasc. Division, Faculty of Medicine, Humboldt-University Berlin, GDR

Metabolic Pattern in the Reperfusion Period of Different Cardiovascular Operations in the Coronary Sinus

G. GOLA,[1] K. KOTHE,[1] K. F. LINDENAU, A. LUN, H. WARNKE and C. WAGENKNECHT[1]

The estimation and prevention of myocardial damage caused by cardiovascular operations is up to now one of the problems in cardiac surgery.

The aim of this investigation was to test,

1. if the degree of alteration of the myocardial metabolism has a reflexion in the metabolite profile of the coronary sinus blood
2. if there exists a dependence of the metabolite profiles on the basic disease.

Inhomogenous distribution of cardioplegic solutions with following inadaequate myocardial protection in the poststenotic areas and bad preoperative conditions, i.e. the severe impaired hemodynamic function of the myocardium with the tendency to negative energy balances are discussed as causes of the myocardial damage, which begins in the reperfusion period. Therefore the arterio-venous differences of lactate, pyruvate, hypoxanthine, K^+, and Ca^{2+} were measured arterially before unclamping the aorta and in the arterial and the coronary sinus blood after unclamping after 1, 3, 5, 10 and 15 min. The data were compared with the postoperative clinical course. Also we looked for the relation between the obtained metabolic data and the preoperative invasive parameters, i.e. the stage of sclerosis and asynergy, decreased ejection fraction, massive hypertrophy and valvar pressure gradients.

Complete data were available in 25 patients. Out of the control group of congenital septal atrial defects, where the heart was not clamped out, all patients had a multidose cardioplegia (after the Buckberg formula).

Lactate and hypoxanthine were the parameters with characteristic changes.

In the control group (5 patients) only slight decreases of lactate extraction in some cases occured, hypoxanthine levels were normal or slightly elevated. In contrast we considered in patients with aorto-coronary veine bypass operations (ACVB) and with prothetic valve replacement (VR) individuell very different profiles which possibly reflect the extent of myocardial metabolic alteration.

The comparison of the lactate and hypoxanthine curves showed, that the effect of total ischaemia on myocardial metabolism in bypass patients even in cases with high sclerosis stages are less pronounced than in VR patients. In Figures 1 and 2 the time course of the metabolites is shown. Patients with cross clamp times over 60 min have over the whole period a higher lactate release; patients with cross clamp times under 60 min tend to normalize early. In the latter group are only bypass patients. The differences are important in the first minute. The hypoxanthine profiles are in coincidence with the lactate curves.

The more pronounced release of lactate and hypoxanthine is not only a function of the longer cross clamp times in these patients — by comparing the ACVB patients and the VR patients in the group with cross clamp times over 60 min one can show, that the VR patients have higher arterial and venous hypoxanthine concentrations and a more negative lactate extraction (Fig. 3). We believe, that the cause for the higher arterial and venous hypoxanthine concentration and

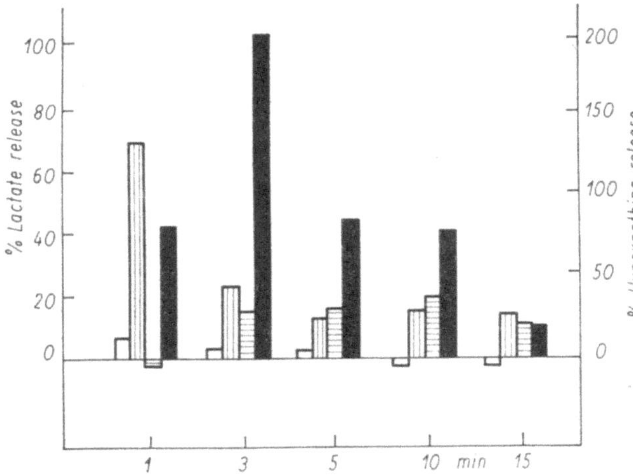

Fig. 1. Comparison of the lactate and hypoxanthine release in the time course of patients with different cross clamp times.
Cross clamp time: lactate □ < 60 min, ▥ > 60 min; hypoxanthine ▤ < 60 min, ■ > 60 min; means ± S.E.M.

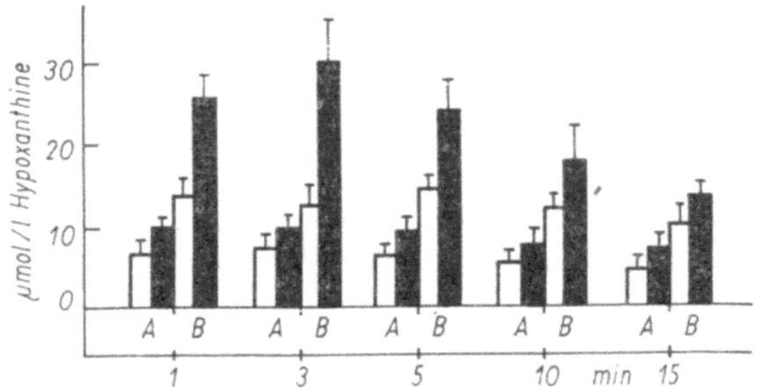

Fig. 2. Comparison of the arterial and venous hypoxanthine concentrations in patients with different cross clamp times. Cross clamp times:
< 60 min: Group A; > 60 mib: Group B. □ arterial, ■ venous; means ± S.E.M.

release of metabolites is the impaired hemodynamic function of our patients with VR. The occurence of massive hypertrophy and generalised hypokinesia as the result of the chronic functional overload causes the restriction of the myocardial function and energy reserves in the reperfusion period and the greater loss of metabolites. We could not demonstrate an influence of the sclerosis stage on the metabolite release in the bypass patient group, indicating that distribution disturbances of the cardioplegic solution are of less importence for the pathogenesis of perioperative myocardial ischaemia.

The comparison of patients with and without hypokinesia showed, that patients with generalized hypokinesia have higher arterial and venous hypoxanthine levels and a delayed normalization of the lactate extraction. Whereas the maximal hypoxanthine liberation in the latter group was over 220%, the liberation rate in patients without generalized hypokinesia was 110%. (Table 1)

In this study the mechanical work of the myocardium in the reperfusion period was not measured — but the mechanical support of the extracorporal circulation may influence the myocardial energy bilance. Allthough in all patients the metabolic peak was seen within the first ten minutes, it is possible, that with the onset of the full mechanical activity drastic changes in the energy

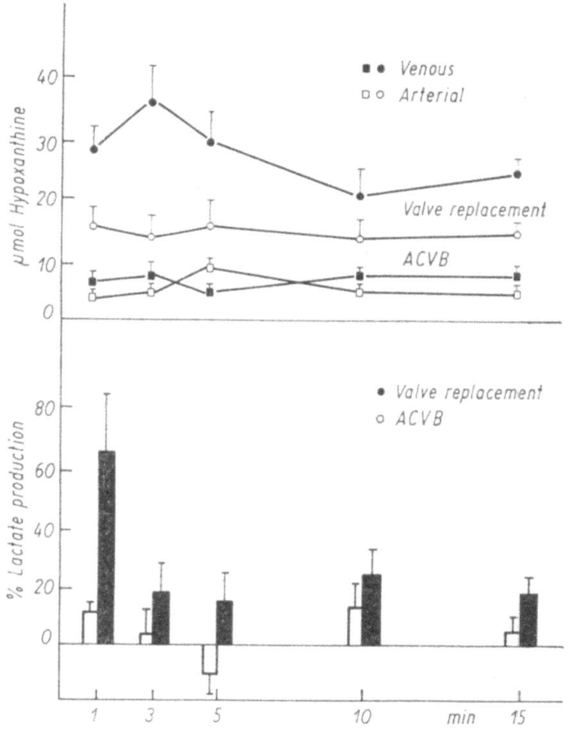

Fig. 3. Hypoxanthine concentrations and lactate release in patients with cross clamp times larger than 60 min.

Table 1

Comparison of the lactate release and the hypoxanthine levels of patients with and without generalised hypokinesia (all data are means)

Generalized hypokinesia	% Lactate extraction 1′	3′	5′	10′	15′
+	−48	−25	−18	−16	−11
−	−84	+13	+1	−2	+4
	art./ven. Hypoxanthine level (µmol/l)				
+	17/27	15/40	17/35	13/25	12/14
−	8/22	6/22	8/13	7/7	7/8

balance may occur. This can be a possible cause for the circumstance,that only a part of our patients showed a relation between the intraoperative metabolite profile and the perioperative clinical course. In these cases the high metabolites have their reflexion in high enzyme activities, which begun to arise already in the reperfusion period, longer phases of hypotension and cardiac insufficiency.

Central Institute of Heart and Circulation Research, Academy of Sciences of the GDR, 1115 Berlin-Buch, GDR

Closing Remarks

A. WOLLENBERGER

Our Symposium is now coming to an end and it is up to me to say a few closing words. First of all, let me extend my heartfelt thanks to all of you here who have participated in this meeting and made it a success and a highly stimulating affair. Particular thanks I owe, together with my colleagues from Berlin-Buch, to those participants who have taken the trouble to come to Berlin from afar. And I think I can speak in the name of all participants, if I express our feelings of gratitude to the members of the Organizing Committee and their helpers, whose diligent work has made it possible that this meeting could proceed smoothly. A personal word of thanks I wish to address to those of you who have wished me well on my 70th birthday, who have presented me with beautiful gifts, and who have said kind words to me. I feel deeply touched by these signs and manifestations of kindness and affection. At the same time I feel greatly honored by having my name associated with this important symposium. Albert EINSTEIN, with whom I had quite a few conversations on the occasions of my staying as a guest in his house in Princeton, once said that birthdays are something for children. Indeed, the fact that my birthday happened to provide a reason for launching this symposium makes me feel happy like a child.

About a year and a half ago, before there was any thought of holding this symposium, I was approached by two of the members of its present scientific board who asked me, whether I would consent to have what we in German call a "Festschrift" dedicated to me in honor of my 70th birthday. I briefly thought it over and then replied, in free English transliteration: "No, thank you. Fest me no Schrift!". Thereupon the idea was born of organizing this symposium. In connection with my birthday a lot of praise has been heaped upon me and I have heard many flattering statements about my work. However, I think it would perhaps have been more useful and instructive, particularly to the young people who had to listen to all the eulogy, if somebody had also pointed out the errors that I have committed in the course of my career and the failures for which I could be blamed. Of course, such frankness would have been contrary to etiquette.

Being not restricted by considerations of this sort may I be allowed to take a minute of your time to relate to you one such case of failure of which I was reminded today by a poster shown downstairs by my good friend Mitja RAPOPORT and his collaborator Miss ZIMMERMANN. In this poster, which is entitled "Ouabain-induced alterations of brain and heart cells", one discerns results that are very similar to those reported in a paper of mine [8] in 1947. (Nineteen forty-seven, i.e. 35 years ago — exactly point of half-life!) My paper, like the just-mentioned poster, dealt with experiments in which the respiration of heart and brain tissue was measured under the influence of the cardiac glycoside ouabain. Most of the work was done with tissue slices, but a few experiments were also conducted with diluted homogenates. Two findings which in my paper were mentioned only in passing were (a) that homogenates of brain (cerebral cortex of guinea pigs) that had been prepared in buffer containing 100 mM NaCl, K^+ ions being present in a concentration of 14 mM, respired at a considerably higher rate than did homogenates that had been prepared in low sodium medium, i.e. without addition of Na^+ ions, and (b) that the increment in the rate of oxygen uptake due to Na^+ was abolished by ouabain. Today one would have no difficulty in finding a correct explanation of these results. The higher tissue respiration due to Na^+ can be attributed to activation of Na^+, K^+-ATPase, with resulting increases in the concentration of the breakdown products of ATP, namely ADP and orthophosphate, both of which are regulators of mitochondrial oxygen consumption. In the same vein the inhibition of the Na^+-dependent O_2 uptake of the brain homogenates by ouabain can be traced to the inhibitory action of the cardiac glycoside on $Na^+ + K^+$-activated splitting of ATP. In fact, in 1964 WHITTAM and BLOND [7] published a curve showing a strictly linear correlation between the rate of ATP breakdown and the rate of O_2 uptake in brain homogenates at different concentrations of ouabain. But in 1947 Na^+, K^+-ATPase had not yet been discovered and I was influenced in the interpretation of my findings by a prominent Canadian biochemist, K.A.C. ELLIOTT from McGill University, whom I had met in April 1947 at a Federation Meeting in Chicago, two months before my 1947 paper was submitted for publication, and according to whom homogenization of brain tissue in solutions rich in Na^+ minimized cytolysis [1]. So I concluded that intactness of the cell architecture was essential to the observed inhibitory effect of ouabain on tissue respiration and that in brain homogenates prepared in high Na^+ buffer this effect was exerted on cells not disrupted by the homogenization process.

Although there had been hints in the pre-war literature that phosphate acceptors and orthophosphate may exert a determining influence on the rate of cellular oxygen consumption, it was not until the early fifties that more convincing evidence for a pace-setting role of ADP and orthophosphate in cellular respiration was forthcoming [3]. A paper by Henry MCILWAIN [4], the renowned British neurochemist, called attention to the fact that brain tissue was not an exception to this rule. In the spring of 1953, after having kept away for a while from the area of cellular energy metabolism, I came to London to work in the laboratory of MCILWAIN on the respiratory metabolism of electrically stimulated brain cortex tissue [9]. This was a golden opportunity to look again at my older data on the respiratory responses of brain homogenates to Na^+ and ouabain and to consider them in the light of the new concept of the control of cellular respiration by the products of ATPase activity. But for one reason or the other I let this opportunity pass by which so easily could have led me to the recognition of the existence of a glycoside-sensitive, Na^+ plus K^+-activated ATPase. The enzyme was discovered 4 years later, in 1957, in crab nerve by SKOU [6].

I am not the only one who missed discovering Na^+, K^+-ATPase. Efraim RACKER [5], in a volume dedicated to Severo OCHOA, recounts how the same misfortune happened to him, at a time when he, too, was working with brain homogenates. To find myself in such distinguished company is at least a consolation. Anyhow, that is the way it can go in science when you are loaded with preconceived notions and do not have a completely open mind. So much in the way of reminiscing and of supplementing my scientific biography.

Let me just make another, brief comment in connection with this symposium. During the last two days we have dealt both with fundamental problems of the regulation of the heart and with the application of basic knowledge to the study of cardiac disease — specifically ischaemic heart disease —, focussing on the myocardium. This dichotomy of attention is well in line with the general research policy of our group in Berlin-Buch ever since it was founded in 1956 and, I think, also with the research programs of similar groups elsewhere, some of which my collaborators and I have the pleasure to see represented here at this meeting. There is no reason to apologize for this division of interest. After all, working in the field of molecular and cellular cardiology and earning a living that way one has a moral obligation to pay close attention to the needs and demands of the clinic. In Berlin-Buch our emphasis had at times been on basic and at other times on applied research and over the years we have been quite happily oscillating in this way in our research activities. We have been preoccupied, too, with other types of oscillations, such as oscillations of glycolytic intermediates in the heart during the aerobic-anaerobic transition [2] and oscillations of myocardial cyclic nucleotide levels during the cardiac contraction cycle [10]. But this is another story.

I trust that everyone in this audience will agree with me if I state that this symposium has fully achieved its aim, namely, fruitful scientific exchange and the establishment and strengthening of ties of friendship among the participants from different countries. We shall return from here to our laboratories more convinced than we were before that molecular and cellular cardiology will for the foreseeable future remain a fertile field of research.

Nineteen eighty-two being a Goethe Year, the 150th year after his death, let me close by quoting from this greatest of German writers. Goethe once said: "Das sicherste Mittel, ein freundliches Verhältnis zu hegen und zu erhalten, finde ich darin, daß man sich wechselseitig mitteile, was man tut." In my English translation this quotation reads: "I find that the surest means to cherish and keep up an amicable relationship is to inform the other side what one is doing." Is this not a good characterization of our Symposium? Thank you again and good luck to everybody.

References

[1] ELLIOTT, K. A. C. and B. LIBET: On the metabolism of brain suspensions. I. Oxygen uptake. J. Biol. Chem. **143** (1942), 227—246.

[2] KRAUSE, E.-G. and A. WOLLENBERGER: Oszillierende Glykolyse im ischämischen Herzmuskel. Stud. Biophys. **1** (1966), 79—82.

[3] LARDY, H. A. and H. WELLMAN: Oxidative phosphorylation: Role of inorganic phosphate and acceptor systems in control of metabolic rates. J. Biol. Chem. **195** (1952), 215—224.

[4] MCILWAIN, H.: Phosphates and nucleotides of the central nervous system. In: Biochemical Symposia No. 8, Metabolism and Function in Nervous Tissue, pp. 27—43, At the University Press, Cambridge, 1952.

[5] RACKER, E.: A pathway from psychiatry to cancer. In: Reflections on Biochemistry, ed. by A. Kornberg, B. L. Horecker, L. Cornudella, and J. Oro, pp. 39—44, Pergamon Press, Oxford, 1976.

[6] SKOU, J. C.: The influence of some cations on an adenosine triphosphatase from peripheral nerve. Biochim. Biophys. Acta **23** (1957), 394—401.

[7] WHITTAM, R. and D. M. BLOND: Respiratory control by an adenosine triphosphatase involved in active transport in brain cortex. Biochem. J. **92** (1964), 147—158.

[8] WOLLENBERGER, A.: Metabolic action of the cardiac glycosides. I. Influence on respiration of heart muscle and brain cortex. J. Pharmacol. Exp Ther. **91** (1947), 39–51.
[9] WOLLENBERGER, A.: Action of protroveratrine on the metabolism of cerebral cortex. 2. Electrically stimulated cerebral-cortex tissue. Biochem. J. **61** (1955), 77–80.
[10] WOLLENBERGER, A., E. B. BABSKII, E.-G. KRAUSE, S. GENZ, D. BLOHM and E. V. BOGDANOVA: Cyclic changes in levels of cyclic AMP and cyclic GMP in frog myocardium during the cardiac cycle. Biochem. Biophys. Res. Commun. **55** (1973), 446–452.

List of contributors

BARTEL, S.: Central Institute of Heart and Circulation Research, Acad. Sci. GDR, 1115 Berlin-Buch, GDR

BLASIG, I. E.: Institute of Drug Research, Academy of Sciences of the GDR, 1136 Berlin, GDR

BRASELMANN, H.: Humboldt-University Berlin, Charité, Institute of Pathology, Cardiological Res. Group, 1040 Berlin, GDR

CAFFIER, G.: Humboldt-University, Berlin, Institute of Physiology, 1040 Berlin, GDR

CARAFOLI, E.: Swiss Federal Institute of Technology (ETH), Laboratory of Biochemistry, 8092 Zürich, Switzerland

DHALLA, N. S.: University of Manitoba, Faculty of Medicine, Department of Physiology, Laboratorium of Experimental Cardiology, Winnipeg, Manitoba R3E OW3, Canada

ENGLAND, P. J.: University of Bristol, Department of Biochemistry Bristol BS8 1TD, England

FERRARI, R.: University of Parma, Faculty of Medicine and Surgery, Dept. Cardiology, I-43100 Parma, Italy

FÖRSTER, W.: Martin-Luther-University, Halle, Institute of Pharmacology, 4020 Halle, GDR

GELLERICH, F.-N.: Med. Acad. Magdeburg, Institute of Physiological Chemistry, 3000 Magdeburg, GDR

GOLA, G.: Inst. of Physiol. and Biol. Chemistry, Clinic of Surgery, Cardiovasc. Division, Faculty of Medicine, Humboldt-University Berlin, GDR

GOOS, H.: Humboldt-University of Berlin, Med. Fac. Charité, Dept. Internal Medicine, 1040 Berlin, GDR

GROSSE, R.: Central Institute of Molecular Biology, Academy of Sciences of the GDR, 1115 Berlin-Buch, GDR

GUDBJARNASON, S.: University of Iceland, Science Institute, IS-107 Reykjavik, Iceland

GÜNTHER, J.: Humboldt-University, Berlin, Institute of Pharmacology, 1040 Berlin, GDR

HERING, S.: Central Institute of Heart and Circulation Research, Academy of Sciences of the GDR, Berlin-Buch, GDR

HERRMANN, H. J.: Central Institute of Heart and Circulation Research, Acad. Sci. GDR, 1115 Berlin-Buch, GDR

HOFFMANN, P.: Martin-Luther-University Halle, Institute of Pharmacology and Toxicology, 4020 Halle, GDR

Holtzhauer, M.: Central Institute of Heart and Circulation Research, Acad. Sci. GDR, 1115 Berlin-Buch, GDR

HYNIE, S.: Charles University Prague, Institute of Pharmacology, CS-12800 Praha, CSSR

KAMMERMEIER, H.: Technical University, Med. Fac., Dept. Physiology, D-5100 Aachen, FRG

KRAUSE, E.-G.: Central Institute of Heart and Circulation Research, Academy of Sciences of the GDR, 1115 Berlin-Buch, GDR

KURSKY, M. D.: A. V. Paladin Institute of Biochemistry, Academy of Sciences of the Ukrainian SSR, Kiev, USSR
LAMERS, J. M.: Erasmus University Rotterdam, Medical Faculty, Department of Biochemistry I, 300 DR Rotterdam, The Netherlands
LEHMANN, I.: Humboldt University Berlin, Charité, Institute of Physiological and Biological Chemistry, 1040 Berlin, GDR
LEVITSKY, D.: USSR Cardiology Research Center, Institute of Experimental Cardiology, Moscow, USSR
LÖWE, H.: Institute of Drug Research, Academy of Sciences of the GDR, 1136 Berlin, GDR
MEERSON, F. Z.: Acad. Med. Sci. USSR, Institute of General Pathology and Pathophysiology, Lab. Pathophysiol. of the Heart, Moscow, USSR
METSÄ-KETELÄ, T.: University of Tampere, Dept, Biomedical Sciences, SF-33101 Tampere 10, Finland
MONTFOORT, A.: Erasmus University Rotterdam, Dept. Exp. Pathology, 3000 DR Rotterdam, The Netherlands
MÖRITZ, K.-U.: Ernst Moritz-Arndt University Greifswald, Institute of Pharmacology and Toxicology, 2200 Greifswald, GDR
MOSINGER, S.: Institute of Clinical and Experimental Medicine, 14622 Prague, 4, CSSR
NILIUS, B.: Martin Luther University of Halle, Julius Bernstein-Institute of Physiology, 4020 Halle, GDR
OŠTÀDAL, B.: Institute of Physiology, Czechoslovak Academy of Sciences, Prague, CSSR
PANAGIA, V.: Experimental Cardiology Section, Department of Physiology, Faculty of Medicine, University of Manitoba, Winnipeg, Canada R3E OW3
PELOUCH, V.: Institute of Physiology, Czechoslovak Academy of Sciences, Prague, CSSR
PFEIFFER, C. H.: Wilhelm-Pieck University Rostock, Institute of Physiology, 2500 Rostock, GDR
POGÁTSA, G.: National Institute of Cardiology, H-1450 Budapest, Hungary
PORZIG, H.: University Bern, Dept. Pharmacology, CH-3008 Bern, Switzerland
RABITZSCH, G.: Central Institute of Heart and Circulation Research, Acad. Sci. GDR, 1115 Berlin-Buch, GDR
RAPOPORT, S. M.: Humboldt-University Berlin, Institute of Physiological and Biological Chemistry, 1040 Berlin, GDR
SAKS, V. M.: USSR Cardiology Research Center, Institute of Experimental Cardiology, Moscow, USSR
SCHIRPKE, B.: Central Institute of Heart and Circulation Research, Acad. Sci. GDR, 1115 Berlin-Buch, GDR
SCHOLZ, H.: University Hospital Eppendorf, Division of General Pharmacology, D-2000 Hamburg 20, FRG
SCHÖNFELD, P.: Medical Academy Magdeburg, Institute of Physiological Chemistry, 3000 Magdeburg, GDR
SCHULZE, W.: Central Institute of Heart and Circulation Research, Acad. Sci. GDR, 1115 Berlin-Buch, GDR
SUKO, J.: Institute of Pharmacology, University of Vienna, A-1090 Vienna, Austria
SWYNGHEDAUW, B.: I.N.S.E.R.M., Unité 127, Hospital Lariborisiére, 75010 Paris; France
SZEKERES, L.: University, Med. School of Szeged, Institute of Pharmacology, H-6701 Szeged/ Hungary
TAKATS, I.: University Medical School of Szeged, Institute of Pharmacology, 6701 Szeged, Hungary
TITLBACH, O.: Karl-Marx-University Leipzig, Medical Clinic, 7010 Leipzig, GDR
VÁGHY, P. L.: University Med. School of Szeged, Institute of Pharmacology, H-6701 Szeged, Hungary
VETTER, R.: Humboldt-University, Berlin, Institute of Physiology, 1040 Berlin, GDR

WALLUKAT, G.: Central Institute of Heart and Circulation Research, Acad. Sci. GDR, 1115 Berlin-Buch, GDR
WETZKER, R.: Friedrich-Schiller-University, Jena, Institute of Physiological Chemistry, 6900 Jena, GDR
WILL, H.: Central Institute of Heart and Circulation Research, Academy of Sciences of the GDR, 1115 Berlin-Buch, GDR
WILL-SHAHAB, L.: Central Institute of Heart and Circulation Research, Acad. Sci. GDR, 1115 Berlin-Buch, GDR
WOLLENBERGER, A.: Central Institute of Heart and Circulation Research, Acad. Sci. GDR, 1115 Berlin-Buch, GDR
WUSSLING, M.: Martin-Luther University, Halle, Julius-Bernstein-Institute of Physiology, 4020 Halle, GDR
ZIEGELHÖFFER, A.: Center of Physiological Sciences of the Slovakian Academy of Sciences, Institute of Experimental Surgery, Bratislava, CSSR

Bei Fragen zur Produktsicherheit wenden Sie sich bitte an:
If you have any questions regarding product safety, please contact:

Walter de Gruyter GmbH
Genthiner Straße 13
10785 Berlin
productsafety@degruyterbrill.com